International Handbook of Occupational Therapy Interventions

Ingrid Söderback
Editor

International Handbook of Occupational Therapy Interventions

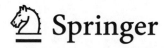 Springer

Editor
Ingrid Söderback
Associate Professor in Occupational Therapy and Rehabilitation
Karolinska Institute, Stockholm, Sweden
and
University Lecturer Emerita
Department of Public Health and Caring Sciences
Uppsala University, Uppsala, Sweden
Home address: Sickla Kanalgata 31 nb
SE 13165 Nacka
E-mail: Ingrid_Soderback@hotmail.com

ISBN 978-0-387-75423-9 (hardcover)   e-ISBN 978-0-387-75424-6
ISBN 978-1-4419-6739-8 (softcover)
DOI 10.1007/978-0-387-75424-6
Springer New York Dordrecht Heidelberg London

Library of Congress Control Number: 2009927464

Printed on acid-free paper

Springer is part of Springer Science+Business Media (www.springer.com)

To be occupied is a fundamental right in every human being's life.
The occupational therapists' main professional role is to encourage the clients' occupational performances.

To occupational therapy students, occupational therapists, and members of rehabilitation and health care teams, who are professionally working to improve their clients' health and wellness, and to stakeholders responsible for the administration of occupational therapy, worldwide.

Foreword

The World Federation of Occupational Therapists (WFOT) estimates that there are over 300,000 practicing occupational therapists (OTs) in 66 countries. The growth of the profession of occupational therapy in the last 50 years is extraordinary. When I first practiced occupational therapy in the Brooklyn Day Hospital in New York City in 1958, there were about 4000 OTs in the United States and a few more thousand in the rest of the world. The countries of the former British Commonwealth, Scandinavia, and the Unites States dominated practice. Most OTs worked in hospitals either in psychiatric or long-term chronic care facilities. Occupational therapy was primarily paired with physical and speech therapies as rehabilitation professions. The modalities used in practice were mainly arts and crafts and creative media. Now, in 2009, the profession of occupational therapy has expanded its concepts, intervention modalities, and scope of practice.

This handbook represents the coming of age in global occupational therapy. The authors are distinguished experts in the diverse practice of occupational therapy from around the world. They describe practice from three perspectives: the healer working directly with the patient in preventing, treating, and restoring function; the teacher training the patient in activities of daily living (ADL) skills, assisting the caregiver and informing individuals at risk about how to prevent illness and disease; and the ergonomist in adapting the home, work, and school environments to increase function and prevent injuries. This handbook is comprehensive, and includes a wide range of occupational therapy modalities such as orthotics, universal design, assistive devices, biofeedback, driver education, sensory integration, horticulture, and music. The authors describe interventions for a wide range of individuals with physical as well as psychological disabilities. The emphasis in the book is pragmatic, keeping with the core values of occupational therapy, to help the individual to maintain or increase functional activities through occupation. Evidence-based practice is the guiding principle in deciding what is the best practice. There are many case examples to help the student or clinician understand in a realistic manner how the interventions work and the precautions in therapy.

This is a book for the 21st century that integrates the global practice of occupational therapy with research evidence. It should serve as a ready reference for the student and OT to apply interventions in a holistic framework.

Franklin Stein, PhD, OTR, FAOTA
Founding Editor, *Occupational Therapy International*

Preface

The *International Handbook of Occupational Therapy Interventions* contains an encyclopedic overview of the theoretical core content of occupational therapy and the occupational therapy interventions that are common and used worldwide. The main theme of the handbook is the occupational therapist's role in *managing, teaching, enabling, and promoting* the clients' potential to be occupied with desired and meaningful occupations, daily activities, and tasks. The purposes of the occupational therapy services are as follows: *adaptation*, in that the clients' internal, temporal, and environmental adaptations are expected to improve; *teaching*, in that the clients learn or relearn to perform daily activities; *recovery*, in that the clients experience themselves as being occupied through participation in meaningful activities and tasks that influence their physiologic and psychological healing; and *health and wellness*, in that motor vehicle accidents and accidents at home and at work are prevented, so as to promote the clients' health. The principles for performing quality assurance and the prerequisites for judging the scientific evidence of the effectiveness of the occupational therapy interventions are presented. The reader is informed about the extensive literature review that constitutes the genesis of this handbook.

Based on 90 authors' expert knowledge, scientific methodology, and my 40 years of professional work outlined in several case studies, this handbook will be a helpful tool for students, occupational therapists, clinicians on rehabilitation and health care teams, stakeholders, and readers who want a survey of the occupational therapy core content and practice.

Åkersberga, Sweden   Ingrid Söderback
September 2008

Acknowledgments

I want to express my sincere gratitude to the chapter authors, without whose efforts this handbook would not have become a reality. Your expert knowledge has enriched this handbook by demonstrating how occupational therapy is practiced worldwide and how our knowledge contributes to rehabilitation and medical services. My hope is that this handbook is the beginning of a continuing process of documenting our profession's clinical work.

I am grateful to the clients and patients whose cases are discussed in this handbook. I also thank all the other clients I have worked with in my 40-year career. They have shared their experience of living with disabilities and therefore in an invaluable way have enriched my professional experiences and my life.

I also want to express my gratitude to my former colleagues at the Rehabilitation Clinic of Danderyd Hospital in Stockholm, Sweden: to Gunilla Myrin, for your boundless support through the years and for your contribution of your research about the case of Marie-Louise Huss; to Anette Erikson, Elisabeth Hultman, Lena Krumlinde Sundholm, and Kerstin Wikell, for your interest in my work; and to Marianne Söderström, in memorium.

My sincere appreciation is offered to Professor Franklin Stein, Madison, Wisconsin, for your foreword to this handbook, for your advice and friendship in our work on the journal *Occupational Therapy International* and for introducing me to the world of publishing; and to Professor Karen Jacobs, Boston, Massachusetts, for your sponsorship, your friendship, and our work on the journal *Work: A Journal of Prevention, Assessment, and Rehabilitation.*

I thank my colleagues in the clinical, education, and research areas, for supporting my work aimed at developing our profession. Special thanks are due to Marina Härtull for your comments based on your wide clinical OT experience. I thank my students through the years, whose critical questions and debates have helped me reflect on the core content of occupational therapy.

My thanks are due to the occupational therapists and pioneers of Swedish occupational therapy who introduced me to the profession, especially Gunnel Nelson and Inga-Britt Bränholm in memorium.

My sincere gratitude is expressed to Tim Crosfield, for your 25 years of sensible advice and your patience in teaching me how to express my thoughts in English. My deepest gratitude is expressed to Naum Purits, for your Russian–English language translations and computer support, for making our work together fun, and for your curiosity and interest in occupational therapy, which supported my efforts in bringing this handbook to fruition.

My deepest gratitude is due to my friends and family: Maria Söderback and Peter, Klara, Anton Disbo, Mårten Söderback, and Sandra Alevärn. Your encouragement, support, and love helped me complete this two-year endeavor. I also express my gratitude to Per Söderback in memorium.

I also want to express my appreciation to Springer Science + Business Media editor Janice Stern, for giving me the confidence to carry out the work of this handbook, and to the editorial assistants Emma Holmgren and Ian Marvinney, for their excellent assistance with author correspondence and for their advice and information that helped make my work easier.

Åkersberga   Ingrid Söderback
October 6, 2008

Contents

Accommodation

Electric Prostheses, Orthotics, and Splints

Assistive Devices

Universal Design

Temporal Adaptation

**Part III   Interventions: The Occupational Therapist Teaches
and the Client Learns**

Introduction

Consultation in the Prevention of Illness

Part VI   Evaluation of Occupational Therapy Interventions

Contributors

Kirsten Avlund, MD
Section of Social Medicine, Department of Public Health,
University of Copenhagen, Copenhagen, Denmark

Anne Bouchez, OT
Université d'Angers, Angers, France

Mary H. Bowman, OTR/L
Department of Psychology, University of Alabama at Birmingham,
South Birmingham, Alabama, USA

Joke Bradt, PhD, MT-BC, LCAT
Arts and Quality of Life Research Center, Temple University, Philadelphia,
Pennsylvania USA

Åse Brandt, PhD, MPT
Research and Development Department, Danish Centre for Assistive Technology,
Århus, Denmark

Wendy Bryant, MSc, Dipcot, PGcort, LTHE
School of Health Sciences and Social Care, Brunel University, Uxbridge,
Middlesex, UK

Patricia C. Buchain, Specialist in Psychiatry and Mental Health
Ovídio Pires de Campos, Sao Paulo, Brazil

Gonca Bumin, PhD
Faculty of Health Sciences, Department of Physical Therapy and
Rehabilitation–Occupational Therapy Unit, Hacettepe University, Ankara, Turkey

Leslie Bunt, Professor of Arts in Health
Faculty of Health and Life Sciences, University of the West of England,
Bristol, UK

Tom Burns, MD
University Department of Psychiatry, Wareford Hospital, Oxford, UK

Cynthia Z. Burton, BA
140 Arbor Drive, San Diego, DA, 92103 USA

Chetwyn C.H. Chan, PhD
Applied Cognitive Neuroscience Laboratory, Department of Rehabilitation
Sciences, Hong Kong Polytechnic University, Hong Kong, China

Sunny Ho-Wan Chan, BSc (OT), PgD (Psychology), MScoSc (Mental Health)
Department of Occupational Therapy, Pamela Youde Nethersole Eastern Hospital,
Hong Kong, China

Lindy Clemson, PhD
Faculty of Health Sciences, University of Sydney, Lidcombe, Australia

Al Copolillo, PhD, OTR/L
Department of Occupational Therapy at Virginia Commonwealth University,
Richmond, Virginia, USA

Jocelyn Cowls, Occupational Therapist Reg. (ON)
Homewood Health Centre, Post Traumatic Stress Recovery Program, Guelph,
Ontario, Canada

B. Cathy Craven, Assistant Professor
Lyndhurst Centre, Toronto Rehabilitation Institute, Toronto, Ontaio, Canada

Shelley Crawford, PhD
Occupational Therapy Department, Mater Hospital, Belfast, Ireland

Norma Daykin, Professor of Music Therapy
Faculty of Health and Life Sciences, University of the West of England,
Bristol, UK

Gabe de Vries, Professor, MD
Department of Psychiatry, Academic Medical Center, University of Amsterdam,
Amsterdam, The Netherlands

Cheryl Dileo, PhD, MT-BC
Arts and Quality of Life Research Center, Temple University, Philadelphia,
Pennsylvania, USA

Marilyn Di Stefano, BAppSc (Occ. Ther.) Grad. Dip. Ergonomics. PhD
Centre for Human Factors and Ergonomics, La Trobe University, Bundoora,
Australia

Megan Edgelow, Associate Professor, Occupational Therapist
School of Rehabilitation Therapy, Queen's University, Kingston, Ontario, Canada

Hélio Elkis, MD, PhD
Ovídio Pires de Campos, Sao Paulo, Brazil

Melanie T. Ellexson, MA, OTR, FA OTA
Chicago State University, Chicago, Illinois, USA

Serge Fanello MD, PhD
Université d'Angers, Angers, France

Elisabetta Farina, MD
Neurorehabilitation Unit, IRCCS Don Gnocchi Foundation, University of Milan,
Milan, Italy

Marcia Finlayson, PhD, OT (C), OTR/L
Department of Occupational Therapy, University of Illinois at Chicago,
Chicago, Illinois, USA

Jennifer Fleming BoccThy (Hons), PhD
School of Health and Rehabilitation Sciences, University of Queensland,
Brisbane, Australia

Sharon Flinn, PhD, OTR/L
Division of Occupational Therapy, School of Allied Medical Professions,
Ohio State University, Columbus, Ohio, USA

Jonathan Garabette, Professor
University Department of Psychiatry, Wareford Hospital, Oxford, UK

Chantal Geusgens, MSc, PhD
Department of Medical Psychology, Atrium Medical Centre, Heerlen,
The Netherlands

Libby Gibson, PhD
School of Health and Rehabilitation Sciences, University of Queensland, Brisbane,
Australia

Laura N. Gitlin, PhD
Department of Occupational Therapy, Jefferson College of Health Professions,
Thomas Jefferson University, Philadelphia, Pennsylvania, USA

Glenn Goodman, PhD, OTR/L
Cleveland State University, Cleveland, Ohio, USA

Maud J.L. Graff, PhD/OT
Research Group for Allied Health Care, Department of Occupational Therapy,
University of Nijmegen Medical Center, Nijmegen, The Netherlands

Sandra Hale, Reg. OT; (BC)
Practice Coordinator Mental Health Rehabilitation, Vancouver Coastal Health,
Vancouver, British Columbia, Canada

Alison Hammond, PhD, FCOT
Centre for Rehabilitation and Human Performance Research,
University of Salford, Salford, Greater Manchester, UK

Thamar Melanie Heijstra, MA, PhD Student in Sociology
Faculty of Social and Human Sciences, Department of Sociology,
University of Iceland Reykjavík, Iceland

Hermie J. Hermens, PhD
Roessingh Research and Development, Faculty of Electrical Engineering,
Mathematics and Computer Science, University of Twente, Enschede,
The Netherlands

Katherine Herron, PhD
Department of Psychology, University of Surrey, Surrey, UK

Brian Hoare, MBBS, FRACP, FAFRM, RACP
Pediatric Rehabilitation Service, Monash Medical Centre, Clayton, Australia

Susanne Iwarsson, PhD
Department of Health Sciences, Lund University, Lund, Sweden

Tal Jarus, PhD, OTR
Department of Occupational Science and Occupational Therapy, CanDo Research
Unit, Faculty of Medicine, University of British Columbia, Vancouver,
British Columbia,
Canada

Hulya Kayihan, PhD
Faculty of Health Sciences, Department of Physical Therapy and
Rehabilitation–Occupational Therapy Unit, Hacettepe University,
Ankara, Turkey

Terry Krupa, Msc (Rehat Science)
School of Rehabilitation Therapy, Queen's University, Kingston,
Ontario, Canada

Lottie F.M. Kuijt-Evers, PhD
TNO Work and Employment, Hoofddorp, The Netherlands

Rodney A. Lambert, DipCOT, CHSM, MA, PhD
School of Allied Health Professions, University of East Anglia, Norfolk,
Norwich, UK

Barbara A. Larson, DHS, MBA, OTR
Private Practice, Duluth, Minnesota, USA

Mindy F. Levin, PhD, PT
Physical Therapy Program, School of Physical and Occupational Therapy,
Faculty of Medicine, McGill University, Montreal, Quebec, Canada

Karen P.Y. Liu, PhD
Applied Cognitive Neuroscience Laboratory, Department of Rehabilitation
Sciences, Hong Kong Polytechnic University, Hong Kong, China

Wendy Macdonald, Bsc (Psychol), Dip Psych, PhD
Centre for Ergonomics and Human Factors, La Trobe University, Bundoora,
Australia

Kinsuk Maitra, PhD, OTR/L
Occupational Therapy, Rush University Medical Center, Chicago, Illinois, USA

Susan M. Maloney, PhD, CHT, OTR/L, LVE
Cleveland State University, Cleveland, Ohio, USA

Victor W. Mark, MD
Department of Physical Medicine and Rehabilitation, University of Alabama
at Birmingham, Birmingham, Alabama, USA

Leonora Nel
Educational Occupational Therapist, Head of the Department at Pretoria School
for Learner with Special Education Needs, the South African Department of
Education, Pretoria, South Africa
Groenkloof, South Africa

Jorge Henna Netto
Specialist in Psychiatry and Mental Health, Ovídio Pires de Campos,
Sao Paulo, Brazil

Sigrid Østensjø, PhD
Associate Professor, Faculty of Health Sciences, Oslo University College,
Oslo, Norway

Tatiana Petrova
Consultant; Social worker, Narcologic Department of the Viborg Region,
St. Petersburg, Russian Federation

Milos R. Popovic
Professor, Rehabilitation Engineering Laboratory, Lyndhurst Centre, Toronto
Rehabilitation Institute, Toronto, Ontario, Canada

Natalia Punanova
Phychiatrist; Expert of narcology; Occupational Therapist, Narcologic Department
of the Viborg Region, St. Petersburg, Russian Federation

Debbie Radloff-Gabriel
Occupational Therapist, Providence Care Mental Health Services,
Kingston, Ontario, Canada

Gudbjörg Linda Rafnsdottir, MA, PhD
Professor in Sociology and Dean of the Faculty of Social and Human Sciences,
Faculty of Social and Human Sciences, Department of Sociology, University
of Iceland, Reykjavík, Iceland

Navah Z. Ratzon
Assistant Professor; Head of Occupational Therapy Department, Department
of Occupational Therapy, Tel Aviv University, Tel Aviv, Israel

Isabelle Richard, MD, PhD
Université d'Angers, Angers, France

Nancy Rickerson, PhD, OTR/L
Snoqualmie Valley Rehabilitation Clinic, Snoqualmie, Washington, USA

Remo N. Russo, BOT
Paediatric Rehabilitation Service, Women's and Children's Hospital,
North Adelaide, Australia

Kersti Samuelsson, PhD, MPH
Clinical Department of Rehabilitation Medicine, University Hospital,
Linköping, Sweden

Jennifer Sanders, MSc
Department of Psychology, University of Surrey, Surrey, UK

Aart H. Schene, MA
Department of Psychiatry, Academic Medical Center, University of Amsterdam,
Amsterdam, The Netherlands

Gul Sener, PhD
Faculty of Health Sciences, Department of Physical Therapy and Rehabilitation–
Occupational Therapy Unit, Hacettepe University, Ankara, Turkey

Robert J. Shannon, MSc
School of Health Sciences, University of Southampton, Southampton, UK

Megan Simons, BOccThy, PhD
Stuart Pegg Paediatric Burns Centre, Royal Children's Hospital, Herston,
Brisbane, Australia

Ingrid Söderback, Associate Professor, DrMedSci, OT/Legitimate
Department of Public Health and Caring Sciences, Uppsala University,
Uppsala, Sweden

Laura Stana, MD
Université d'Angers, Angers, France

Franklin Stein, PhD, OTR, FAOTA
Professor Emeritus, University South Dakota and Editor
Occupational Therapy International, John Wiley & Sons, Ltd.,
The Atrium Southern Gate, Chichester, West Sussex PO 19 8 SQ, UK

Annette Sterr, BSc
Department of Psychology, University of Surrey, Surrey UK

May Stinson, PhD
School of Health Sciences, University of Ulster, Antrim, UK

Edward Taub, PhD
Department of Psychology, University of Alabama at Birmingham, Birmingham,
Alabama, USA

Elizabeth W. Twamley, PhD
Department of Psychiatry, University of California, San Diego
and
Psychology Service, VA San Diego Health Care System
San Diego, California, USA

Mine Uyanik, PhD
Faculty of Health Sciences, Department of Physical Therapy and Rehabilitation–
Occupational Therapy Unit, Hacettepe University, Ankara, Turkey

Colette van der Westhuyzen l
Educational Occupational Therapist,
The Department at Pretoria School for Learner with Special Education Needs,
The South African Department of Education, Pretoria, South Africa
Gezina, South Africa

Caroline van Heugten, MSc, PhD
Department of Psychiatry, Maastricht University, Maastricht, The Netherlands

Mikkel Vass, DrMedSci, MD
Section of General Practice, Department of Public Health,
University of Copenhagen, Copenhagen, Denmark

Lea Vella, MPH
San Diego State University/University of California Davis San Diego Joint
Doctoral Program in Clinical Psychology
San Diego, California, USA

Fabiana Villanelli, PhD
Neurorehabilitation Unit, IRCCS Don Gnocchi Foundation, University of Milan,
Milan, Italy

Adriana D.B. Vizzotto, MD, PhD
Ovídio Pires de Campos, Sao Paulo, Brazil

Miriam M.R. Vollenbroek-Hutten, MD
Roessingh Research and Development, Enschede, The Netherlands

Daniel Wever, MD
Roessingh Research and Development, Enschede, The Netherlands

Josephine Man Wah Wong, MScHC(OT), MSc
Adjunct Assistant Professor, Founding Chair
Hong Kong Society for Hand Therapy
Occupational Therapy Department, Prince of Wales Hospital, Hong Kong, China

Midori Yasukawa, PhD, RN
Department of Nursing, College of Medical and Pharmaceutical and Health
Sciences, Kanazawa University, Kanazawa, Ishikawa, Japan

Part I
Introduction

Chapter 1
The Genesis of the Handbook: Material and Methods

Ingrid Söderback*

Abstract The *International Handbook of Occupational Therapy Interventions* came about through extensive literature searches on occupational therapy and medical rehabilitation. These searches also helped is selecting the authors of the chapters in this book, who are experts on clinical interventions in occupational therapy. The searches also identified four major roles for the occupational therapist (OT[1]): (1) to manage adaptations applied to the clients' environment; (2) to teach clients how, through occupation, to regain functioning and daily living skills; (3) to enable clients to perform purposeful and meaningful occupations that may help their recovery; and (4) to promote health and well-being in preventive interventions. These four roles overlap, as is illustrated in the case study of a woman with a femur fracture.

Keywords Femur fracture • Scientific methods • Origin • The occupational therapist's • role

Core Content of Occupational Therapy

The interventions presented in this book elucidate the professional core content of occupational therapy. These occupational therapy interventions are commonly used in clinical practice and are documented by research. My purpose in compiling this handbook was to increase our understanding of how the occupational therapy contributes to clients' health and well-being.

In the late 1960s, the occupational therapy profession was relatively sparsely represented at acute hospitals in my country—Sweden. I was in my first professional job on neurologic and orthopedic wards, and in those days physicians made patient referrals verbally, not in writing. I was responsible for a referral case from a respected physician, an expert in orthopedics. The record contained the descriptive phrase: "Sixty-eight-year-old woman with right femur fracture, at present

---

* Söderback is the Swedish spelling and Soderback is the English spelling of the author's family name.

[1] Occupational Therapist is shortened as OT or OTs throughout the Handbook.

I. Söderback (ed.), *International Handbook of Occupational Therapy Interventions,*
DOI: 10.1007/978-0-387-75424-6_1, © Springer Science+Business Media, LLC 2010

having her leg in traction for at least 2 weeks." The prescription was: "A teddy bear—thank you." What did this mean? After interviewing the patient it became clear that she wanted something to do while waiting for her femur fracture to heal. She wanted to make a teddy bear, which was to be a gift to her newborn grandchild. Thus, the occupational therapist (OT[1]) was able to offer the patient the opportunity to do something that was meaningful and useful for her. This type of recovery intervention is the primary origin of occupational therapy.

Finding a useful project for this patient also provided me with the incentive to explain and disseminate knowledge about occupational therapy, as there are now many other cost-effective measures that would have been appropriate for this patient. Today, the physicians' prescription would have included a postoperative occupational training program. During the hospital stay, the interventions would have comprised an individualized learning process to improve the patient's ability to ambulate indoors, to perform light housework, and get into and out of an automobile.

As for environmental adaptations, the OT would have prescribed assistive devices, such as a reacher, a raised toilet seat, a raised bed, and stocking pullers. These devices would make the patient independent in self-care, such as personal hygiene, bathing, and toileting. There is now considerable evidence to support such interventions for people suffering from hip fractures (Hagsten et al., 2004, 2006; Hagsten and Söderback, 1994).

To assess health promotion and risk, a home visit aimed at preventing further accidental falls (Avlund et al., 2007) would have taken place after the patient's discharge from the hospital (Söderback, 2008).

The four major factors exemplified above—adaptive interventions, recovery interventions, interventions using the teaching–learning process, and measures of health promotion and risk assessment—constitute the core content of the occupational therapy interventions presented in this handbook.

Method and Material

Study Design

An extensive review of the literature (Stein and Cutler, 2000) determined which occupational therapy interventions should be included and which scientists and clinicians should be invited to contribute chapters to this handbook.

The inclusion criteria for occupational therapy interventions were as follows:

- Keywords: occupational therapy.
- Articles containing in the title or suggesting in the text an identifiable occupational therapy intervention.
- Articles published in referee-examined scientific journals.
- Publications describing types of case reports, clinical trials, consensus, developmental conference reports, comparative studies, evaluation studies, literature reviews, meta-analyses, randomized control trials, research reports, and research supports according to the PubMed database classification (National Library of Medicine and Health, 2006).

- Publications based on studies of clients or literature.
- The selected intervention is described in more than one published study.
- The publications contain a complete abstract in English.
- The author names and email addresses or postal addresses are identifiable through an Internet search.
- Recent articles were chosen over older ones.
- An international distribution of the publications was desirable.

Exclusion Criteria

- Publications concerning psychometric investigations and validation of occupational therapy assessment instrument and of occupational therapy theories and models.
- Publications concerning interventions known from textbooks, such as the Bobath neurodevelopment reflex inhibition therapy (Bobath and Bobath, 1950), are not represented in this handbook, since no study thereof was found connected with occupational therapy, or no author was available, or the method had no proved evidence of its efficacy for patients (e.g., stroke patients) (Kappelle et al., 2007).

Selection of Interventions and Authors

To obtain an overview of the occupational therapy interventions presented in textbooks, I reviewed the 27 textbooks (Table 1.1) that I have used during my 40-year career, searching for occupational therapy interventions. This overview and the inclusion criteria listed above served to validate the choice of interventions for this handbook. The overview also demonstrated the four major occupational therapy intervention factors that characterize the interventions as illustrated in Fig. 1.1: the therapist manages the patient's adaptation (Chapter 2), the therapist teaches and the patient learns (Chapter 3), the therapist enables the patient's recovery (Chapter 4), and the therapist promotes health and wellness (Chapter 5).

Data searches of scientific publications were performed with the PubMed database as the primary source. Additional sources were the OT seeker (http://www. otseeker.com/), and the following *Journal of Occupational Therapy, Occupational Therapy International*, and *Work, A Journal of Prevention, Assessment, and Rehabilitation* (Shawn, 2007).

The primary PubMed search with the keywords "occupational therapy" and the inclusion and exclusion criteria generated 4456 items (about 50% of the available items) published from 1960 to July 2006, and 225 items published from August 2006 to December 2007. The abstracts of these publications were saved on the EndNote database (EndNote, 1998–2000). Publications before 2002 were saved for possible future documentation of the history of the interventions if they were to be

Table 1.1 Textbooks used for identification and an overview of occupational therapy interventions

1. Allen, C. (1985). Occupational Therapy for Psychiatric Diseases: Measurement and Management of Cognitive Disabilities. Boston, MA: Little, Brown.
2. Christiansen, C. (1994). Ways of Living. Self-Care Strategies for Special Needs. Bethesda, MD: AOTA Director of Nonperiodical Publications.
3. Christiansen, C., and Baum, C. (1991). Occupational Therapy. Overcoming Human Performance Deficits. Thorofare, NJ: Slack.
4. Christiansen, C., and Baum, C. (1997). Occupational Therapy. Enabling Function and Well-Being. Thorofare, NJ: Slack.
5. Cynkin, S., and Robinson, A. M. (1990). Occupational Therapy and Activities Health: Toward Health Through Activities. Boston, MA: Little, Brown.
6. Ellergård, K., and Nordell, K. (1997). Att bryta vanmakt mot egenmakt (To Break Powerlessness Against Arbitrariness) (In Swedish). Borås: Johnsson & Skyttes Förlag.
7. Fleming Cottrell, R.P. (1993). Psychosocial Occupational Therapy. Bethesda, MD: AOTA
8. Hagedorn, R. (1995). Occupational Therapy. Perspectives and Process. Edinburgh: Churchill Livingstone.
9. Hopkins, H.L., and Smith, H.D. (1993). Willard and Spackman's Occupational Therapy, 8th ed. Philadelphia: J.B. Lippincott.
10. Jacobs Gold, K. (1993). The nature and quality of optimal flow experience. A form of job satisfaction, in a selected occupation. The case of occupational therapy practitioner. Doctoral Dissertation. Faculty of the college of education, University of Massachusetts, Lowell.
11. Johnson, J.A., and Yerxa, E.J. (1989). Occupational Science: The Foundation for a New Model of Practice. London: Haworth.
12. Katz, N. (1992). Cognitive Rehabilitation. Models for Intervention in Occupational Therapy, 1st ed. Boston: Andover Medical Publishers.
13. Kielhofner, G. (1985). A Model of Human Occupation. Theory and Application. London: Williams & Wilkins.
14. Kielhofner, G. (1992). Conceptual Foundations of Occupational Therapy. Philadelphia: F.A. Davis.
15. Kielhofner, G. (1995). A Model of Human Occupation: Theory and Application, 2nd ed. Baltimore, MD: Williams & Wilkins.
16. Lamport, N.K., Coffey, M.S., and Hersch, G.I. (1989). Activity Analysis. Handbook. Thorofare, NJ: Slack.
17. Macdonald, E.M. (1964). Occupational Therapy in Rehabilitation. A Handbook for OTs, Students and Others Interested in This Aspect of Reablement. London: Ballière, Tindall and Cox.
18. Mann, W.C., and Lane, J.P. (1991). Assistive Technology for Persons with Disabilities. The Role of Occupational Therapy. Bethesda, MD: AOTA.
19. Miller, R.J., Sieg, K.W., Ludwig, F.M., Denegan Shortridge, S., and van Deusen, J. (1988). Six Perspectives on Theories for the Practice of Occupational Therapy. Rockville, MD: Aspen.
20. Miller, R.J., and Walker, K.F. (1993). Perspectives on Theory for Practice of Occupational Therapy, Vol. 1. Gaithersburg, MD: Aspen.
21. Mosey, A.C. (1973). Activities Therapy. New York: Raven.
22. Mosey, A. C. (1986). Psychosocial Components of Occupational Therapy. New York: Raven.
23. Neistadt, M.E., and Crepeau, E. B. (1998). Willard & Spackman's Occupational Therapy, 9th ed. Philadelphia: Lippincott Raven.
24. Pedretti, L.W., and Early, M. B. (2001). Occupational Therapy. Practice Skill for Physical Dysfunction, 5th ed. London: Mosby.
25. Read, C., and Sanderson, S. R. (1980). Concepts of Occupational Therapy. Baltimore, MD: Williams & Wilkins.
26. Stein, F., and Roose, B. (2000). Pocket Guide to Treatment in Occupational Therapy. San Diego, CA: Singular Publishing Group.
27. Stein, F., Söderback, I., Cutler, S.K., and Larson, B. (2006). Occupational Therapy and Ergonomics. Applying Ergonomic Principles to Everyday Occupation in the Home and at Work, 1st ed. London/Philadelphia: Whurr/Wiley.

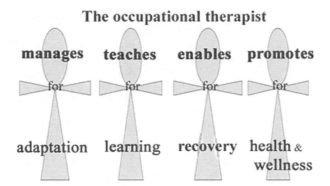

Fig. 1.1 Four major occupational therapy intervention factors.

included. Publications from 2002 to 2007 (n = 959) were chosen for primary categorization.

The abstracts of the articles were carefully reviewed. The articles that did not fulfill the inclusion/exclusion criteria were discarded, leaving 352 in the original file. These articles were critically evaluated and classified by (1) the intervention factor, (2) the subjects of the interventions (children, adolescents, adults, frail elderly), (3) the diagnoses, and (4) the titles and database references (authors' names, addresses, and publication facts). Four copies of the original file, one for each intervention factor, were used for further identification of the interventions.

Many of the interventions identified had no author name, title, or other designation. However, the authors had explained their aims in terms of body function, body structure, activity and participation, environmental factors, or diagnoses. I therefore could use the concepts of the International Classification of Functioning, Disability, and Health (ICD) (World Health Organization, 2007) for further classification. With the ICD definitions in mind, the articles in each of the four files were again carefully reviewed and categorized.

The definitions of the interventions were validated by a comparison according to the *Thesaurus of Occupational Therapy* subject headings (American Occupational Therapy Foundation, 2004) and the PubMed MeSH database (National Library of Medicine and Health, 2006). The content of each intervention was reviewed based on the definitions, and the intervention was labeled according to the authors' suggestions.

For interventions represented by more than one published study, a scale was constructed, giving priority to randomized studies, to the newest publications, to authors with OT qualifications, and to wide geographic distribution. Identification continued until a saturation point was reached; that is, the same articles or authors turned up irrespective of the search method. A descriptive meta-analysis and an annotated bibliography showing the interventions presented in the handbook are given for each of the four major intervention factors.

Authors were suggested for each identified intervention, and they were contacted by email, letter, or telephone call. Fourteen of those contacted declined, and addresses for another 14 were not found.

Results

By July 2008, the handbook contained 61 chapters by 90 authors from around the world (Fig. 1.2 and Table 1.2), who are affiliated with 59 universities or hospitals or in private practice. The chapters discuss the selected occupational therapy interventions (Fig. 1.1).

Discussion

The chapters of the handbook may be viewed as a sample of the available occupational therapy interventions.

The selection of the chapters presented in this handbook is the result of an attempt to apply scientific methodology. However, this process of identification of authors was somewhat restricted by language barriers, as we strived to select mainly English-speaking authors. In addition, there are doubtless more occupational therapy interventions in clinical use that are not presented in published studies and therefore are not represented in this handbook.

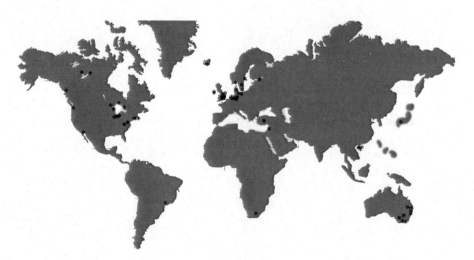

Fig. 1.2 An approximate map of where the authors of the chapters in this book live.

Table 1.2 The worldwide distribution of the authors' chapters

Chapter no.	Hospital/institution/university	City	Country
4 and 18	Thomas Jefferson University	Philadelphia, PA	USA
5	Lund University	Lund	Sweden
6	Cleveland State University	Cleveland, OH	USA
6	Ohio State University	Columbus, OH	USA
7	University of Ulster	Antrim, Ulster	Northern Ireland
7	Mater Hospital	Belfast	Northern Ireland
8	Danish Centre for Assistive Technology	Århus	Denmark
8	Linköping University Regional Hospital	Linköping	Sweden
9	University of Toronto	Toronto, ON	Canada
10	Prince of Wales Hospital	Shatin, New Territories, Hong Kong	China
56	University of British Columbia	Vancouver	Canada
11	Royal Children's Hospital	Herston, Queensland	Australia
12	Oslo University College	Oslo	Norway
13	Department of Occupational Therapy at VCU	Richmond, VA	USA
14	Snoqualmie Valley Rehab Clinic	Snoqualmie, WA	USA
15	TNO Work and Employment	AS Hoofddorp	The Netherlands
16	Queen's University	Kingston, ON	Canada
19	University Nijmegen Medical Center	Nijmegen	The Netherlands
20	The University of Queensland	Brisbane	Australia
21	The Hong Kong Polytechnic University	Hong Kong	China
22	Maastricht University	Maastricht	The Netherlands
23	University of Illinois at Chicago	Chicago, IL	USA
24	Homewood Health Centre	Guelph, ON	Canada
24	Vancouver Coastal Health	Vancouver	Canada
25	Pamela Youde Nethersole Eastern Hospital	Hong Kong	China
26	University of São Paulo	Sao Paulo	Brazil
27	University of East Anglia	Norfolk	United Kingdom
28	St. Petersburg	St. Petersburg	Russia
29	McGill University	Montreal, QC	Canada
30	University of Alabama at Birmingham	Birmingham, AL	USA
31	University of Surrey	Guildford, Surrey	United Kingdom
32	Rush University Medical Center	Chicago, IL	USA
33	University of Salford	Great Manchester	United Kingdom
34	Hacettepe University	Ankara	Turkey
35	Women's and Children's Hospital	Adelaide	Australia
35	Monash Medical Centre	Clayton	Australia
36	Rehabilitation centre Het Roessingh	Enschede	The Netherlands
36	Roessingh Research and Development	Enschede	The Netherlands
37	Université d'Angers	Angers	France
38	Chicago State University	Chicago, IL	USA

(continued)

Table 1.2   (continued)

Chapter no.	Hospital/institution/university	City	Country
38	Private practice	Duluth, MN	USA
39	University of Amsterdam	Amsterdam	The Netherlands
40	University of California	San Diego, CA	USA
41	University of Oxford	Oxford	United Kingdom
42	Pretoria School for Learners with Disabilities	Gezina and Groenkloof, Pretoria	South Africa
44	Brunel University	Isleworth, Middlesex	United Kingdom
45	University of Milan	Milan	Italy
46	Kanazawa University	Kanazawa, Ishikawa	Japan
47	Temple University	Philadelphia, PA	USA
48	University of the West of England (UWE)	Bristol	United Kingdom
50 and 52	University of Copenhagen	Copenhagen	Denmark
51	The University of Sydney	Lidcombe, Sydney	Australia
53	La Trobe University	Bundoora, Melbourne, Victoria	Australia
54	The University of Iceland	Reykjavík	Iceland
55	University of Queensland	Brisbane	Australia
56	Tel Aviv University	Tel Aviv	Israel
57	University of Southampton	Southampton	United Kingdom

The final presentation of occupational therapy interventions has thus been affected by the rapid publication of new and innovative interventions during the 2 years in which this handbook was written.

My intention was to find authors from a wide range of countries. But the occupational therapy interventions included here are largely from Australia, Europe, and the United States. There are none from Africa (apart from South Africa), South America, and Asia (apart from Russian Federation). Occupational therapy/rehabilitation in these countries, if available as a public clinical practice, is very sparsely represented both here and in the literature, possibly because of political decisions and national economical scarcity that limit the funding of public rehabilitation.

The chapters in this handbook provide evidence-based interventions that can be clinically applied. It is hoped that this handbook will contributes to the future development of occupational therapy worldwide.

References

American Occupational Therapy Foundation. (2004). Thesaurus of occupational therapy subject headings. A subject guide to OT search. Binderman M, ed. 3rd ed., vol. 1998–2007). Bethesda, MD: American Occupational Therapy Foundation. http://www.aotf.org/html/thesaurus.shtml

Avlund, K., Vass, M., Kvist, K., Hendriksen, C., and Keiding, N. (2007). Educational intervention toward preventive home visitors reduced functional decline in community-living older women. J Clin Epidemiol, 60(9), 954–962.

Bobath, L., and Bobath, B. (1950). Spastic paralysis treatment of by the use of reflex inhibition. Br J Phys Med, 13(6), 121–127.

EndNote. (1998–2000). EndNote 4. Bibliographies and Now Manuscripts Made Easy (Version 6) [Database]. New York: Thomson ISI ResearchSoft.

Hagsten, B.E., and Söderback, I. (1994). Occupational therapy after hip fracture: A pilot study of the clients, the care and the costs. Clin Rehabil, 8(2), 52–58.

Hagsten, B., Svensson, O., and Gardulf, A. (2004). Early individualized postoperative occupational therapy training in 100 patients improves ADL after hip fracture: a randomized trial. Acta Orthop Scand, 75(2), 177–183.

Hagsten, B., Svensson, O., and Gardulf, A. (2006). Health-related quality of life and self-reported ability concerning ADL and IADL after hip fracture: a randomized trial. Acta Orthop, 77(1), 114–119.

Kappelle, J., Grypdonck, M.H., and Algra, A. (2007). Effects of Bobath-based therapy on depression, shoulder pain and health-related quality of life in patients after stroke. J Rehabil Med, 39(8), 627–632.

United States National Library of Medicine, National Institutes of Health. (2006). PubMed Entrez; journal, author, title search and the MeSH database. Retrieved 2006/04/03, from www.ncbi.nlm.nih.gow/sites/entrenz?db = PubMed and www.ncbi.nlm.nih.gow/sites/entrenz?db = mesh

Shawn, T. (2007). Neurotransmitter.net Journal Directory. http://www.beyritrabsnutter.bet/hiyrbaks/cat_016.html

Söderback, I. (2008). Hospital discharge among frail elderly people: a pilot study in Sweden. Occup Ther Int, 15(1), 18–31.

Stein, F., and Cutler, S. K. (2000). Clinical Research in Occupational Therapy, 4th ed. San Diego, CA: Singular Publishing Group/Thomson Learning.

World Health Organization. (2007). ICF introduction. http://www.who.int/classifications/icf/site/intros/ICF-Eng-Intro.pdf.

Chapter 2
Occupational Therapy: Emphasis on Clinical Practice

Ingrid Söderback

Abstract This chapter surveys the classification systems for identifying candidates for occupational therapy. Clients[1] are diagnosed with medical conditions causing functional limitations and restrictions in activities of daily living, such as self-care, and in home, work, and leisure activities. Occupational therapy core contents, purposes, and goals are defined. The theoretical basis, fundamental principles, ethical considerations, and therapeutic media are outlined, and the occupational therapist's (OT's) role is clarified.

Keywords Clients • clinical reasoning • Disability • goals • Health • ICF • International Classification of Functioning • interventions • Need for occupational therapy • Occupational therapy • purpose • statements • theoretical base and therapeutic media.

Statements of Definitions of Occupational Therapy Core Contents

Occupation is the core content and the most basic concept of occupational therapy.

> Occupations is everything people do to occupy themselves, including looking after themselves...enjoying life...and contributing to the social and economic fabric of their communities.... (Law et al., 1997)

Occupations deal with the equality of the interventions in occupational therapy.

> Occupation or goal-directed activity is a method to improve human performance in self-care, work, and play/leisure pursuits. These methods are originated in theory and research that links the physical, psychological, cognitive, and emotional factors (capabilities) of human performances to the individual's attitudes, motivation, values, interests, habits, living environment, and present culture. (Levine and Brayley, 1991)

---

[1] Client is the chosen term throughout the Handbook. However, it is interchangeable with the term patient.

I. Söderback (ed.), *International Handbook of Occupational Therapy Interventions*,
DOI: 10.1007/978-0-387-75424-6_2, © Springer Science+Business Media, LLC 2010

Thus,

> Occupational therapy is any activity, mental, or physical, medically prescribed and profes-
> sionally guided to aid a patient (client) in recovery from disease or injury. (McNary, 1947)

In occupational therapy, occupation is thus both the mediator and the goal of the intervening process (Royeen, 2002).

In other words, purposeful and meaningful activities are used in occupational therapy (Stein and Roose, 2000) to *restore* people's functioning and to *prevent* disability. Environmental barriers frequently need to be removed to *facilitate* people's *participation* in social life (World Health Organization, 2007a).

Core elements of the work of occupational therapists (OTs) are (1) the production of tasks and activities and the time it takes to do them; (2) the "doing" process itself; and (3) clients' motivation for "doing," their experience of meaning and satisfaction while doing, and the results (Nelson, 1988, 1996).

How a therapeutic occupation is performed depends strongly on the individuals' functional capability, will, interests, habits, roles, and what is socially common and acceptable in the individual's culture (Kielhofner, 2007). These factors deeply influence how the OT conducts an intervention.

This facts are illustrated: Many years ago, an OT from South Africa met a Swedish colleague of mine during a conference. In his presentation, my colleague explained how to adapt the knobs on an electric stove if the patient has weak handgrips, and how to arrange for a person in a wheelchair to be able to reach the knob when cooking. The South African's comment after the lecture:

> This is not relevant, possible, or appropriate in my country: you know, most women, even
> if they are not disabled, sit on the ground and do their cooking over an open fire.

Professional Titles in Occupational Therapy

Some European countries use the terms *ergotherapy* and *ergotherapist* instead of occupational therapy and occupational therapist (World Federation of Occupational Therapists (WFOT), (2008a).

The ancient Egyptian *ankh symbol* is the professional sign adopted by OTs working in the United States and Sweden. The symbol (Fig. 2.1) represents "everlastingly life, contributing to good health and protecting from negative active influence" (Ellison, 2008; Wikipedia, 2008a).

Throughout this handbook, a stylized ankh is used to symbolize the OTs' therapeutic roles (Fig. 2.1) in health care and social welfare.

Classifying Those Who May Need Occupational Therapy

Clients who participate in occupational therapy may do so at (1) a hospital; (2) a care institution, such as a nursing home, senior citizens' home, or health center; (3)

Fig. 2.1 The Ankh sign. A wall at the Temple of Karnak, Luxor, Egypt. (Photo: Ingrid Söderback.).

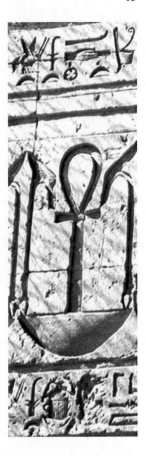

a wide range of workplaces; and (4) in their homes. Students may participate in occupational therapy at their schools (WFOT, 2008a).

Classification systems are used to define and describe strengths and deficits of people who may need occupational therapy. The following are used alone or in combination:

- *International Classification of Functioning, Disability, and Health (ICF)* is "used to understand and measure health conditions." This is a system for classifying health and health-related domains that describes body functions and structures, activities, and participation. The ICF also includes a list of environmental factors. The term *functioning* is the catchall term for "body functions, activities, and participation," and *disability* is the catchall term for "impairments, activity limitations, or participation restrictions" (World Health Organization, 2007a).

According to the ICF, people may be helped by occupational therapy if they meet the following criteria:

- Have impairments due to changed body functions or structures concerning (1) mental functions, (2) sensory functions, (3) neuromusculoskeletal and movement-related functions, or (4) functions of the skin and related structures. They *seldom have impairments due to* (1) voice and speech functions; or (2) functions of the cardiovascular, hematologic, immunologic, and respiratory systems. They

The occupational therapist

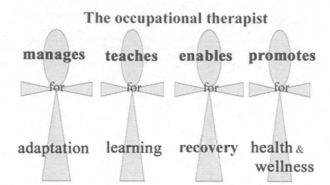

Fig. 2.2 The occupational therapist's roles are as follows: To manage internal, temporal, occupational, and environmental adaptations that affect occupational behavior and performance and that influence patterns of daily occupation. To teach activities of daily living so that that clients learn to accomplish desired and expected tasks at home, at work, at school, in leisure time, and in the community. To enable the client to perform meaningful and purposeful occupations, which then promotes his or her recovery and well-being. To promote health and wellness, i.e., prevent accidents and illness (Soderback, 2008). The figures are stylized Ankh signs (see page 3).

very seldom have impairments due to functions of the digestive, metabolic, and endocrine system, and they *almost never have impairments due to* genitourinary and reproductive functions.

- Have a combination of impairments and disabilities or solely disabilities concerning performances of (1) learning and applying knowledge, (2) general tasks and demands, (3) communication, (4) mobility, (5) self-care, and (6) domestic life.
- Have restricted participation in (1) personal interaction and relationships; or (2) community, social, and civic life.

  - *The Occupational Therapy Framework: Domain and Process ("The Framework")* (American Occupational Therapy Association (AOTA), (2002) describes occupational therapy in general. It shows how clients have strengths and deficits in occupational spheres, performance skills/patterns in relation to context, what an activity demands, body functions and body structures, and other factors affecting the occupation. According to the Framework, candidates for occupational therapy have performance limitations when conducting needed or desired occupations (see, for example, Chapter 44).
  - The *Diagnostic and Statistical Manual of Mental Disorders DSM-IV-TR* (American Psychiatric Association, 2008).
  - Other country-specific systems for classifying care interventions and used in several care professions, include, for example, for use in Sweden, "Classification of Care Interventions" (National Board of Health and Welfare [Socialstyrelsen], 2008).
  - Occupational therapy interventions may depend on the client's age. (For children, see Chapters 35 and 42; for adults, older adults, and frail elderly, see Chapters 18 and 52.)

– The *Statistical Classification of Diseases and Related Health Problems* 10th Revision, Version for 2007 (ICD[10th]) contains 22 chapter blocks classifying diseases and disorders (World Health Organization, 2007b) resulting from illness or injury.

The diagnoses represented in this handbook are classified according to the ICD, and are presented in Table 2.1. They correspond relatively well to those in occupational therapy textbooks, such as that by Pedretti and Early (2001).

While the ICD might not be considered the most appropriate system for describing strengths and deficits among occupational therapy clients, it has the overwhelming advantage of being well known among health professions and stakeholders internationally, for which reason it is used here.

As long as there is no consensus among OTs worldwide regarding what classification system has the desired validity for identifying people needing therapy, it is of less significance what system is used—either one of those mentioned above, or a locally used system. Similar shortcomings in "agreement between the definitions of the Framework and the clinical application" have been demonstrated by Butts and Nelson (2007). Consequently, epidemiologic knowledge of which people need and participate in occupational therapy should be further developed by conducting research on needs assessment (Soriano, 1993). These considerations also influence the public's knowledge of the discipline of occupational therapy.

The Occupational Therapist

An occupational therapist is a health care practitioner who analyzes the impact of occupation on health and quality of life in order to restore a functional interaction between the person and the environment. (School of Physical and Occupational Therapy McGill University, 2008)

The Occupational Therapist's Main Roles

The OT's main roles are as follows:

1. The *therapeutic role:* responsibility for collaborating with clients so that they reach the goals of engagement in meaningful and purposeful activities of daily living (ADL).
2. The *team-member role:* acting together with other health professionals in habilitation, medical rehabilitation, geriatric, or social welfare teams to attain the client's expected health goals.
3. The *consulting role:* cooperating with the client's family, friends, coworkers, and others (landlords, architects) who can play a significant role in helping the client attain his or her goals. These roles entail interpersonal relationships, requiring the OT's cooperation and management (Yerxa, 2001), meaning that OTs guide, advise, recommend, and coach to solve problems (Glantz and Richman, 1997).

Table 2.1 Examples of diseases/disorders represented in this handbook, thus describing the candidates who may participate in occupational therapy

ICD-RHP Blocks	Title	Disease	Exemplified in the handbook Disease/disorder specified	Chapter no.
F10–F19	Mental and behavioral disorders	Due to psychoactive substance use	Alcoholisms and drug abuse	28
F20–F29	Mental and behavioral disorders		Severe mental illness	41
F20–F29	Mental and behavioral disorders	Schizophrenia, schizotypical, and delusional disorders	Schizophrenia	16
F20–F29		Schizophrenia, schizotypical, and delusional disorders	Schizophrenia	24
F20–F29		Schizophrenia, schizotypical, and delusional disorders	Schizophrenia	25
F20–F29		Schizophrenia, schizotypical, and delusional disorders	Schizophrenia	26
F20–F29			Depressive disorders	40
F30–F39	Mental and behavioral disorders	Mood: state of depression	Dementia	19
F30–F39		Mood: anxiety and panic disorder	Anxiety and panic disorder	27
F70–F79	Mental and behavioral disorders	Disorders of adult personality and behavior	Mental retardation	34
G80	Diseases of the nervous system	Cerebral palsy and other paralytic syndromes	Cerebral palsy	35
G82	Injury, poisoning, and certain other consequences of external causes	Paresis/paralysis in the lower limb	Paraplegia, tetraplegia, and muscle weakness	8
G83	Injury, poisoning, and certain other consequences of external causes	Injury, poisoning, and certain other consequences of external causes	Several various diseases, e.g., cerebral paresis	29
G83		Paralysis of upper limb	Stroke	31
G00–G09	Diseases of the nervous system	Inflammatory diseases of the central nervous system	Musculoskeletal pain and fatigue	38
G82	Injury, poisoning, and certain other consequences of external causes	Paralysis of upper limb	Cumulative trauma disorders	6
G82		Paresis/paralysis in the lower limb	Paraplegia and tetraplegia	7
G83	Injury, poisoning, and certain other consequences of external causes	Paresis/paralysis in the lower limb	Stroke, hemiparesis	9
H00–H59	Visual disturbances and blindness	Low vision on both eyes	Various eye diseases	13
LF30–LF39	Mental and behavioral disorders	Schizophrenia, schizotypical, and delusional disorders	Alzheimer's disease	45
M00–M99	Diseases of the musculoskeletal system and connective tissue	Neck and back pain	Musculoskeletal pain	36

ICD code	Category	Description	Condition	No.
M00–M99		Neck and back pain	Chronic low back pain disorder	37
M00–M99			Neck and back pain	38
M00–M99			Neck and back pain	55
M00–M99			Neck and back pain	56
M05–M14	Inflammatory polyarthropathies		Rheumatoid arthritis	33
M15–M19	Inflammatory polyarthropathies		Arthrosis	33
S00–T98	Injuries, poisoning, and certain other consequences of external causes	Injuries to the wrist and hand, fractures, burns	Hand trauma, hand arthritis	10
S00–T98		Injuries to the wrist and hand, fractures, burns	Burn injury	11
S10–S19	Injuries to the neck; spinal cord injury	Injuries to the neck; spinal cord injury	Musculoskeletal pain	36
S6	Intracranial injury (brain injury) (brain damage)	Acquired brain injury	Stroke	20
S6			Acquired brain injury, stroke	21
S6			Acquired brain injury, stroke: apraxia	22
S6			Multiple sclerosis	23
S6			Stroke	30
S6			Parkinson's disease	32

The classification is according to the International Classification of Diseases and Related Health Problems (ICD-RHP), 10th Version, for the World Health Organization (2007b).

During this interaction, OTs focus on strategies that (1) create a relationship built on confidence with their client, (2) support goal setting that makes use of the client's experience, and (3) motivate the client's interdependent living (Guidetti and Tham, 2002).

The Therapeutic Aspect of the Occupational Therapist's Role in Health Care

In the clinical cooperation between the client and the OT, the OT is the partner who possesses the pedagogic, psychological, and medical knowledge and professional skill to conduct interventions. She or he is (1) *the manager of adaptations* (see Part II), (2) *the teacher of functioning* (see Part III), (3) *the enabler of occupations* (see Part IV), and (4) *the promoter of health prevention* (see Part V) (Fig. 2.2).

This four-factor classification of the therapeutic content of occupational therapy differs from earlier approaches. It was framed early on in the development of this handbook (see Chapter 1) as a way of considering the discipline as a whole. It is based partly on the author's 40 years of clinical experience as an OT and partly on occupational therapy textbooks. It may usefully be refined and needs further research to be valid for future use.

The Purposes of Occupational Therapy

The main purposes (Fig. 2.2) of occupational therapy are (1) to help clients learn or relearn activities they want and need to master for the conduct of their daily lives, (2) to help clients adapt to their disability so as to develop effective occupational performance, (3) to help clients by providing environmental adaptations that facilitate increased participation in social life, (4) to ensure that clients are occupied in ways that promote feelings of recovery, and (5) to work to prevent disease and trauma and thus promote health and wellness.

The Occupational Therapy Discipline

The academic discipline of occupational therapy may be divided into basic research and applied research:

- The newly developing *basic research area* is termed *occupational science*. This area concerns mainly studies of how occupations affect human health and vice versa (Clark et al., 1991; Zemke and Clark, 1996).
- The *applied research area* includes studies of (1) needs assessment (Müllersdorf and Soderback, 2000; Soriano, 1995); (2) clinical reasoning (Schell and Schell,

2007); (3) marketing (Soderback and Frost, 1995); (4) controlled studies of evidence for the intervention's effectiveness; and (5) cost effectiveness (Graff et al., 2008).

The applied research focuses on interventions—the area with which the handbook is mainly concerned (Parts II to V).

The Theoretical Base of Occupational Therapy Interventions

Clinical practice is guided by the occupational therapy's theoretical and applied knowledge consisting of the following:

- *Axioms* and *theories* that describe the human as an occupied being
- *Values and beliefs* about people's capacity to alter their performance of daily occupations toward health
- *Ethical considerations*
- *Clinical reasoning* about how to manage specific interventions with clients
- *Experience of conducting interventions*

Axiom

An axiom is a fundamental statement that "commends itself to general acceptance" (Oxford English Dictionary). Axioms include a presumption that truth is not susceptible of proof with currently available scientific methodology.

The axioms used in occupational therapy all concern hypotheses about the relationship between the occupied human being and his or her health. Meyer (1922), a psychiatrist and neurobiologist who worked with people with mental illness, is widely considered the "father of occupational therapy." He stated this axiom:

> Man learns to organize time and he does it in terms of doing things. (Meyer, 1922; quoted in Christiansen and Baum, 1997, p. 33)

This may be understood to mean that occupation provides the human being with "a sense of reality, achievements, and temporal organization" (Christiansen and Baum, 1997, p. 33).

Another often quoted and well-known axiom was stated by Reilly (1962):

> Man, through the use of his hands as they are energized by mind and will, can influence the state of his own health. (p. 2)

Through creativity and doing tasks a person can "deploy his thinking, feelings, purposes to make himself at home" (van Deusen, 1993, p. 159).

Axioms that include statements such as the above are criticized for lacking connection with the OT's everyday role and clinical practice. Elizabeth Yerxa (1967) recognized this gap between occupational science and clinical practice. She emphasizes the role of the OT in "assisting the individual to cope with problems of everyday living and to adapt to limitations that interfere with competent role performance" (Baum and Christiansen, 1997, p. 34).

A typical axiom for this handbook is that *occupational therapy interventions influence clients' states of activity health*, which include the experience of (1) being in a state of occupied equilibrium, (2) conveniently, and with feelings of (3) meaningfulness, (4) well-being, (5) satisfaction, and (6) optimal quality of life.

Activity health means that experience and feelings when performing occupations of daily life meet a person's expected goals and appropriate sociocultural norms (Cynkin and Robinson, 1990; Soderback, 1999). This experience is a possible outcome factor of occupational therapy.

Theories and Models

Occupational theories and models describe *people as occupied beings living in their social and cultural environments*. Among many promising approaches, the predominate models, in my view, are as follows:

- The *Model of Human Occupation* (Kielhofner, 1985, 1995, 2002, 2005, 2007)
- The *Occupational Science* (Johnson and Yerxa, 1989; Zemke and Clark, 1996)
- The *Person–Environment Occupational Performance: A Conceptual Model for Practice* (Christiansen and Baum, 1997)[2]

These models have made invaluable contributions to the development of the discipline and to OTs' clinical reasoning (see page 11).

Values and Beliefs

The following prominent values permeate OTs' thinking in their work with clients:

- People have the capacity to find *alternative ways* of performing occupations to gain competence and master their desired and expected roles in life. This may entail changes toward a state of *occupied equilibrium*, meaningfulness, and well-being. This positively influences quality of life and health.
- *Participation* in occupational therapy, where clients are occupied in various purposeful or meaningful ways, *influences* their *occupational capability*.
- OTs seek to apply *client-centered interventions* (Sumsion, 2006). Here the client is *valued* as his or her own expert. Therefore, it is the client's knowledge of how to arrange his or her daily habits, and choice of meaningful and purposeful activities, that influences the OTs intervention plans.

---

[2] For extensive accounts of the contents and the pros and cons of these Models reference is to the original literature.

- The client is the actor, the occupied partner during all therapy sessions. The OT acts as a guide, *helping the client to self-help.*
- The habilitative/rehabilitative aspect is highly valued, focusing on the client's future ability to move from *dependence to interdependence to independence.*

Ethical Considerations

Ethical considerations operate in all clinical situations in which OTs need to decide on what is right or wrong. They may involve the following:

- *Autonomy:* the clients' right to determine the contents of and their participation in the interventions.
- *Justice:* the clients' right to well-balanced resources employed in scientific and evidence-based professional practice.
- *Beneficence:* the OT's obligation always do the best for the client, with an interest in the client's personality and life history, and to avoid doing harm, injury, or damages (nonmaleficence).
- *Equity:* the OT's way of treating all clients equally irrespective of their age, impairment, disability, social class, race, sex, religion, or cultural values.
- *Fidelity:* the OT's legal responsibility to maintain confidentiality (Hansen, 1993; Peloquin, 1998).

Clinical Reasoning

Clinical reasoning is a chain of theories of the occupied human being, scientific knowledge, and evidence-based practice. The chain may be viewed as the art of managing occupational therapy interventions (Hagedorn, 1995) and the emphatic and ethical ways of meeting the client.
Clinical reasoning entails the following:

- The OT's ideas of optimal clinical practice are compatible with the needs of the client. Clinical practice embraces all that happens during an interactive intervention process.
- The OT has the knowledge and experience to conduct therapy. OTs must respect clients' narratives about their experience of disability and life in order to understand and make decisions about interventions that may also be applied with future clients. OTs use this information to explain intervention choices, motivate the client to participate, and make the final decisions about the therapy.
- The OT makes use of available information about the client when planning, directing, and reflecting on a client's proposed participation. The following questions help: Who is the client? What is his or her occupied status? What does the client want in relation to what occupational therapy can offer and the community can afford? What are the goal and expected outcome? What would be the

most effective and appropriate intervention? Is the stipulated intervention evidence-based and cost-effective? (Early, 2001).

Conducting Occupational Therapy Interventions

Intervention refers to what occurs during an occupational therapy session. It is the OT's application of methods used to adapt, teach, enable occupations, and promote activity health (Fig. 2.2; see also the accounts in Parts II to V).

Interventions are made based on the OT's professional management skills, which constitute a *case management process*. The process involves evaluation, intervention, and outcome (American Occupational Therapy Association, 2007). The seven aims of the process are (1) to evaluate the client's occupational performance status, (2) to set realistic and appropriate goals in accordance with the client's wishes and expectations, (3) to judge whether available interventions may contribute to the client's activity health, (4) to select and implement appropriate intervention(s), (5) to use appropriate therapeutic media, (6) to give the client information that may boost motivation and participation (see Chapter 57), and (7) to discharge the patient and assess the outcome (see Part VI).

This process is described as linear (Reed and Sanderson, 1980). However, in clinical practice the steps are interactive and may be used as an integrative case management process, as described by Hagedorn (1995). This interactive process where the various steps were used simultaneously has been demonstrated in a clinical study of six outpatients (Soderback et al., 1994).

The Goals of Occupational Therapy

In occupational therapy, a goal is a concise statement of what is expected to occur over the short term or a long term (Hagedorn, 1995). Goal setting is based on assessments[3].

The OT states appropriate goals for the intervention depending on the client's occupational and medical statuses. The direction of the medical prognosis may be as follows:

- *Improvement.* Recovery is possible, such as after a hip replacement. The goal is to *develop* or *restore* the clients' functioning and occupational performance.
- *Status quo.* The client's condition is a permanent state, such as paraplegia. The intervention goals are to *maintain* present functional status of (regained) abilities, allowing the performance of needed and desired daily occupations.

---

[3] For an extensive overview of available assessments, see the Index of Assessments, Approaches and Instruments" (C Christiansen & Baum, 1997) and use a database search, e.g., Entrez PubMed (National Library of Medicine, 2008).

- *Deterioration.* A decrease in functional status is expected, such as with Alzheimer's disease clients. The intervention goals are to *compensate* for lost disability by adapting occupations and environments and to *prevent* risks of ill health that restricted occupational performance incurs (American Occupational Therapy Association (AOTA), 2002).

Summarizing, the main goals of occupational therapy interventions are to optimize function, activity, and participation, to enable/improve the performance of ADL tasks, and to express feelings of being occupied.

Subgoals may be to acquire new ways of doing daily occupations, change behavior toward a healthier lifestyle, overcome internal or external obstacles to occupation, obtain or keep paid employment, and maintain daily occupations (Reed and Sanderson, 1980).

Therapeutic Media Used in Interventions

Occupational therapy interventions include combinations of therapeutic media, also termed *professionally legitimized tools* (Mosey, 1986). The most commonly used therapeutic media are discussed in the following subsections.

Deliberate Therapeutic Conscious Use of Self

The use of self is the professional way that OTs meet and communicate with clients, team members, and other health professionals and people involved in the clients' care and habilitation/rehabilitation. It is the OT's "planned use of personality, insights, perceptions, and judgments [that contribute to] the therapeutic process" (Rogers, 2007). Engagement and knowledge should mark the OT's cooperation with and management of the client. This cooperation should comprise an understanding of the client's personal circumstances. The OT should show empathy and respect for the client's life situation, and maintain ethical behavior (see page 11) (Hagedorn, 1995; Schwartzberg, 1993).

Activity Analysis and Activity Synthesis

These analyses focus on the tasks that constitute the performances of an occupation or activity. Activity synthesis is the integration of some or all of these performance components with an appropriate theory that is consistent with the client's goals and present status (Crepeau, 1998). Activity analysis and synthesis are prerequisites for using purposeful and meaningful occupations as legitimate tools (Mosey, 1986).

Activity analysis is the OT's detailed examination giving information about the inherent qualities and requirements of an occupation, an activity, or a task. This examination is required if the occupation is to be usable as a therapeutic medium. Through it, the OT may understand (1) the performance components and sequential steps that complete a task; (2) the tools, equipment, material, and other sources needed for the "doing"; (3) how the task's difficulty level can be adapted to various degree of difficulties; (4) the time necessary for completion; (5) ergonomically and environmental prerequisites of effective and optimal performance; and (6) elements of risk or danger in the doing process. Results of an activity analysis also give OTs information about the clients' feelings about what they are doing (e.g., not everyone enjoys washing dishes) (Lamport et al., 1989; Stein and Roose, 2000).

Activity analysis also underlies *job analysis*, showing what a job requires of a worker in terms of functions, characteristics, components, temperament, and environmental conditions (Scaaerfl, 2003; U.S. Department of Labor, 1996; U.S. Department of Labor, Employment and Training Administration, and Service, 1991). Such analysis is used in connection with simulated work tasks in occupational rehabilitation (VALPAR, 1993), to modify work tasks so that they match the worker's ability and to prevent occupational injuries (Soderback, 2006; Soderback et al., 2000; Stein et al., 2006).

Activity synthesis consists of the integrative processes among the client, the actual occupation, and the appropriate theory [i.e., frames of reference (Mosey, 1986)]. Activity synthesis leads to the development of *strategies* with which the client learns desirable new ways of performing occupations. This learned-performance approach is expected to be able to generalize to new occupations or new situations. Thus, activity syntheses may be used for selecting which performance components should be stressed during an intervention, and how the occupation should be graded and adapted (Creapeau, 1998; Hagedorn, 1995).

Activity synthesis requires of the OT specific knowledge of the biomechanical, ergonomic, neurodevelopmental, cognitive–perceptual, and psychosocial theories that may be the focus of the intervention. Activity syntheses are a part of the OT's professional knowledge base, though they seldom are distinctly explicit.

Activity synthesis is the base for the following:

- *Intervention approaches* (see Part III) used for teaching functional training for remediating (see Chapters 20 to 22). An example is cognitive teaching of the dialogue technique approach.
- *Constructing occupational therapy assessments.* For example, the Intellectual Housework Assessment (IHA) consists of integration between the analysis of housework tasks, where work sequences are selected and integrated with Luria's neuropsychological functional reorganization theory (Soderback, 1988).

Purposeful Activities Used Therapeutically

This therapeutic medium comprises the clients' performance of (1) ADL, such as self-maintenance and housework; (2) real or simulated work tasks; (3) tasks used for training functional performances, such as movement of a paralytic arm/hand; and (4) doing arts and crafts (Levine and Brayley, 1991).

Quite simply, the OT selects an activity that is effective for reaching the client's goal. The OT (1) determines degree of difficulty of performance, (2) chooses what tools and materials should be used, and (3) expresses other requirements for performance. These professional decisions are made in relation to the clients' present functional ability, will, and motivation for participation (Mosey, 1973; Schwartzberg, 1993).

Therapeutic Uses of Meaningful Activities

These activities comprise the clients' performance of *things that he or she wants to do*. OTs in various ways enable clients to perform occupations otherwise barred to them by their current status. Doing meaningful activities is a way of meeting the client's need for acceptance, achievement, creativity, autonomy, and social relations. The meaningfulness of the activity should help the clients to feel that they are productive, contributing, and needed members of the community (see case of Marie-Louise, Chapter 43).

Therapeutic Uses of Problem Solving

These uses include (1) how OTs may suggest unusual ways of performing occupations; problem solving in this context is closely related to adaptive interventions (see Chapter 3); and (2) a training strategy for managing common social situations (Liberman et al., 1998).

Therapeutic Uses of Group Dynamics

Mosey (1986) stated: "A group is an aggregate of people who share a common purpose and are interdependent in the achievement of that purpose." Group dynamics as a legitimate tool is often used (1) to create spirit of community, (2) to express feelings among clients who have a similar experience of disability, (3) to foster a healthy lifestyle, and (4) to develop social skills (Mosey, 1986).

A great range of purposeful and meaningful activities, such as arts and crafts, housework, and leisure-time activities, is used to mediate group dynamics. The OT's responsibility for creating a therapeutic group is (1) to plan, analyze, synthesize, and adapt the occupation to be performed; (2) to recommend the constellation and number of group members; (3) to set the goal for the group; (4) to outline norms for the group; and (5) to establish how the environment should be arranged to encourage interaction among the group members. Here the OT's professional leadership skills come into play, in particular managing communication with and among group members, since this is often directed at modeling clients' behavior or facilitating the expression of clients' feelings (Hagedorn, 1995; Schwartzberg, 1998).

Therapeutic Use of Ergonomics and Environmental Factors

Ergonomics is how the environment meets the person's needs for overcoming disability and restricted social participation (see Parts II and V). Environmental factors include the person's immediate surroundings and social interaction with others.

Environmental factors are used deliberately in most occupational therapy interventions aimed at adapting the environment and preventing trauma and ill health in the home and at the workplace.

Ergonomics include applications of (1) *ergonomic physical principles*, such as actions with joints in neutral positions to avoid constant muscle strain and pain (see Chapter 56); (2) *ergonomic psychological principles*, such as organizational factors at work that affect workers' stress levels, possibly leading to stress-related ill health, exhaustion, or depression (see Chapter 54); and (3) *the use of universal design* (Stein et al., 2006) to achieve the best fit between the individual and the tools used (see Chapter 15).

Origin

The term *occupational therapy* originated in the United States in 1914. Occupational therapy is often stated as having originated in the philosophical ideas of the *moral treatment* movement. This movement valued work as having a positive influence on patients' health. However, other influences were from social movements such as the *settlement movement*, which aimed to ameliorate daily life especially among women. The *arts-and-crafts movement* originated in England and was adopted in the U.S. by the founding physicians of occupational therapy, Adoph Meyer, Herbert Hall, and William Dunton, around 1920. Their philosophical believe was that "creative and manual work could help reconstruct one's sense of self and therefore help to counteract the negative effects of industrialization" (Clark et al., 1998, pp. 14–15). In 1925 in Aberdeen, Scotland, the first American-educated OT was employed. Thus, the philosophical beliefs that influenced the origin of occupational therapy were an enriching exchange between the U.S. and the United Kingdom in the early 1920s (Baum and Christiansen, 1997; Clark et al., 1998; Hagedorn, 1995).

The first federation for promoting occupational therapy was founded in 1917 in the U.S. Occupational therapy as a modern *health profession* was established there during the early 1920s and was at first practiced mainly in psychiatric hospitals.[4] A more detailed account of the origin of occupational therapy in USA

---

[4] The following references are recommended for full information about occupational therapy's origins in the USA: "The Occupational Therapy Context" (Baum & Christiansen, 1997) and in the USA and Great Britain "Occupational Therapy: A Retrospective" (Hagedorn, 1995).

and Great Britain, respectively, is depicted by Baum and Christiansen (1997) and Hagedorn (1995).

Where one places the roots of occupational therapy depends on the country. For example, in Sweden the first official training of occupational therapists was conducted in Stockholm in 1947.[5]

The World Federation of Occupational Therapists (WFOT) was established in 1952 in Stockholm, and it runs an international congress every fourth year.

Occupational Therapy During the Past 40 Years

Occupational therapy has undergone several vicissitudes in the past 40 years according to my interpretation of the context of our textbooks (see, Chapter 1, Table 1.1). During the 1960s, the interventions were linked to medical diagnoses, such as the management of neurologic conditions (Macdonald, 1964). This brought about a reductionist perspective on the human being, with the consequence that the core content of occupational therapy was diminished.

During the 1980s and 1990s, emphasis shifted to descriptions of the development of occupational therapy programs, centering on how the OT contributes to teamwork in, for example, psychosocial rehabilitation (Fleming Cottrell, 1993). This view of occupational therapy frequently caused it to be confused with the contributions of other health care professions, especially physiotherapy.

The late 1970s and the 1980s was a period in many countries, Sweden among them, where political trends required the training of health care professionals, including OTs, to be expanded from a vocational base to an academic university discipline. This opened the way for OTs to earn PhDs and to perform research that revolutionized the scientific bases of occupational therapy.

Professional demarcation and development of the concepts of the core content, especially "occupation," was the order of the day. One consequence of the raised educational level was that developing an academic discipline required theoretical approaches. These theories were expected to contribute to (1) the application of educational curricula, (2) the production of basic knowledge concerning how the human being is occupied, (3) research, and (4) scientific evidence. Occupational therapy gained from this development.

Between 1980 and 1997 many theories (i.e., abstract descriptions of phenomena) and models (i.e., descriptions of conceptual systems) were developed.

---

[5] Personal communication to Inga-Britt Lindström, chair-woman of the Swedish Federation of Occupational Therapists; Gunilla Myrin, former head of the occupational therapy department, the Rehabilitation Clinic, Danderyd hospital, Stockholm Sweden and Kerstin Wikell, former colleague ibid. clinic.

However, there is still a gap between these theories/models/frames of reference and how occupational therapy is clinically applied, as stated by Kielhofner (2005): "Produced by academics … they are not consistently translated into occupational therapy practice." Kielhofner's suggested a solution might be a more effective dialogue between researchers and practitioners. Hopefully, this might contribute to the building of bridges of "generative discourse" and creating demonstration sites (Kielhofner, 2005).

Applications of the above-mentioned theories and models, together with many other theoretical ideas from the psychological–pedagogic–medical–technical sciences constitute *frames of reference* (Dutton et al., 1993; Mosey, 1986) with behavioral, biomechanical, cognitive, and developmental approaches. Their purposes are to provide the OTs with a knowledge base for clinical reasoning concerning the practical use of assessments and interventions (Christiansen, 1991). The authors of this handbook give accounts of the relevant theory/model/frame of reference that contribute to the knowledge base of the interventions they present (see Parts II to V).

The 20th century provided a holistic perspective on the human being. The focuses now are on (1) "occupation" as the core content of occupational therapy interventions, (2) applied research concerning *client-centered practical models* describing the client–therapist interactions (Mortenson and Dyck, 2006); this research was expected to attain the *goals* of developing, maintaining, or improving clients' health and well-being and avoiding ill health; and (3) evidence-based research, which provides the community with information about the outcomes, cost-effectiveness, and value of OT interventions (Pierce, 2001). These perspectives on occupational therapy interventions approximate the contents of this handbook (see Parts II to V). Thus, this handbook may be considered to be one of many generative discourses for education and a source for the development of occupational therapy.

Occupational Therapy: A Worldwide Profession

Statistics and Figures

Currently, OTs are working in health care and social welfare in at least the 73 countries represented in the World Federation of Occupational Therapists (WFOT) (2008b), that is, about one third of the world's 244 states (Wikipedia, 2008). The European Network of Occupational Therapy in Higher Education (ENOTHE) represents 48 European states in which OTs are trained and occupational therapy services exist.

The figures suggest that occupational therapy has a very shifting representation among the world's states. Available figures from Europe show that there are 74 OTs per 100,000 inhabitants in Germany, England, and Denmark, and 62 per 100,000 in Sweden, but only four per 100,000 in Spain and none in Italy.

In most of the Western industrialized world, occupational therapy is now an established service in health care and welfare. Moreover, in many countries it is a university discipline. However, in Eastern and Central Europe the presence of occupational therapy is minimal (European Network of Occupational Therapy in Higher Education, 2008). For example, in some Eastern European countries, such as Russia, OT is a rather new service. In Russia OT training was first conducted as late as 2002, in St. Petersburg.[6] The Swedish Association of Occupational Therapists (2008) conducted and guaranteed the quality of this 2-year program.

This handbook's authors were chosen partly in attempt to produce a worldwide representation of occupational therapy (see Chapter 1). They represent 56 universities, institutions, and hospitals, distributed worldwide as shown in Fig. 1.1 in Chapter 1.

Factors Influencing the Existence, Need for, and Evolution of Occupational Therapy Services

Over the years, *the medical health panorama* has strongly influenced occupational therapy. Here are some examples:

- As a consequence of the polio epidemic of the 1950s, people survived with serious disabilities. To assist these people, rehabilitation clinics were started, for example at Danderyd Hospital in Stockholm, Sweden, in 1962. In the countries to which people returned from the battlefields of the Second World War with physical disabilities, the need for medical rehabilitation and occupational therapy grew both in the U.S. and the U.K.
- During the tuberculosis epidemic of the 1920s, sanatoria were established in Sweden, where occupational therapy was included in the recovery treatment. However, because medical treatment has drastically reduced the number of patients with tubercular diagnoses, rehabilitation/occupational therapy is no longer needed. Thus, when medicine makes revolutionary progress, the panorama of candidates participating in occupational therapy changes.

Political and Economical Factors

The medical care organization and policy of individual countries determines the extent of health and medical care and social welfare, including whether occupational therapy is a part of the system. The portion of gross national product that a country chooses to allocate to health care is also significant. The social insurance system also affects how much occupational therapy a client is entitled to.

---

[6] Personal communication to Natalia Ponanova, author of Chapter 27.

Legal Factors

Legislation affects the status of occupational therapy and the respect in which the profession is held. Thus, for example, certification in Sweden has positively affected the respect for occupational therapy.

Cultural Factors

Cultural factors affect the content of occupational therapy. For example, the extent to which arts and crafts are used as a legitimate tool varies extensively around the world. Furthermore, traditional ideas of how health care should be conducted in various countries also influence the therapy, which is reflected in this handbook (see also p. 2).

Marketing

Marketing is a decisive factor in the existence and development of occupational therapy. Information on the discipline must be conveyed in terms of professional competence, current research, and the proven effects of participation. It is the moral duty of every OT to contribute to this marketing so that it may contribute to the health and well-being of present and future clients and to the advancement of health care and social care.

Conclusion

This chapter provided a short overview of the extensive knowledge that constitutes occupational therapy. The content presented here is what is judged necessary to understand the content of Parts II to VI. However, it is strongly recommended that the reader study the references and follow the development of occupational therapy through available scientific articles and textbooks.

References

American Occupational Therapy Association (AOTA). (2002). Occupational therapy practice framework: domain and process. In: The Reference Manual of the Official Documents of the American Occupational Therapy Association, Inc. (Vol. 56, pp. 211–236, 609–634). Bethesda, MD: AOTA.

American Occupational Therapy Association. (2007). AOTA classification codes for continuing education activities. Category 2. Occupational therapy process. http://www.aota.org/Practitioners/ProfDev/CE/WebFind/38453.aspx

American Psychiatric Association. (2008). Diagnostic and Statistical Manual of Mental Disorders (DSM-IV-TR). http://www.allpsych.com/disorders/dsm.html

Baum, C., and Christiansen, C. (1997). The occupational therapy. Context. Philosophy–principles–practice. In: Christiansen, C., and Baum, C., eds. Occupational Therapy. Enabling Function and Well-Being (pp. 33–35). Thorofare, NJ: Slack.

Butts, D.S., and Nelson, D.L. (2007). Agreement between occupational therapy practice framework classifications and occupational therapists' classifications. Am J Occup Ther, 61(5), 512–518.

Christiansen, C. (1991). Occupational therapy. Intervention for life performance. In: Christiansen, C., and Baum, C., eds. Occupational Therapy. Overcoming Human Performance Deficits (pp. 4–43, 12, 49). Thorofare, NJ: Slack.

Christiansen, C., and Baum, C. (1991). Occupational Therapy. Overcoming Human Performance Deficits. Thorofare, NJ: Slack.

Christiansen, C., and Baum, C. (1997). Person–environment occupational performance. A conceptual model for practice. In: Christiansen, C., and Baum, C., eds. Occupational Therapy. Enabling Function and Well-Being, 2nd ed. Thorofare, NJ: Slack. pp. 607–608.

Clark, F.A., Parham, D., Carlson, M.E., et al. (1991). Occupational science: Academic innovation in the service of occupational therapy's future. Am J Occup Ther, 45(4), 300–310.

Clark, F., Wood, W., and Larson, E.A. (1998). Occupational science: Occupational therapy's legacy for the 21st century. In: Niestadt, M.E., and Crepeau, E.B., eds. Willard and Spackman's Occupational Therapy, 9th ed. (pp. 14–15). Philadelphia: Lippincott.

Crepeau, E.B. (1998). Activity analysis: a way of thinking about occupational performance. In: Niestadt, M.E., and Crepeau, E.B., eds. Willard and Spackman's Occupational Therapy, 9th ed. (pp. 135–147). Philadelphia: Lippincott.

Cynkin, S., and Robinson, A.M. (1990). Occupational Therapy and Activities Health: Toward Health Through Activities. Boston: Little, Brown.

Dutton, R., Levy, L.L., and Simon, C. J. (1993). Frames of references in occupational therapy: Introduction. In: Willard and Spackman's Occupational Therapy, 8th ed. (pp. 62–63). Philadelphia: Lippincott.

Early, M.B. (2001). The occupational therapy process—an overview. In: Pedretti, L.W., and Early, M.B., eds. Occupational Therapy. Practice Skills for Physical Dysfunction. London: Mosby.

Ellison, T.R. (2008). The ancient ankh symbol. http://www.touregypt.net/featurestories/ankh.htm.

European Network of Occupational Therapy in Higher Education. (2008). Organisation: ENOTHE members. http://www.enothe.hva.nl/org/members-eng.htm.

Fleming Cottrell, R.P. (1993). Psychosocial Occupational Therapy. Bethesda, MD: AOTA.

Förbundet Sveriges Arbetsterapeuter. (2008). The Swedish association of occupational therapists—FSA. http://www.fsa.akademikerhuset.se/.

Glantz, C.H., and Richman, N. (1997). OTR–COTA collaboration in home health: Roles and supervisory issues. Am J Occup Ther, 51(6), 446–452.

Graff, M.J., Adang, E.M., Vernooij-Dassen, M.J., et al. (2008). Community occupational therapy for older patients with dementia and their care givers: cost effectiveness study. BMJ, 19(336–337), 134–138.

Guidetti, S., and Tham, K. (2002). Therapeutic strategies used by occupational therapists in self-care training: A qualitative study. Occup Ther Int, 9(4), 257–276.

Hagedorn, R. (1995). Occupational Therapy. Perspectives and Process. Edinburgh: Churchill Livingstone.

Hansen, R. A. (1993). Ethics in occupational therapy. In: Hopkins, H.L., and Smith, S.L., eds. Willard and Spackman's Occupational Therapy (8th ed.). Philadelphia: Lippincott.

Johnson, J.A., and Yerxa, E.J. (1989). Occupational Science: The Foundation for New Model of Practice. London: Haworth.

Kielhofner, G. (1985). A Model of Human Occupation. Theory and Application. London: Williams & Wilkins.

Kielhofner, G. (1995). A Model of Human Occupation: Theory and Application, 2nd ed. Baltimore, MD: Williams & Wilkins.

Kielhofner, G. (2002). A Model of Human Occupation: Theory and Application, 3rd ed. Baltimore, MD: Williams & Wilkins.

Kielhofner, G. (2005). Scholarship and practice: Bridging the divide. Am J Occup Ther, 59(2), 231–239.

Kielhofner, G. (2007). A Model of Human Occupations: Theory and Application, 4th ed. Baltimore, MD: Williams & Wilkins.

Lamport, N.K., Coffey, M.S., and Hersch, G.I. (1989). Activity Analysis. Handbook. Thorofare, NJ: Slack.

Law, M., Polatajko, H., Baptiste, W., and Townsend, E. (1997). Core concepts of occupational therapy. In: Townsend, E., ed. Enabling Occupation. An Occupational Therapy Perspective (pp. 29–56). Ottawa: Canadian Association of OTs. (Quoted from Canadian Occupational Therapy Association, 2002. http://www.aota.org/Practitioners/Official/Guidelines/41089.aspx.)

Levine, R.E., and Brayley, C.R. (1991). Occupation as a therapeutic medium. In: Christiansen, C., and Baum, C., eds. Occupational Therapy. Overcoming Human Performances Deficits, Vol. 1 (pp. 597, 616–618). Thorofare, NJ: Slack.

Liberman, R.P., Wallace, C.J., Blackwell, G., Kopelowicz, A., Vaccaro, J.V., and Mintz, J. (1998). Skills training versus psychosocial occupational therapy for persons with persistent schizophrenia [see comments]. Am J Psychiatry, 155(8), 1087–1091.

Macdonald, E.M. (1964). Occupational Therapy in Rehabilitation. A Handbook for Occupational Therapists, Students and Others Interested in This Aspect of Reablement. London: Ballière, Tindall and Cox.

McNary, H. (1947). Quoted in Hopkins, H.H. An Introduction to Occupational Therapy. Scope of Occupational Therapy (p. 3). Hopkins and Smith, 1993.

Meyer, A. (1922). The philosophy of occupational therapy. Arch Occup Ther, 1(1), 1–10.

Mortenson, W.B., and Dyck, I. (2006). Power and client-centred practice: an insider exploration of occupational therapists' experience. Can J Occup Ther, 73(5), 261–274.

Mosey, A.C. (1973). Activities Therapy. New York: Raven.

Mosey, A.C. (1986). Psychosocial components of occupational therapy. In: Mosey, A.C., ed. Psychosocial Components of Occupational Therapy (pp. 16–18, 450–476)., New York: Raven.

Müllersdorf, M., and Soderback, I. (2000). Assessing health care needs. The actual state of self-perceived activity limitation and participation restrictions due to pain in a national-wide Swedish population. Int J Rehabil Res, 23, 201–207.

National Board of Health and Welfare (Socialstyrelsen). (2008). Klassifikation av vårdåtgärder (KVA). [Classification of care interventions.] (in Swedish). http://www.socialstyrelsen.se/Om_Sos/organisation/Epidemiologiskt_Centrum/Enheter/EKT/KVA.htm.

National Library of Medicine. (2008). Entrez-PubMed. http://www.nslij-genetics.org/search_pubmed.html. Retrieved 12/03/2009.

Nelson, D. L. (1988). Occupation: form and performance. Am J Occup Ther, 42(10), 633–641.

Nelson, D.L. (1996). Therapeutic occupation: a definition. Am J Occup Ther, 50(10), 775–782.

Oxford English Dictionary. The definitive record of the English language. http://www.oed.com/.

Pedretti, L.W., and Early, M. B. (2001). Occupational Therapy. Practice Skill for Physical Dysfunction, 5th ed. London: Mosby.

Peloquin, S. M. (1998). The therapeutic relationship. In: Niestadt, M.E., and Crepeau, E.B., eds. Willard and Spackman's Occupational Therapy, 9th ed. (pp. 105–119). Philadelphia: Lippincott.

Pierce, D. (2001). Occupation by design: Dimensions, therapeutic power, and creative process. Am J Occup Ther, 55(3), 249–259.

Reed, K., and Sanderson, S.R. (1980). Concepts of Occupational Therapy. London: Williams & Wilkins.

Reilly, M. (1962). Occupational therapy can be one of the great ideas of the 20 century medicine. The Eleanor Clarke Slagle lecture. Am J Occup Ther, 16, 1–9.

Rogers, S. (2007). Occupation-Based Intervention in Medical-Based Settings (pp. 1–8). Thorofare, NJ: AOTA's OT JobLink.

Royeen, C.B. (2002). Occupation reconsidered. Occup Ther Int, 9(2), 111–120.

Scaaerfl, R.A. (2003). Dictionary of Occupational Titles. http://www.dictionay-occupationalaltitles.net/index.html.

Schell, B.A., and Schell, J.W. (2007). Clinical and Professional Reasoning in Occupational Therapy. London: Lippincott Williams & Wilkins.

School of Physical and Occupational Therapy, McGill University. (2008). Occupational therapy program. http://www.mcgill.ca/spot/ot

Schwartzberg, S.L. (1998). Group process. In: Niestadt, M.E., and Crepeau, E.B., eds. Willard and Spackman's Occupational Therapy, 9th ed. (pp. 120–131). Philadelphia: Lippincott.

Schwartzberg , S.L. (1993). Therapeutic use of self. In: Hopkins, H.L., and Smith, H.D., eds. Willard and Spackman's Occupational Therapy, 8th ed. (pp. 269–274). Philadelphia: Lippincott.

Soderback, I. (1988). Intellectual Function Training and Intellectual Housework Training in Patients with Acquired Brain Damage. A Study of Occupational Therapy Methods. Stockholm: Karolinska Institute.

Soderback, I. (1999). Validation of the theory: satisfaction with time-delimited daily occupations. Work, 12(2), 165–174.

Soderback, I. (2006). Vocational counselling. In: Schmidt, R.F., and Willis, W.D., eds. Encyclopaedia of Pain, 1st ed. (pp. 2651–2654). Berlin: Springer.

Soderback, I., and Frost, D. (1995). Transfer of knowledge in occupational therapy. A case of work ability assessment. Work, 5(3), 157–165.

Soderback, I., Krakau, I., Gruvsved, Å., et al. (1994). The quality of occupational therapy evaluated in six outpatients. Occup Ther Int, 1(2), 122–138.

Soderback, I., Schult, M.-L., and Jacobs, K. (2000). A criterion-referenced multidimensional job-related model predicting capability to perform occupations among persons with chronic pain. Work, 15(1), 25–39.

Soriano, F.I. (1995). Conducting Needs Assessments. A Multidisciplinary Approach. London: Sage.

Stein, F., and Roose, B. (2000). Pocket Guide to Treatment in Occupational Therapy. San Diego, CA: Singular.

Stein, F., Soderback, I., Cutler, S.K., and Larson, B. (2006). Occupational Therapy and Ergonomics. Applying Ergonomic Principles to Everyday Occupation in the Home and at Work, 1st ed. London/Philadelphia: Whurr/Wiley.

Sumsion, T. (2006). Client-Centered Practice in Occupational Therapy: A Guide to Implementation, 2nd ed. London: Churchill Livingstone.

U.S. Department of Labor. (1996). JIST's Electronic Enhanced Dictionary of Occupational Titles (JIST's DOT). Indianapolis, IN: JIST Work.

U.S. Department of Labor, Employment and Training Administration, and Service. (1991). Dictionary of Occupational Titles. Indianapolis, IN: JIST Work.

VALPAR. (1993). VALPAR Component Work Samples (VCWS). Tucson: VALPAR.

van Deusen, J. (1993). Mary Reilly. In: Miller, R.J., and Walker, K.F., eds. Perspectives on Theory for the Practice of Occupational Therapy (pp. 155–178). Gaithersburg, MD: Aspen.

Wikipedia. (2008). List of countries. http://sv.wikipedia.org/wiki/Lista_%C3%B6ver_l%C3%A4nder.

World Federation of Occupational Therapists (WFOT). (2008a). What is occupational therapy? http://www.wfot.org/information.asp.

World Federation of Occupational Therapists (WFOT). (2008b). Country profiles. http://www.wfot.org/information.asp.

World Health Organization. (2007a). International classification of functioning, disability and health. ICF introduction (homepage). http://www.who.int/classification/icf/site/icftemplate.cfm?myurl = home.

World Health Organization. (2007b). International statistical classification of diseases and related health problems. http://www.who.int/classifications/apps/icd/icd10online/.

Yerxa, E.J. (1967). 1966 Eleanor Clarke Slagle lecture. Authentic occupational therapy. Am J Occup Ther, 21(1), 1–9.

Yerxa, E.J. (2001). The social and psychological experience of having a disability: Implications for occupational therapists. In: Pedretti, L.W., and Early, M.B., eds. Occupational Therapy. Practice Skills for Physical Dysfunction (pp. 487–488). London: Mosby.

Zemke, R., and Clark, F. (1996). Occupational Science: The Evolving Discipline. Philadelphia: F.A. Davis.

Part II
Interventions: The Occupational Therapist Manages and Facilitates the Client's Adaptation

Chapter 3
Adaptive Interventions: Overview

Ingrid Söderback

Abstract This chapter surveys the intrinsic, occupational, temporal, and environmental adaptive interventions used in occupational therapy. Therapeutic media are outlined, and the occupational therapist's role is clarified. The chapters of this part of the handbook exemplify how OTs manage the clients' various adaptations aimed at facilitate his or her (Fig. 3.1) occupational performance. The clinical applications of the four major factors of adaptations are illustrated through the case of John, a man suffering from paraplegia.

Keywords Adaptive interventions • Environmental • Intrinsic • Occupational • Paraplegia • Temporal • Therapeutic media.

Case Study

An accident at work left John paraplegic and wheelchair-bound. He had been a manager of a large farm. He lived in a first-floor apartment in an old building on the farm that came with the job, but the bathroom was on the ground floor.

John had very firm opinions on everything in his life. Thus, for example he refused, most unreasonably, to wear shoes since he could not walk. John had come to the rehabilitation department many months previously and should have left weeks ago. He was bored and refused to participate in almost all activities, particularly occupational therapy.

The primary opinion of the rehabilitation team was that John could not move back to his apartment at the farm. The owner judged it impossible to render the apartment wheelchair-friendly. John had been offered an apartment for people with disabilities in an apartment building, but he refused to move to any other place. The rehabilitation team was very concerned: what would happen to John?

My job was being John's contact person. I managed to persuade him to wear boots when he went out for some fresh air in the winter, so that his feet wouldn't freeze. If the boots were put between the wheelchair's foot supports, they stood firm enough for him to lift his paralyzed leg into the leg of the boot; gravity did the rest.

I. Söderback (ed.), *International Handbook of Occupational Therapy Interventions,*
DOI: 10.1007/978-0-387-75424-6_3, © Springer Science+Business Media, LLC 2010

The occupational therapist

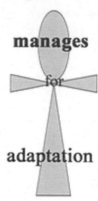

manages

for

adaptation

Fig. 3.1 The figure shows the OT's role in managing the occupational therapy interventions aimed at adaptation of the client's internal and external environment. The figure is a stylized Ankh-sign.

This way of putting on his boots allowed John to be less afraid of losing his balance and falling out of the wheelchair, thus giving him a feeling of independence.

When our patients were outdoors, I sat next to John. I talked to him, sometimes without getting an answer. I put a deck of cards in my pocket and one day I asked John if he could play cards. John was happy to be able to show me something he was good at: playing poker. We had established contact at last.

I asked John if he had visited his home since the accident (I knew that he had not). Spring came and a week or so later John asked me if I could take him to visit his home. He wanted to see the apple blossoms on the farm. I got permission from his physician, and a taxi was ordered for the next day. It was the first time John had been outside the hospital grounds. When we reached the farm, John wanted me to go in and fetch a few things for him. There were stairs up to the front door and just inside there were 14 steep steps up to the apartment. To the right was the bathroom with a door that was too narrow to admit a wheelchair.

I could not find the things John wanted. Then he decided to "walk" up to the apartment himself. At the bottom stair, he raised himself from the wheelchair and sat on the second stair. He then lifted himself, facing backward, up to the apartment. I carried the folded wheelchair and John raised himself first onto a stool and then into his wheelchair. He went into his kitchen and bedroom without a problem.

Following a telephone call to the hospital, John decided to stay home until the next day. I brought him a special raised toilet seat combined with a latrine bucket. When I visited him the next day, John had spent 24 hours at home without any problems.

The rehabilitation team planned to discharge John to his apartment at the farm—a very cost-effective measure. I organized the necessary contacts for home adaptation and a discussion with the farm's owner to explain what changes in the apartment were absolutely necessary. A stair-lift was installed, plus handrails at suitable points. John received daily help from a home help service.

In professional terms, what occupational-therapy interventions were effective in enabling John to live independently at home?

The main intervention was *adaptation*, which is the changing process aimed at fitting different human conditions into various environments. In John's case, this meant his interaction with his home environment. Because this interaction went well, there were improvements in John's behavior (Barris et al., 1985), in his ability to perform tasks independently, rationally, and effectively, and in his will to live at home. This interactive human balance may be changed by using *intrinsic, occupational, temporal,* and *environmental* adaptations.

Intrinsic Adaptations

Intrinsic adaptations address cognitive factors: (1) *ability* to acquire general or special types of knowledge (National Library of Medicine and Health, 2006); (2) *skills*, indicating at what level of competence tasks are performed; and (c) *capacity*, the current potential to perform. Ability, skills, and capacity are affected by the individual's functional status: (1) *self-efficacy*, meaning one's perception of and belief in one's ability to perform tasks successfully; and (2) *motivation*, the innate drive to master challenges. These personality factors generate the emotional reactions that affect the individual's occupational performances (Matheson, 1997) and hence constitute the individual's intrinsic adaptation.

The occupational therapist (OT) uses environmental stimuli to bring about changes in intrinsic adaptation. Another term for intrinsic adaptation is *occupational adaptation*, which Bontje et al. (2004) defined as people's attempt at overcoming disabling influences on occupational functioning.

John's paraplegia impaired his ability to perform daily activities. He had lost his capacity to walk, let alone work. In this situation John was very vulnerable to the environmental demands, as his social role had changed completely (Hansen et al., 2005; Matheson, 1997), stifling all initiative, energy, motivation, and drive. The consequences of this were loss of self-efficacy and motivation to be independent and occupied. John's innate and intrinsic needs to master occupational challenges were severely disturbed. In Levine and Brayley's (1991) words, the optimal fit between intrinsic adaptation and social and environmental demands was in imbalance. The occupational therapy goal was to effect a positive change in motivation and self-efficacy.

The Occupational Therapist's Role

In situations like John's, the OT's role is to establish communication based on the client's psychosocial status, will, wishes, and interests (Bränholm, 1992; Kielhofner, 1985). The OT may use his or her knowledge, experiences, understanding, engagement, empathy, and respect to motivate the client to perform self-initiated, self-chosen, purposeful, and meaningful activities. The *therapeutic use of self* is the medium for bringing about the change in the client's intrinsic adaptation (Schwartzberg, 1993).

John's intrinsic adaptation was initially influenced through the way the OT presented poker playing. John became engaged in an occupation within his sphere of interest. As against his present role as an impaired person, he could feel himself as being a more competent and skilled person, doing something he was good at and that was meaningful to him. Presenting tasks in ways that engage clients may prompt them to act as their own agent of change (Dunn, 1997).

The terms *internal adaptation* and *coping* are closely related. Schultz (1997) stated that coping is the individual's specific emotional reaction to a particular condition, while adaptation is the individual's reaction to how far environmental demands are within his or her capacities.

My database search prior to inviting authors to contribute to this handbook found numerous studies addressing the relationship between coping and stress, and descriptions of the *progress* of intrinsic adaptation among several diagnostic groups, for example the elderly (Bontje et al., 2004), patients with craniocerebral trauma (Dumont et al., 2007), and patients with poliomyelitis sequelae (Jönsson et al., 1999). However, few studies addressed therapeutic approaches aimed at improving clients' intrinsic adaptation. Therefore, this subject is not further included in this handbook.

Occupational Adaptation

Occupational adaptation of tasks and activities makes use of tools and materials (Schwartzberg, 1993). It addresses how to help clients adjust to perform a task in the most functional, rational, practical, effective, and ergonomically appropriate way (Stein et al., 2006). Examples include (1) determining the most practical direction for peeling potatoes—toward you or away from you, (2) determining the most ergonomically and labor-saving way of opening a jar—with one hand or by fixing the jar in place, (3) using a tool that requires less force, (4) determining which hammer and what type of nails are most effective for a particular task, and (5) determining the most practical way of cutting slices of a tomato to show a "fleur-de-lis" pattern and to prevent the seeds from spilling out.

Adapting clients' task performance may follow a natural development (Bontje et al., 2004), potentially observed among people born with impaired nervous systems (e.g., cerebral paresis), or those who slowly develop such impairments (e.g., degenerative muscular dystrophy diseases) (Nätterlund, 2001).

Motivation prompts the client to adapt to the performance of an task. This internal prompt is affected by the client's perception of how meaningful the task is and how satisfied he or she will feel upon its completion. The various ways of performing a task depend on (1) *personal factors*, such as habits, skills, and experience; (2) what *task* is expected to be performed, and the form and function of the result; and (3) the *context for the performances*, for example, the process, available time, and cultural norms (Knox, 1993).

John was motivated to be outdoors every day. This habit was originated from his farm work. During this work, he normally wore boots, not shoes. Because of his impaired neuromusculoskeletal and movement-related function, he had two options: either to remain dependent on another person to help him put on his boots every time he wanted to go outdoors, or learn to put on his boots in a different way than he did before he was injured.

In a therapeutic perspective, clients adapting the performance of an task always choose a method or procedure that differs from their regular habits or from the general manner in which most people perform the task. These alternative methods and procedures permit people to accomplish a part of or the complete task.

People who are suddenly disabled, like John, may have difficulty adapting to the performances of tasks and therefore need professional help.

The Occupational Therapist's Role

The role of the OT is a *supporting and educational* one (see chapter 17). The OT promotes the client's attempt to carry out the task in a way that suits his or her personality and the environmental context. The OT draws on his or her experience and imagination to create the optimal adaptation for the occupation (task) to be performed. The occupational adaptations include the following principles (Nätterlund, 2001; Nätterlund and Ahlström, 1999; Stein et al., 2006):

- *Problem solving*, which includes steps to identify, develop, plan for, and implement an appropriate and meaningful solution for the client. For John, the solution to the problem of toileting was the special raised seat combined with a latrine bucket.
- *Using an unusual body part* for performing an activity, such as using the toes for gripping and handling a paint brush (Mouth-and-Feet Artists, 2007). This is exemplified by how John used his back to *walk* upstairs.
- Using *gravity as a force*. Hence, John used the weight of his leg to help in putting on his boot.
- *Holding an object* or keeping an object still by using unusual body parts, such as holding a bowl between the knees. Alternatively, holding an object still by external arrangements, such as putting the bowl on an anti-slip mat, fixing the work object in place with clamps, or holding a boot between the footrests of a wheelchair, as John did.
- The muscle strength required for opening, lifting, bending, pushing, filling, or pouring can be decreased by *using both hands* or by using tools with leverage.
- *Optimal body positioning*. People with a hemiparetic arm can learn to put on a shirt, blouse, or cardigan by turning the neckline in position away from the body, holding the wrong side of the garment up, and taking the paretic arm to cross the middle line of the body. When drawing the sleeve over the hand, the hand and arm will turn into the garment. Then it is easy to draw it over the shoulder (Eggers, 1991).

The above-mentioned principles for adaptation of tasks need to be addressed in clinical studies, as there is little documentation, which is why this topic is not further represented in this handbook.

Temporal Adaptation

Temporal adaptation is the process of assessing and adjusting one's use of time during performances, and how this time use arouses feelings (Szalai and Converse, 1973; Soderback, 1996; van Deusen, 1993). Temporal adaptation varies depending on the task and activity, such as daily self-care, sleep, work, recreation, and rest (Kielhofner, 1977; Kielhofner et al., 1980; Nurit and Michal, 2003). The *temporal balance* should mirror the client's realistic adaptation to scheduled and organized time, in which the client gives priority to occupations that are desired or expected. Adolph Meyer (1922), the "father of occupational therapy," stated, "A suitable balance among individuals' daily activities, self-maintenance, work, leisure time activities, rest and sleep is important for remaining in good mental health" (see also Weeder, 1986).

The way people manage their *temporal balance* is expressed in unique *temporal activity patterns* or idiosyncratic configurations.

A temporal activity pattern consists of time-cycles of occupational performance. These patterns include *when* (timing), *how long* (duration), sequential *order*, and *frequency* of performance. Temporal activity patterns appear in daily routines that are rational and suitably managed and common in the culture in which the individual lives (Kielhofner, 1977). The patterns are configured by the individual's self-perception of his/her efficacy level, values, interests, and goals. Temporal activity patterns are influenced by the individual's intrinsic adaptation, seeking to structure and organize activity to overcome stress. Therefore, when an individual experiences balance within the temporal activity pattern, comfortable feelings may be aroused.

McKenna et al. (2007) demonstrated a habitual average temporal activity pattern among 195 Australian people, 75 years of age or older. The participants spent "most of their time on sleep (8.4 h/day), solitary leisure (4.5 h/day), instrumental activities of daily living (3.1 h/day), social leisure (2.7 h/day), and basic activities of daily living (2.6 h/day)." Such outcomes of the temporal activity patterns are expected to determine people's *activity health,* well-being, and satisfaction (Cynkin and Robinson, 1990; Nieistadt, 1993). Activity health is promoted when the individual has control over available time within a time frame and is able to properly organize time into a balance of occupations.

Activity ill-health may be seen as imbalances or disorganizations of the temporal activities patterns (Kielhofner, 1977; Rosenthal and Howe, 1984; Soderback, 1996). Activity ill-health has been demonstrated, for example, among people suffering from paraplegia (Yerxa and Locker, 1990) and stroke (Soderback and Lilja, 1995), and among the elderly (Nystrom, 1974). Activity ill-health interferes with an individual's ability to manage time to accomplish occupations in sequential order or as a daily routine. When disruption of regularly cycles occurs, it often leads to a feeling of disorientation and confusion, a feeling of being unsettled of being in a somewhat chaotic state, and being unable to set goals that give meaning to the performance of activities. This condition appears commonly when social roles are changed (Kielhofner, 1977). Individuals may feel (1) that they have too much time, because they are no longer employed; or (2) that they have too little time, because physical, cognitive, or social limitations make activities of daily living very time-consuming, or

(3) that social limitations lead to stress, which can lead to taking sick-leave from work.

In the case of John, activity ill-health occurred in terms of temporal maladaptations, which were observed because he did not want to participate into the offered rehabilitative activities.

An *activity configuration log* (Cynkin and Robinson, 1990; Soderback, 1996; Yerxa and Locker, 1990) or diaries (Ellergård and Nordell, 1997) are a either paper-and-pen or a computerized[1] self-assessment instrument (e.g., Soderback, 1996). This assessment instrument is used to measure clients' temporal balance between activity health and activity ill-health in terms of activity patterns. Temporal adaptation, that is, the configuration of the client's occupational patterns, might be shown in the outcome factors of *satisfaction* (Sandqvist and Eklund, 2007) and *meaningfulness* in relation to the client's perception of the amount of *effort* needed to accomplish the activities and of the quality of the *results*. These outcome factors are assessed by a four-point Likert scale (1 = negative value; 4 = positive value) (Soderback, 1996).

Soderback (1996) made an attempt to validate the Activity Configuration Log among 142 employees (21 to 60 years of age) divided into four groups of those who were on sick-leave 4%, 21%, 52%, or 97% of the 135 observation days. The result showed a weak support for the discriminative validity between the group of the participants with the most extensive sick-leave time and the three other groups, regarding the amount of time used for self-care ($p = 0.02$) and work ($p = 0.00$) activities and for the group's perception of how much effort they used in the performance of daily activities. Further research in this area is required. However, clinical application of this study might be used for investigation of employees in order to prevent sick-leave.

The use of a temporal adaptive intervention is further discussed in Chapter 16.

The Occupational Therapist's Role

The OT plays a supporting role in temporal adaptation, eliciting the client's feedback. The interventions directed at client's temporal adaptation are aimed at improving the balance of the temporal activity patterns, and are guided by the following principles:

- The OT *supports* the client's opportunities to participate in activities that correspond to his or her interests and values. The interventions may bring about a reorientation of the client's pattern of interests or habits, framed by how the client uses his or her time (van Deusen, 1993).

In John's case the OT supported his interest in playing poker. During these sessions, an interaction began between John and his spectrum of time-related activities. This might have supported communication and promoted healthy behavior on an ongoing

---

[1] A computerized version of the activity configuration log is available from the author.

daily basis that in turn might have influenced his development of a changed social role.

- The OT *offers clients meaningful occupations* that structure their day and enable social networking (see Chapter 44).

Environmental Adaptation

Environment is the "external elements and conditions which surround, influence, and affect the life and development of an organism or population" (National Library of Medicine and Health, 2008), and that may impede or facilitate live.

The social, attitudinal, cultural, and physical factors that make up the environment include settings such as home, workplace, school, and community. The environment includes products and technology for personal use in daily living, communications, transportation, and recreational facilities (World Health Organization, 2007a, b). The *social environment* is characterized by norms and routines. The *cultural environment* includes economic considerations, customs, beliefs, activity patterns, and societal expectations. The *physical environment* contains all objects that are natural or fabricated. Examples are plants, animals, landscape, buildings, furniture, tools, devices, and clothes. All objects are systems of products, equipment, and technology that are gathered, created, produced, or manufactured (Stein et al., 2006; World Health Organization, 2007b).

General Environmental Adaptations

Environmental adaptations involve modifications of the clients' physical environments that facilitate and enable occupational performance and promote occupational health and well-being. The interventions concern how client's occupational performance is influenced by modifications within the person-environment-occupational transactional system (Christiansen and Baum, 1997a; Kohlmeyer and Ericsson Lewin, 1993; Schult, 2002). Thus, the environment contains the interactive relationship between the time dimensions, active use of space, and changes in people's micro- and macroenvironments that facilitate occupational performance. The general principles of occupational therapy intervention address adaptations of the home and the public environment and are discussed in Chapters 4 and 5.

The Occupational Therapist's Role

The role of the OT is to be a *facilitator* of the client's occupational performance by managing the removing of environmental barriers.

In the case of John, modification of the physical environment—the indoor stair—and adding the supporting handles and handrails enabled John to move back to his apartment and perform the necessary daily activities. The OT facilitates environmental adaptations, taking into account the client's cultural, social, financial, and environmental circumstances. This work is performed in cooperation with architects, landlords, and living partners.

The prerequisites for effective environmental adaptations are that the client accepts and is satisfied with the modification and feels it is meaningful and useful (Early, 2001). This was true for John, who wanted to return to his apartment on the farm.

The effectiveness of the adaptation is also influenced by external circumstances. For example, the owner of the building where John lived felt it was impossible to make the apartment accessible by a wheelchair. Here the OT is working as a *moderator* until a solution that is acceptable for all partners can be found.

Environmental Adaptations: Accessibility and Accommodation

The environmental adaptive interventions include two major factors: accessibility and accommodation. *Accessibility* is aimed at eliminating physical, architectural, or communicative barriers from the environment of the home and the community, and from transportation (Smith, 2001). People deserve access to their physical environment, irrespective of how they transport themselves, be it by walking, by using crutches, a walker, or a wheelchair, or by driving.

Accessibility entails the design of an environment that removes physical barriers and other problems (Nygren et al., 2007). Good accessibility fosters the client's trust and privacy, and offers affordable and usable transportation (Coughlin et al., 2007). These factors affect clients' satisfaction with their living arrangements. Moreover, Nygren et al. showed that the more accessible the elderly perceived their homes to be, the more useful and meaningful it was in relation to their routines and everyday activities.

Computer workstation adaptation (see Chapter 6) is an example of accessibility adaptation. Here, the ergonomic principles and environmental changes are aimed at reducing the occurrences of work-related injuries associated with intensive computer use.

Accommodation is aimed at facilitating people's well-being and independent living. Accommodating interventions are used (1) to change the position or placement of objects in the physical environment (Cook and Hussey, 2002); (2) to apply objects to body structures related to movement, the nervous system, and the skin, that protect joints and enable performance of daily activities; and (3) to provide tools that facilitate activities of daily living.

Occupational therapy interventions that use accommodation principles are adjusted to meet the clients' need for the following:

- *Optimal positioning* and comfortable seating in a wheelchair (see Chapter 7).
- Wheelchair use: finding the most suitable wheelchair, adjusted to the client's anatomic dimensions, movement-related functions, and the environment where it will be used (see Chapter 8).
- *Electrical neuroprosthetics*, which are used as an intervention tool during electrical therapy to increase grasping movements among people suffering from a spinal cord or other neuromuscular injury causing arm/hand pareses. (see Chapter 9).
- An *orthosis* for the hand, which is an "apparatus used to support, align, prevent, or correct deformities or to improve the function of movable parts of the body" (National Library of Medicine, 2008). The functional aims are to decrease abnormal muscle tone, assist functioning in clients with weak muscles, and prevent or correct deformity.
- *Splints*, which are "rigid or flexible appliances used to maintain in position a displaced or movable part or to keep in place and protect an injured part" (National Library of Medicine, 2008). The aims of splints are preventive and corrective, and they provide stabilization. Splints are commonly used for the hand as well as other parts of the body. Splints help attain the best functional movements. Splints are used by people who had (1) hand surgery due to rheumatoid arthritis, (2) a traumatic hand injury (see Chapter 10), or (3) a burn injury (see Chapter 11).
- An *assistive device* (also called *assistive technologies, adaptive equipment,* or *equipment for self-help devices;* http://www.adaptivemall.com) is "not affixed to the body, [and is] designed to help persons having musculoskeletal or neuromuscular disabilities to perform activities involving movement" (National Library of Medicine, 2008).

As for intervention media, environmental adaptive interventions for accessibility and accommodation are mediated by the following factors:

- *Physical arrangement of the home environment*, which includes arranging furniture to provide accessibility, prevent falls, and facilitate dressing (Kratz and Soderback, 1990; Kratz et al., 1997; Stein et al., 2006). When the physical arrangement is optimal, it may improve people's skills (Christiansen and Baum, 1997b) and activity patterns (Niva and Skär, 2006).
- *Biomechanical principles*, which include gravity, force, pressure, and laws of motion. These principles are used to help maintain a functional body posture and reduce stress to the spine. For example, biomechanical principles are used to design a wheelchair.
- *Ergonomic principles*, which include (1) physical factors, such as taking microbreaks, using energy-conservation methods, and placing joints in a neutral position; and (2) psychological principles that reduce stress and increase participation. These principles are used to adapt the environment to the individual's ability and capacity, and to promote energy-saving (see Chapter 23) and injury-preventing performance of tasks.
- Universal design, which entails seven principles that are applied to people's occupational performance (see Chapter 14).

- Ergonomic principles, which pertain to the design of hand tools so as to facilitate work performance. The principles address tools, equipment, consumer products, machine systems, and workstations (see Chapter 15)
- *Human factor ergonomics*, which is used to improve technology and to promote workers' comfort and safety (Stein et al., 2006).
- *Usability testing*, which provides consumers with information about safety testing results and procurement of assistive devices (Swedish Institute of Assistive Technology, 2008).

The Occupational Therapist's Role

The OT's role includes gathering information, selecting and prescribing the most appropriate devices, adapting the devices to the client, and teaching the client how to use them effectively. This role entails an interactive process with the physical, social, and cultural environment (Kohlmeyer, 1993; Trefler, 1997). The use of assistive devices by children is discussed in Chapter 12. The OT's role of prescribing and integrating low vision assistive devices (LVADs) into daily routines by older people is discussed in Chapter 13.

References

Barris, R., Kielhofner, G., Levine, R., and Neaville, A. (1985). Occupation as interaction with the environment. In: Kielhofner, G., ed. A Model of Human Occupation, Theory and Application, 1st ed., Vol. 1 (pp. 42). Baltimore: Williams & Wilkins.

Bontje, P., Kinébanian, A., Josephsson, S., and Tamura, Y. (2004). Occupational adaptation: the experiences of older persons with physical disabilities. Am J Occup Ther, 58(2), 140–149.

Bränholm, I. (1992). On Life Satisfaction, Occupational Roles and Activity Preferences. Occupational Therapy Aspects. Umeå University, Umeå.

Christiansen, C., and Baum, C. (1997a). Person-environment occupational performance. A conceptual model for practice. In: Christiansen, B.C., ed. Occupational Therapy. Enabling Function and Well-Being, 2nd ed. Thorofare, NJ: Slack.

Christiansen, C., and Baum, C. (1997b). Occupational Therapy. Enabling Function and Well-Being. Thorofare, NJ: Slack.

Cook, A.M., and Hussey, S.M. (2002). Technologies that enable mobility. In: Cook, A.M., and Hussey, S.M., ed. Assistive Technology: Principles and Practices (pp. 329–373). St. Louis: Mosby.

Coughlin, J., D'Ambrosio, L.A., Reimer, B., and Pratt, M.R. (2007). Older adult perceptions of smart home technologies: implications for research, policy and market innovations in healthcare. In: Conference Proceedings of the Institute of Electrical and Electronic Engineers, Vol. 1 (pp. 1810–1815). Medical and Biological Society.

Cynkin, S., and Robinson, A.M. (1990). Occupational Therapy and Activities Health: Toward Health Through Activities. Boston: Little, Brown.

Dumont, C., Fougeyrollas, P., Gervais, M., and Bertrand, R. (2007). The adaptation process of adults who sustained craniocerebral trauma. Can J Occup Ther, 74(1), 48–60.

Dunn, W. (1997). Assessing sensory performance enablers. In: Christensen, C., and Baum, C., eds. Occupational Therapy. Overcoming Human Performance Deficits (pp. 476). Thorofare, NJ: Slack.

Early, M.B. (2001). Occupational performances. In: Pedretti, L.W., and Early, M.B., eds. Occupational Therapy. Practice Skills for Physical Dysfunction, 5th ed. (pp. 122). St. Louis: Mosby.

Eggers, O. (1991). Occupational Therapy in the Treatment of Adult Hemiplegia, 7th ed. Chippenham, Wiltshire: Butterworth-Heinemann.

Ellergård, K., and Nordell, K. (1997). Att bryta vanmakt mot egenmakt [To break powerlessness against arbitrariness.] (In Swedish) Borås: Johnsson and Skyttes Förlag.

Hansen, A., Edlund, C., and Bränholm, I. (2005). Significant resources needed return to work after sick leave. Work, 25(3), 231–240.

Jönsson, A., Möller, A., and Grimby, G. (1999). Managing occupations in everyday life to achieve adaptation. Am J Occup Ther, 53(4), 353–362.

Kielhofner, G. (1977). Temporal adaptation: a conceptual framework for occupational therapy. Am J Occup Ther, 31(4), 235–242.

Kielhofner, G. (1985). A Model of Human Occupation. Theory and Application. London: Williams & Wilkins.

Kielhofner, G., Burke, J.P., and Igi, C.H. (1980). A model of human occupation, part 4. Assessment and intervention. Am J Occup Ther, 34(12), 777–788.

Knox, S.H. (1993). Play and leisure. In: Hopkins, H.L., et al., eds. Willard and Spackman's Occupational Therapy, 8th ed. (pp. 260–268). Philadelphia: Lippincott.

Kohlmeyer, K.M. (1993). Assistive and adaptive equipment. In: Hopkins, H.L., et al., eds. Willard and Spackman's Occupational Therapy, 8th ed. (pp. 316–320). Philadelphia: Lippincott.

Kohlmeyer, K.M., and Ericsson Lewin, J. (1993). Environmental adaptation. In: Hopkins, H.L., et al., eds. Willard and Spackman's Occupational Therapy, 8th ed. (pp. 320–325). Philadelphia: Lippincott.

Kratz, G., and Soderback, I. (1990). Individualised adaptation of clothes for impaired persons. Scand J Rehabil Med, 22, 163–170.

Kratz, G., Soderback, I., Guidetti, S., Hultling, C., Rykatkin, T., and Söderström, M. (1997). Wheelchair users' experience of non-adapted and adapted handicap clothes during sailing, quard rugby or wheel-working. Int Disabil Stud,19(1), 26–34.

Levine, R.E., and Brayley, C.R. (1991). Occupation as a therapeutic medium. In: Christensen, C., and Baum, C., eds. Occupational Therapy: Overcoming Human Performances Deficits, Vol. 1 (pp. 616–618). Thorofare, NJ: Slack.

Matheson, L.N. (1997). Occupational competence across the life span. In: Christensen, C., and Baum, C., eds. Occupational Therapy: Enabling Function and Well-Being, 2nd ed. (pp. 431–436). Thorofare, NJ: Slack.

McKenna, K., Broome, K., and Liddle, J. (2007). What older people do: time use and exploring the link between role participation and life satisfaction in people aged 65 years and over. Aust Occup Ther J, 54(4), 273–284.

Meyer, A. (1922). The philosophy of occupation therapy. Arch Occup Ther, 1(1), 1–10.

Mouth-and-Feet Artists. (2007). Mun-och fot målande konstärers förlag AB. [The publishing association of mouth-and-feet artists.] http://www.munochfotkonst.se/content3.html.

National Library of Medicine (2008). PubMed: MeSH is NLM's controlled vocabulary used for indexing articles in PubMed. http://www.ncbi.nlm.nih.gov/entrez/query.fcgi?db = PubMed.

National Library of Medicine and Health (2006, 2008). PubMed and the MeSH databases. www.ncbi.nlm.nih.gow/sites/entrenz?db and www.ncbi.nlm.nih.gow/sites/entrenz?db.

Nätterlund, B. (2001). Living with muscular dystrophy. Illness experience, activities of daily living, coping, quality of life and rehabilitation. Uppsala, Sweden: Uppsala University.

Nätterlund, B., and Ahlström, G. (1999). Problem-focused coping and satisfaction in individuals with muscular dystrophy and post-polio. Scand J Caring Sci, 13(1), 26–32.

Nieistadt, M.E. (1993). Stress management. In: Hopkins, H.L., and Smith, H.D., eds. Willard and Spackman's Occupational Therapy, 6th ed. (pp. 594). Philadelphia: Lippincott.

Niva, B., and Skär, L. (2006). A pilot study of the activity patterns of five elderly persons after a housing adaptation. Occup Ther Int, 13(1), 21–34.

Nurit, W. and Michal, A. B. (2003). Rest: a qualitative exploration of the phenomenon. Occup
    Ther Int, 10(4), 227–238.
Nygren, C., Oswald, F., Iwarsson, S., et al. (2007). Relationships between objective and perceived
    housing in very old age. Gerontologist, 47(1), 85–95.
Nystrom, E.P. (1974). Activity patterns and leisure concepts among the elderly. Am J Occup Ther,
    28(6), 337–345.
Rosenthal, L.A., and Howe, M.C. (1984). Activity patterns and leisure concepts: a comparison of
    temporal adaptation among day versus night shift workers. Ocup Ther Ment Health, 4(2), 59–79.
Sandqvist, G., and Eklund, M. (2007). Women with limited systemic sclerosis. Disabil Rehabil, 8,
    1–9.
Schult, M.-L. (2002). Multidimensional Assessment of People with Chronic Pain. A Critical
    Appraisal of the Person, Environment, Occupation Model. Unpublished Monograph. Uppsala,
    Sweden: Uppsala University.
Schultz, S. (1997). Adaptation. In: Christensen, C., and Baum, C., eds. Occupational Therapy:
    Enabling Functioning and Well-Being (pp. 459–460). Thorofare, NJ: Slack.
Schwartzberg, S.L. (1993). Tools of practice. In: Hopkins, H.L., and Smith, H.D., eds. Willard and
    Spackman's Occupational Therapy (pp. 269). Philadelphia: Lippincott.
Smith, P. (2001). Americans with disabilities act: accommodating persons with disabilities. In:
    Pedretti, L.W., and Early, M.B., eds. Occupational Therapy. Practice Skills for Physical
    Dysfunction, 8th ed. (pp. 237–248). Philadelphia: Mosby.
Soderback, I. (1996). Temporal adaptation. A predictor of being working or sicklisted. Paper
    presented at the IVth European Congress on Occupational Therapy. Certificado di comunica-
    cion oral, Madrid, Spain.
Soderback, I., and Lilja, M. (1995). A study of activity in the home environment among individuals
    with disability following a stroke. Neurorehabilitation, 6(4), 347–357.
Stein, F., Söderback, I., Cutler, S.K., and Larson, B. (2006). Occupational Therapy and Ergonomics.
    Applying Ergonomic Principles to Everyday Occupation in the Home and at Work, 1st ed.
    London/Philadelphia: Whurr/Wiley.
Swedish Institute of Assistive Technology (2008). http://www.hi.se/templats_132.apx.
Szalai, A., and Converse, P.E. (1973). The Use of Time. Daily Activities of Urban and Suburban
    Populations in Twelve Countries. The Hague: Mouton and Converse.
Trefler, E. (1997). Assistive technology. In: Christensen, C., and Baum, C., eds. Occupational
    Therapy: Enabling Function and Well-Being (pp. 489–492). Thorofare, NJ: Slack.
van Deusen, J. (1993). Mary Reilly. In: Miller, R.J., and Walker, K.F., eds. Perspectives on Theory
    for the Practice of Occupational Therapy (pp. 155–178). Gaiterhburg, MD: Aspen.
Weeder, T.C. (1986). Comparison of temporal patterns and meaningfulness of the daily activities
    of schizophrenic and normal adults. Occup Ther Ment Health, 6(4), 27–48.
World Health Organization (2007a). International Classification of Functioning, Disability and
    Health. http://www.who.int/classification/icf/site/icftemplate.cfm?myurl = home..
World Health Organization (2007b). International Classification of Functioning, Disability and
    Health. http://www.who.int/classification/site/intros/ICG-Eng-intro.pdf.
Yerxa, E., and Locker, S.B. (1990). Quality of time use by adults with spinal cord injures. Am J
    Occup Ther, 44(4), 318–326.

Chapter 4
Environmental Adaptations for Older Adults and Their Families in the Home and Community

Laura N. Gitlin

The OT provided various items that made my life easier and comforted me. It gave me a new outlook. I realized I don't have to succumb to my physical difficulties and I won't.

—An 84-year-old woman living alone at home

Abstract Environmental adaptation is an important intervention to help older adults remain at home independently and ease the burden of care on their families. A range of adaptations can be considered, including removing or rearranging objects, special equipment, and adaptive tools. Providing an environmental adaptation involves assessment of a person's needs and capabilities and the environment's physical properties; choosing an adaptation; ordering and installing it; and training the older adult and family member in its use. This chapter provides an overview of environmental adaptation as an intervention for the elderly, clinical principles, and the evidence to support this approach.

Keywords Adaptive equipment • Assistive devices • Frailty • Home modification

Definitions

Environmental adaptations refer to strategies that modify the physical environment, with the goal of supporting and enhancing everyday competencies of persons with physical or cognitive functional challenges (Gitlin, 2001). There are three basic forms of environmental adaptations: assistive technology, structural changes or home modifications, and material adjustments.

Assistive technology (AT), also referred to as special equipment or assistive devices, reflects a wide range of equipment and device choices of varying complexity and cost. Special equipment includes various attachments to a home structure (handrails, grab bars, stair glides). Assistive devices refer to "any item, piece of equipment, or product system, whether acquired commercially off the shelf, modified or customized, that is used to increase, maintain, or improve functional capabilities of individuals with disabilities" (Technology Related Assistance for Individuals with Disabilities Act of 1988). An assistive device can be attached to the home structure or applied to or directly manipulated by a person, such as a wheelchair, walker, cane, or reacher.

Structural alterations or home modifications refer to changes to the original home structure (widening doors, lowering cabinets), including electrical or plumbing work (installation of first-floor powder room).

Material adjustments include alterations to the nonpermanent features of a home (e.g., clearing pathways, removing throw rugs, tacking down carpets, adjusting lighting, rearranging furniture, and color coding or labeling objects.

Use of an environmental adaptation typically requires a behavioral adjustment or a change in the way a person interacts with his or her physical environment. Behavioral adjustments, for example, may include changing footwear, modifying task performance (e.g., sitting on a high stool when preparing meals), simplifying tasks (e.g., pacing self, planning ahead), or changing the function of a living area, such as converting a living room to a bedroom (Gitlin, 1998).

As a therapeutic modality to enhance competencies in older adults, an environmental adaptation is grounded in a Competence-Press Model (Lawton and Nahemow, 1973; Wahl and Gitlin, 2007). This model provides a broad, overarching framework allowing different types and levels of competence such as sensory loss, physical mobility loss, or cognitive decline, and environmental factors including housing standards, neighborhood conditions, or public transport, to be considered. The fundamental assumption of this model for aging persons is that there is an optimal combination of (still) available competence and environmental circumstances, leading to the relative highest possible behavioral and emotional functioning for that person. The model also suggests that it is at the lower levels of competence that older people become the most susceptible to their environment such that low competence in conjunction with high "environmental press" or demands negatively impacts an individual's autonomy, affect, functional capacity, and well-being. A related point is that as competencies decline, the zone of adaptation narrows such that environmental choices that can promote well-being become increasingly more limited, although there is always an option. Within this framework, adjustments to the environment are designed to obtain the right *person-environment fit* to maximize competence.

The role of environmental adaptation as a therapeutic intervention is also supported by prevailing models of disablement, which posit a pathway or trajectory from pathology (a disease state) to performing everyday living tasks with disability. In these models, disability reflects a gap between a person's capability, the demands of a particular task, and the social and physical environment. Verbrugge and Jette's (1994) disablement model suggests the environment is highly relevant to two related aspects of competency: an individual's ability regardless of context, which is referred to as intrinsic ability; and an individual's ability as supported or constrained by the person's physical and social environment, referred to as actual disability.

Here the implication is that the interaction between a person's intrinsic abilities and the built environment, including both its physical and social characteristics, yields actual disability. One conclusion from this model is that disability can be conceptualized as representing an outcome of potentially modifiable environmental factors and can therefore be minimized (Wahl and Gitlin, 2007). Hence, the role of the living environment and its adaptation is paramount in prevailing models of disability and well-being.

Purposes

Environmental adaptations have multiple purposes including a prevention role, such as the use of grab bars for reducing the risk of a fall in the bathroom; a maintenance role, such as the use of task lighting to enable continued participation in a valued activity; or a compensatory role, such as the use of a mobility aid (e.g., cane) to compensate for an underlying impairment. Additionally, adaptation can enhance the ease, safety, and efficiency of everyday performance.

Method

Environmental adaptations are used with increasing frequency by older adults themselves and by health professionals to address age- and health-related functional consequences that compromise daily participation in valued activities (Mann et al., 1995). As a therapeutic modality, it is typically integrated in rehabilitation and home care therapies. Care systems for this therapeutic intervention vary worldwide, with some countries integrating the approach in a sophisticated network of home and community-based services (as for example in Sweden or England). However, in the United States, most older adults who live at home with a functional difficulty do not have access to environmental modification services unless they have a need due to an acute condition, are referred for rehabilitation by a physician, or seek such assistance themselves and pay out-of-pocket. Access to modification services varies widely regionally and there is a complex web of funding mechanisms and no uniformity in assessment, type of modifications available, and training.

Candidates for the Intervention

Environmental adaptations can be helpful to older adults in a wide range of settings (e.g., home, community-based centers) and with varying health and functional challenges including cognitive loss, physical limitations, or sensory changes. Individuals with cognitive impairment may benefit from adaptations involving simple changes to the living environment and ways of performing everyday tasks (Gitlin et al., 2003). Examples of useful adaptations for individuals with cognitive impairment may include, but are not limited to, memory boards, labeling or use of other visual cues including color coding, and removal of clutter or unnecessary objects to promote way finding and in specified areas in which particular tasks are performed (e.g., eating at the kitchen table). Devices such as tub benches, grab bars, and commodes are useful as well. However, more complex technologies (e.g., medication monitoring devices, stair glides) that require new learning may not always be appropriate and need to be determined on a case-by-case basis. Older adults with vision impairments can also benefit from a range of adaptations including, but not limited to, optical devices, color coding, environmental simplification, task lighting, or enlarged clocks, telephones, and reading materials (Horowitz et al., 2006; Wahl et al., 1999).

Recent research suggests that older adults with even subtle physical functional changes such as getting in and out of the tub, or carrying out the garbage, warrant the use of this intervention approach (Gitlin et al., 2006b). Individuals at most risk for functional decline such as those who are over 80 years of age, women, or those of low education, benefit even more than their counterparts from learning and using environmental adaptations (Gitlin et al., 2008). Thus, even the oldest old can improve by using environmental compensatory strategies, and hence this group of elderly persons in particular who are at most risk of frailty should be targeted for this type of service. Although most older adults are willing to make changes to their living environment to address physical limitations, in general this population, particularly in the United States, is relatively unaware of the range of modifications possible and tends to have limited access to services involving assessment and training in the use of equipment, nor are such services typically available or paid for through third-party payers or health insurance programs.

The Role of the Occupational Therapist in Applying the Intervention

Effective use of environmental adaptations requires an occupational therapist (OT) to makes an assessment of the person and the living environment, coordinate or identify a process for obtaining and installing equipment or the home modification, and then instruct the client in its use. In implementing this intervention, OTs may need to work with other professionals including a care manager is coordinating care for the individual, a contractor who may need to install the device (e.g., grab bar, hand rail, or stair glide) or construct the modification (e.g., widening a door), and a family member who may need to learn how to assist or support the older adult in using the modification.

Results

Clinical Application

Providing Environmental Modifications

Providing an environmental modification is a skilled intervention requiring knowledge of an individual's functional, cognitive, and sensory processes, an understanding of the effect of the physical environment on behavior, and an understanding of person–environment dynamics as they unfold in the performance of everyday activities of living (Hagedorn, 2000).

Assessment

Numerous environmental assessments have been developed to evaluate dimensions of settings including the private home, nursing home, or special care unit, and with specific populations, such as residents with dementia, or the physically frail (Gitlin, 2006). Although there is growing recognition of the importance of home assessment, the conceptualization and measurement of living environments remains complex. Moreover, there is not an agreed upon or uniform approach, nor has environmental assessment been incorporated into routine geriatric or traditional home care in the United States.

Existing environmental assessments differ as to their measured characteristics, response formats, and source (self-report, direct observation, proxy) from which ratings are derived. Assessments are either descriptive, in which specific features are identified and described, or evaluative, in which measured dimensions represent desirable attributes, or a combination of the two. Examples of measured dimensions are physical characteristics (lighting, distances, and space); safety; affordance of daily activities (accessibility, prosthetic aids); support of orientation (way-finding); social interaction (privacy and socialization); and support of novelty, stimulation, and challenge. Response formats tend to be nominal (presence or absence of a condition), although ordinal and interval ratings have been developed to reflect the extent to which a desirable attribute is present. Ratings can be obtained through self-report, observation, or both. There is some evidence to suggest, however, that older adults do not accurately report their environmental conditions, and that professional observation yields more reliable information particularly when it concerns home safety and environmental modification needs (Carter et al., 1997; Ramsdell et al., 1989).

Environmental assessments of private residences date back over 30 years in gerontology, with an initial focus on neighborhood and dwelling features. Recent efforts focus on home safety (Johnson et al., 2001) for physically frail older adults (Gitlin et al., 2002; Oliver et al., 1993; Westmead Home Safety Assessment) and are designed and used primarily by health professionals for discharge planning, rehabilitation, or functional maintenance purposes. The Home Environmental Assessment Protocol (HEAP; Gitlin et al., 2002), is an observational tool designed for use in homes of persons with dementia to assess safety, and home modifications in support of function and orientation. Only one assessment, the Housing Enabler, uses a transactional approach in which a person-environment fit index is derived by rating physical features of homes based on a person's capabilities (Iwarsson and Isacsson, 1996). The derived score reflects accessibility or extent to which an individual can access different home features.

Clinical Principles

The provision of an environmental adaptation must be based on certain clinical principles common to the provision of geriatric services overall (Table 4.1). First is that the therapist must assume a client-centered approach. That is, the therapist must involve the client's perspective in problem identification, decision-making, and identification and implementation of specific modifications. Individuals tend to be selective in the types of adaptations that are accepted and may choose one strategy over another based on a wide range of considerations that are not well understood in the research literature. Understanding and respecting a client's preferences is an essential ingredient in this approach.

Another core principle is that since adaptations occur in people's private living space, sensitivity to the meaning of objects and environmental configurations is essential. Objects and environmental setups reflect cultural preferences, long-standing values, and hidden meanings (Oswald and Wahl, 2005). What may appear as a simple alteration that may be helpful to an individual (such as rearranging furniture to enhance way-finding) may disrupt a person's sense of normalcy and long-standing preferred environmental placements. Furthermore, the process of identifying environmental solutions involves problem solving with clients as to their performance difficulties and occupational goals, barriers and supports to performance, and potential environmental solutions. Yet another principle is tailoring. Solutions must be customized to the particular person–environment and cultural and occupational context, with the most effective training actively involving the client through use of demonstration and hands-on practice sessions. Each of these treatment principles is informed by evidence and reflect best practices.

The implementation of a particular environmental solution involves five basic considerations (Table 4.2). These include making small incremental changes to an environment so as not to overwhelm clients and facilitate their adaptation to the change, involving family members when appropriate to support new learning and sustained safe use of modifications, providing only those adaptations that are agreed upon, and providing education about resources for obtaining other adaptations that may be necessary in the future.

Table 4.1 Core principles guiding practice involving environmental interventions with older adults

Core principle	Description	Select eviden-tiary support
Client-driven	Collaborative approach to identify older adult's valued activities and specific performance challenges and explore environmental solutions. Older adult should be viewed as a partner who has valued information about his or her daily challenges and personal functional goals. Client preferences need to be identified and respected. Not every adaptation will be acceptable or perceived as useful to the client such that a range of adaptations should be offered and discussed with only those that are acceptable implemented.	Toth-Cohen et al. (2001)
Cultural relevance and under-standing	View of home as a microculture reflecting values, beliefs, and preferred approaches to carrying out daily activities of self-care. Therapist must identify and understand the specific cultural influences shaping older adult's daily participation choices and what changes in the environment would be acceptable.	Brach and Fraser (2000)
Problem solving	Process of helping older adult identify performance difficulties, environmental barriers, and explore potential environmental solutions. Also, serves as an approach to modeling for older adult to address environmental barriers to effective functioning.	Davis (1973)
Customization	Tailoring of specific environmental strategies to match environmental specifications, person-identified concerns, capabilities, and culturally appropriate solutions.	Richards et al. (2007)
Active engagement	Use of active strategies to instruct older adult in use of adaptations. Use of demonstration, role play, and observed practices are effective.	Chee et al. (2007)

Table 4.2 Key clinical considerations

Make small or incremental changes in the environment, particularly for individuals with cognitive impairments.

Only make those changes acceptable to and agreed upon by the client and family members.

Use catalogues, pictures ,or sample devices as exemplars so that client has realistic understanding of the possibilities.

Allow ample opportunities for practice and refinement of the adaptation if necessary.

Include family members if so desired by the older person in the assessment, adaptation selection process, and training.

Evidence-Based Practice

Knowledge about the evidence of environmental adaptations is emerging. There are several different data sources that support this approach. First, large-scale epidemiologic research consistently shows a relationship between increasing frailty and use of adaptations, suggesting that this is one of the preferred approaches for compensating for decline (Manton et al., 1997). Similarly, studies using population-based samples have shown that use of special equipment is associated with enhanced self-efficacy, whereas reliance on help is not (Verbrugge et al., 1997). Another source of supportive evidence for this approach is from randomized clinical trials with family caregivers and frail elders in which environmental supports are one of the treatment components. While there are few of these studies, they consistently show positive treatment outcomes including reduced falls in fall-risk elders (Cumming et al., 1999), enhanced functioning (Gitlin et al., 2006b; Mann et al., 1999), reduced fear of falling reduced risk of mortality (Gitlin et al., 2006a), and enhanced caregiver self-efficacy and the dementia patient's quality of life (Gitlin et al., 2003). As environmental adaptations tend to be embedded in multicomponent interventions, it is difficult to tease out the specific effects of any one adaptation on a particular behavior or health outcome. Nevertheless, there is a growing consensus that environmental adaptations are an important component of multifactorial approaches to address the complex consequences of chronic illness in older adults.

Discussion

Environmental adaptations mitigate impairment and disability by reducing the press in the environment or demands that exceed a person's capabilities. Of importance is that adaptations be designed to enable an individual to continue participation in a valued occupation.

Existing environmental adaptation services have several limitations that must be noted. First, in many countries, and particularly the United States, there is a lack of funding and necessary supports for the delivery of this therapeutic approach. Existing community-based programs typically have eligibility requirements or programs are specific to a region, or are limited in scope with monetary caps or restrictions on the types of environmental modifications that are available. Second, there is the lack of awareness among consumers and health professionals as to the importance of involving OTs in the assessment and training process for such adaptations. As a skilled intervention, OTs have the requisite knowledge and skill for matching persons and environments with adaptive strategies. Third, this approach requires not only an assessment by an OT but also follow-up training. Often, training and follow-up are not provided due to agency budgetary considerations. Fourth, limited research is available on the relative benefits of any one type of adaptation for specific person–environment configurations so that therapists must often depend on their own experience or collective wisdom. Finally, the evidence is mixed as to whether environmental adaptations prevent falls, whereas there is stronger evidence of its benefits for reducing functional difficulties and enhancing the ability to engage in valued occupations (Mann et al., 1999; Wahl et al., in press).

Acknowledgement This work was supported in part by funds from the National Institute of Mental Health, National Institute on Aging grants RO1 AG22254 and R01 AG13687, and the Pennsylvania Department of Health, Tobacco Funds SAP 4100027298.

References

Brach, C., and Fraser, I. (2000). Can cultural competency reduce racial and ethnic health disparities A review and conceptual model. Med Care Res Rev, Suppl 1, 181–217.

Carter, S.E., Campbell, E.M., Sanson-Fisher, R.W., Redman, S., and Gillespie, W.J. (1997). Environmental hazards in the homes of older people. Age Aging, 26(3), 195–202.

Chee, Y., Gitlin, L.N., Dennis, M.P., and Hauck, W.W. (2007). Predictors of caregiver adherence to a skill-building intervention among dementia caregivers. J Gerontol Med Sci, 62(6), 673–678.

Cumming, R.G., Thomas, M., Szonyi, G., Salkeld, G., O'Neill, E., Westbury, C., and Frampton, G. (1999). Home visits by an occupational therapist for assessment and modification of environmental hazards: a randomized trial of falls prevention. J Am Geriatr Soc, 47, 1397–1402.

Davis, G.A. (1973). Psychology of Problem Solving: Theory and Practice. New York: Basic Books.

Gitlin, L.N. (1998). Testing home modification interventions: issues of theory, measurement, design, and implementation. In: Schulz, R., Lawton, M.P., and Maddox, G., eds. Annual Review of Gerontology and Geriatrics. Intervention Research with Older Adults (pp. 190–246). New York: Springer.

Gitlin, L.N. (2001). Assistive technology in the home and community for older people: psychological and social considerations. In: Scherer, M, ed. Assistive Technology and Rehabilitation Psychology: Shaping an Alliance (pp. 109–122). Washington, DC: American Psychological Association.

Gitlin, L.N. (2006). Environmental assessment. In: Schulz, R, ed. The Encyclopedia of Aging, 4th ed. (pp. 374–375). New York: Springer.

Gitlin, L.N., Hauck, W.W., Winter, L., Dennis, M.P., and Schulz, R. (2006a). Effect of an in-home occupational and physical therapy intervention on reducing mortality in functionally vulnerable elders: preliminary findings. J Am Geriatr Soc, 54(6), 950–955.

Gitlin, L.N., Schinfeld, S., Winter, L., Corcoran, M., and Hauck, W. (2002). Evaluating home environments of person with dementia: interrater reliability and validity of the home environmental assessment protocol (HEAP). Disabil Rehabil, 24(3), 59–71.

Gitlin, L.N., Winter, L., Corcoran, M., Dennis, M., Schinfeld, S., and Hauck, W. (2003). Effects of the home environmental skill-building program on the caregiver-care recipient dyad: Six-month outcomes from the Philadelphia REACH initiative. Gerontologist, 43(4), 532–546.

Gitlin, L.N., Winter, L., Dennis, M., Corcoran, M., Schinfeld, S., and Hauck, W. (2006b). A randomized trial of a multi-component home intervention to reduce functional difficulties in older adults. J Am Geriat Soc, 54(5), 809–816.

Gitlin, L.N., Winter, L., Dennis, M.P., and Hauck, W. (2008). Variation in response to a home intervention to support daily function by age, race, sex, and education. J Gerontol Med Sci, 63A(7), 745–750.

Hagedorn, R. (2000). Tools for Practice in Occupational Therapy: A Structured Approach to Core Skills and Processes. Oxford, UK: Churchill Livingstone.

Horowitz, A., Brennan, M., Reinhardt, J. P., and MacMillan, T. (2006). The impact of assistive device use on disability and depression among older adults with age-related vision impairments. J Gerontol [B]: Psychol Sci Social Sci, 61B(5), S274–S280.

Iwarsson, S., and Isacsson, A. (1996). Development of a novel instrument for occupational therapy assessment of the physical environment in the home—a methodologic study on "The Enabler." Occup Ther J Res, 16(4), 227–244.

Johnson, M., Cusick, A., and Chang, S. (2001). Home-screen: A short scale to measure fall risk in the home. Public Health Nurs, 18(3), 169–177.

Lawton, M.P., and Nahemow, L.E. (1973). Ecology and the aging process. In: Eisdorfer, C., and Lawton, M.P., eds. The Psychology of Adult Development and Aging (pp. 619–674). Washington, DC: American Psychological Association.

Mann, W.C., Hurren, D., Tomita, M., and Charvat, B.A. (1995). The relationship of functional independence to assistive device use of elderly persons living at home. J Appl Gerontol, 14(2), 225–247.

Mann, W.C., Ottenbacher, K.J., Fraas, L., Tomita, M., and Granger, C.V. (1999). Effectiveness of assistive technology and environmental interventions in maintaining independence and reducing home care costs for the frail elderly. Arch Fam Med, 8, 210–217.

Manton, K., Corder, L., and Stallard, E. (1997). Chronic disability trends in elderly United States populations: 1982–1994. Proc Natl Acad Sci, 94, 2593–2598.

Oliver, R., Blathwayt, J., Brackley, C., and Tamaki, T. (1993). Development of the safety assessment of function and the environment for rehabilitation (SAFER) tool. Can J Occup Ther, 60(2), 78–82.

Oswald, F., and Wahl, H.W. (2005). Dimensions of the meaning of home. In: Rowles, G.D., and Chaudhury, H., eds. Home and Identity in Late Life: International Perspectives (pp. 21–45). New York: Springer.

Ramsdell, J.W., Swart, J., Jackson, E., and Renvall, M. (1989). The yield of a home visit in the assessments of geriatric patients. J Am Geriat Soc, 13, 17–24.

Richards, K.C., Enderlin, C.A., Beck, C., McSweeney, J.C., Jones, T.C., and Roberson, P.K. (2007). Tailored biobehavioral interventions: a literature review and synthesis. Res Theory Nurs Pract, 21(4), 271–285.

Technology-related assistance for individuals with disabilities act of 1988 as amended in 1994. Public laws 100–407 and 103–218.

Toth-Cohen, S., Gitlin, L.N., Corcoran, M., Eckhardt, S., Johns, P., and Lipsett, R. (2001). Providing services to family caregivers at home: challenges and recommendations for health and human service professions. Alzheimer's Care Q, 2(4), 23–32.

Verbrugge, L.M., and Jette, A.M. (1994). The disablement process. Soc Sci Med, 38(1), 1–14.

Verbrugge, L.M., Rennert, C., and Madans, J.H. (1997). The great efficacy of personal and equipment assistance in reducing disability. Am J Public Health, 87, 384–392.

Wahl, H.W., Fange, A., Oswald, F., Gitlin, L.N., and Iwarsson, S. (in press). The home environment and disability related outcomes in aging individuals: What is the empirical evidence? The Gerontologist.

Wahl, H.W., and Gitlin, L.N. (2007). Environmental gerontology. In: Birren, J.E., ed. Encyclopedia of Gerontology, 2nd ed. (pp. 494–502). ElsevierOxford, UK: .

Wahl, H.W., Oswald, F., and Zimprich, D. (1999). Everyday competence in visually impaired older adults: A case for person-environment perspectives. Gerontologist, 39(2), 140–149.

Chapter 5
Housing Adaptations: Current Practices and Future Challenges

Susanne Iwarsson

When I signed the contract for this apartment, they said that it was suitable for an older woman like me, with a husband who had had a stroke. But it wasn't at all.

—Client

Abstract Housing adaptation (or home modification) has been an important and common intervention in occupational therapy practice worldwide, based on the notion that occupational performance is the outcome of person–environment–occupation (P-E-O) transactions. Housing adaptation is applicable with all kinds of clients with occupational performance problems in the home setting, since most clients are older people (Iwarsson, 2005). Measures such as removal of thresholds, installation of shower stalls instead of bathtubs, and installation of handrails and grab bars are among the most common. However, based on considerable differences across countries, the possibility of providing such solutions as well as the role of the occupational therapist in the processes of performing housing adaptation vary considerably. A growing body of scientific evidence has the potential to strengthen this part of occupational therapy practice, with the ultimate goal of creating home environments supporting occupational performance.

Keywords Accessibility • Environmental modification • Environmental adaptation • Home modification • usability

Background

Housing adaptation has been an important and common intervention in occupational therapy practice worldwide. It is based on the theoretical notion that occupational performance is the outcome of the person–environment–occupation model (Christiansen and Baum, 1997) transactions (Fänge and Iwarsson, 2007).

Environmental intervention has its roots in a post–World War II philosophy, when clients and rehabilitation practitioners discovered that despite successful functional training, war victims were not able to live independently outside the hospital setting without environmental modification (Steinfeld and Tauke, 2002). Such intervention aims at reducing the demands of the physical environment in the home and its close surroundings, in order to enhance activity and participation and to promote independence (Fänge and Iwarsson, 2005; Gitlin, 1998).

Definitions

The term *housing adaptation* is often used interchangeably with *home modification*, although the latter tends to be used as a broader term, including housing adaptation and other interventions in the home environment, such as home-hazard counseling and provision of assistive technology. Wahl et al. (in press) defined *home modification* as "all efforts to improve a given physical home environment with the aim to make it better suitable to the functional needs of a given person." Thus, to differentiate among different kinds of interventions in the home, the following definition has been suggested for *housing adaptations*, that is, modifications to the built and natural environment:

> The alteration of permanent physical features in the home and the immediate outdoor environment; i.e., the objective is to reduce the demands of the physical environment in the home and its close surroundings, in order to enhance daily activities, and promote the ability to lead an independent life. (Fänge, 2004, pp. 8–9)

The *housing adaptation* may sometimes entail an intervention. The concepts of accessibility, design for all, universal design, and usability, are used interchangeably and without explicit definition and differentiation (Iwarsson and Ståhl, 2003). These concepts have different roots (Steinfeld and Tauke, 2002). To nurture the development of consistent terminology, the following definitions should be used:

Universal Design

> Universal design is synonymous with "design for all" and represents an approach to design that incorporates products as well as building features which, to the greatest extent possible, can be used by everyone. Universal design is the best approximation of an environmental facet to the needs of the maximum possible number of users. Universal design is ultimately about changing attitudes throughout society, emphasizing democracy, equity, and citizenship. Universal design denotes a process more than a definite result.
>
> (Mace, 1985, cited in Iwarsson and Ståhl, 2003)

Accessibility

> Accessibility is a relative concept, implying that accessibility problems should be expressed as a person–environment relationship. In other words, accessibility is the encounter

between the person's or the group's functional capacity and the design and demands of the physical environment. Accessibility refers to compliance with official norms and standards, thus being mainly objective in nature.

(Iwarsson and Ståhl, 2003)

Usability

The concept of usability implies that a person should be able to use, i.e., to move around, be in, and use, the environment on equal terms with other citizens. Accessibility is a necessary precondition for usability, implying that information on the person–environment encounter is imperative. However, usability is not only based on compliance with official norms and standards; it is mainly subjective in nature, taking into account user evaluations and subjective expressions of the degree of usability. Usability is a measure of effectiveness, efficiency, and satisfaction. Most important, there is a third component distinguishing usability from accessibility, viz. the activity component.

(Iwarsson and Ståhl, 2003)

Among these terms *usability* is the most appropriate for the primary outcome of housing adaptation that is based on analysis of person–environment–occupational transactions in order to support the clients' occupational performance.

Purpose

The purpose of housing adaptation is to adapt the housing environment to the clients' needs, given their functional capacity and needs and wishes for optimal occupational performance.

Method

Candidates for the Intervention

Housing adaptation is applicable to all clients with disabilities who have problems performing daily activities in their home setting, where the interventions are aimed at alternation of the environment.

Epidemiology

Research and available statistics show that the vast majority of housing adaptation clients are older people (Boverket, 2005), most often with functional limitations due to the normal process of aging, such as difficulty in bending, difficulty in kneeling, poor balance, and limitations in stamina, in turn leading to dependence on mobility devices (Fänge, 2004).

Housing adaptations for older people are normally not expensive in each case. However, because of current population compositions the cost may aggregate to huge total sums (Fänge and Iwarsson, 2007).

Younger adults living with disabilities caused by neurologic diseases or injuries (e.g., multiple sclerosis or spinal cord injuries) or rheumatic diseases (e.g., rheumatoid arthritis) often need quite expensive housing adaptations (Fänge, 2004).

Children who are disabled due to cerebral paresis, juvenile rheumatoid arthritis, or muscular dystrophy often require extensive and expensive housing adaptations, which entails repeated interventions as they grow and develop.

Settings

Housing adaptations are initiated by occupational therapists (OTs) in all kinds of settings, and the adaptations vary from country to country. In countries where community-based practices are well developed, such interventions are most commonly effectuated by practitioners employed in primary health care, and are run by county councils or municipalities. In countries where OTs run their own enterprises, housing adaptations are often part of their intervention arsenal.

The Role of the Occupational Therapist in Applying the Intervention

Housing adaptation is an intervention for which the prerequisites depend greatly on the national legislative framework. Therefore, it is not feasible to propose basic recommendations that can be generally applicable, and a globally accepted description of the clinical application is not feasible.

Hence, the role of the OT in performing the housing adaptation processes varies considerably. For example, in Sweden, if a health care professional (often an OT) certifies the housing adaptation, the municipality will provide a grant to finance it. The client is the formal applicant and receiver of the grant, and municipality officials administer all applications (Fänge and Iwarsson, 2007). In such a system, the OT's role is well established but contradictory, combining that of an official issuing a certificate of needs for an application process governed by specific legislation, and that of a registered health care professional delivering different kinds of measures intertwined in a client-centered rehabilitation process.

In contrast, delivering housing adaptation interventions in countries where housing adaptation grants do not exist, or depend entirely on whether the client has Medicare insurance, naturally poses quite different demands on the OT.

In current practice, the use of systematic procedures for housing adaptations is scarce (Fänge and Iwarsson, 2005, 2007), and the intervention, which depends very much on the individual therapist, is largely "a black box" (Fänge and Iwarsson, 2007).

Results

Clinical Application

Housing adaptation interventions start with the systematic collection of data for identification of the client's problem. This identification should preferably be based on person–environment–occupational transactions. Analysis of the data leads to the planning of the housing adaptation, which requires the active involvement of the client and his or her family.

Measures such as removal of thresholds, installation of shower stalls instead of bathtubs, and installation of handrails, grab bars, and ramps (Fig. 5.1) are among the most common.

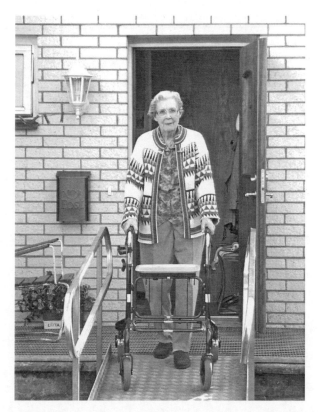

Fig. 5.1 Installation of ramps at entrances is among the most common housing adaptation measures. (Photograph: S. Iwarsson; reproduced with the subject's approval.).

It is necessary to consider the ergonomic working-environment aspects for clients where formal or informal helpers are involved.

Housing adaptation as intervention places great demands on OTs, because they are acting upon the most private domain of a person's living environment. Potential conflicts of interest are inherent in the process.

Evidence-Based Practice

It is hard to evaluate the literature for scientific evidence regarding housing adaptations. The quite diverse systems across countries make comparisons between studies difficult. The majority of published housing-adaptation evaluations lack theory-based definitions of core concepts and outcomes. According to the Cochrane reports (Gillespie et al., 2003; Lyons et al., 2003), the scientific evidence of the effects of housing adaptations is limited, yet a recent literature review including studies with mainly older people (Wahl et al., in press) shows substantial evidence of positive effects. Positive effects were indicated on (1) functional decline (Mann et al., 1999), (2) fear of falling (Cumming et al., 1999; Heywood, 2004), (3) pain and depression (Heywood, 2004), (4) satisfaction and performance in daily activities (Gitlin et al., 2001; Stark, 2004), and (5) costs of health care and social services (Mann et al., 1999).

Discussion

Housing adaptation should be recommended as an important tool for maintaining activities of daily living (Wahl et al., in press) and occupational performance in general (Fänge and Iwarsson, 2007; Gitlin, 1998). Still, there are critical methodologic challenges for practice and future research. As the quotation at the start of this chapter demonstrates, another challenge is to present scientific evidence that would make some individual housing adaptations unnecessary. Applying such a health promotion approach, and using experience and knowledge generated from individual housing adaptation cases, could be translated into recommendations for housing provision as part of the process of planning a society for all (Iwarsson, 2005).

References

Boverket. (2005). Housing Adaptation Grants 2004. Karlskrona, Sweden: Boverket.
Christiansen, C., and Baum, C. (1997). Person-environment occupational performance. A conceptual model for practice. In: Christiansen, B.C., ed. Occupational Therapy. Enabling Function and Well-Being, 2nd ed. Thorofare, NJ: Slack.

Cumming, R.G., Thomas, M., Szonyi, G., Salkeld, G., O'Neill, E., and Westbury, C. (1999). Home visits by occupational therapists for assessment and modification of environmental hazards: a randomized trial of falls prevention. J Am Geriatr Soc, 47, 1397–1402.

Fänge, A. (2004). Strategies for Evaluation of Housing Adaptations—Accessibility, Usability and ADL Dependence. Doctoral dissertation, Faculty of Medicine, Lund University, Sweden.

Fänge, A., and Iwarsson, S. (2005). Changes in ADL dependence and aspects of usability following housing adaptation—a longitudinal perspective. Am J Occup Ther, 59, 296–304.

Fänge, A., and Iwarsson, S. (2007). Challenges in the development of strategies for housing adaptation evaluations. Scand J Occup Ther, 14(3), 140–149.

Gillespie, L.D., Gillespie, W.J., Robertsson, M.C., Lamb, S.E., Cumming, R.G.,Rowe, B.H. (2003). Interventions for preventing falls in elderly people. Cochrane Database of Systematic Reviews, 4, CD000340.

Gitlin, L.N. (1998). Testing home modification interventions: Issues of theory, measurement, design, and implementation. Ann Rev Gerontol Geriatr, 18, 190–246.

Gitlin, L.N., Corcoran, M., Winter, L., Boyce, A., and Hauck, W.W. (2001). A randomized, controlled trial of a home environmental intervention: effect on efficacy and upset in caregivers and on daily function of persons with dementia. Gerontologist, 41, 4–14.

Heywood, F. (2004). The health outcomes of housing adaptations. Disabil Soc, 19, 129–143.

Iwarsson, S. (2005). A long-term perspective on person-environment fit and ADL dependence among older Swedish adults. Gerontologist, 45(3), 327–336.

Iwarsson, S., and Ståhl, A. (2003). Accessibility, usability, and universal design—positioning and definition of concepts describing person-environment relationships. Disabil Rehabil, 25, 57–66.

Lyons, R.A., et al. (2003). Modification of the home environment for the reduction of injuries. Cochrane Database of Systematic Reviews, 4, CD003600.

Mann, W., Ottenbacher, K.J., Fraas, L., Tomita, M., and Granger, C.V. (1999). Effectiveness of assistive technology and environmental interventions in maintaining independence and reducing home care costs for the frail elderly. A randomized controlled trial. Arch Fam Med, 8, 210–217.

Stark, S. (2004). Removing environmental barriers in the homes of older adults with disabilities improves occupational performance. Occup Participation Health, 24, 32–39.

Steinfeld, E., and Tauke, B. (2002). Universal designing. In: Christophersen, J., ed. Universal Design. 17 Ways of Thinking and Teaching. Oslo, Norway: Husbanken.

Wahl, H.W., Fange, A., Oswald, F., Gitlin, L.N., and Iwarsson, S. (in press). The home environment and disability-related outcomes in aging individuals: What is the empirical evidence? The Gerontologist.

Chapter 6
Ergonomic Interventions for Computer Users with Cumulative Trauma Disorders

Glenn Goodman, Sharon Flinn, and Susan M. Maloney

The number of computer keyboard workers with cumulative trauma disorders is as much as 12 times that of non-keyboard users.

(Weiss and Chan, 2008)

Abstract This chapter examines ergonomic interventions for computer users who experience cumulative trauma disorders (CTDs) in the workplace. CTDs are defined. The complex nature of these disorders and the need for holistic and comprehensive evaluation is discussed. Statistics of prevalence and incidence are reviewed. The role of occupational therapy in the management of these disorders is examined. Examples of interventions for these disorders are cited, and a systematic review of the effectiveness of the ergonomic interventions is provided. Finally, recommendations for occupational therapy practice and further research are provided.

Keywords Computers • Cumulative trauma disorders • Ergonomics • Musculoskeletal disorders

Definition

Cumulative trauma disorders (CTDs) are disorders that are caused, precipitated, or aggravated by repeated exertions or movements of the body (Loy, nd). Work-related CTDs are complex in terms of etiology, pathophysiology, prevention, and effectiveness of interventions.

Background

A combination of factors can result in CTDs. Factors reported in the literature include ergonomic and environmental (prolonged positioning in awkward postures, repetitive movements, force, sustained exertion, temperature, lighting, mechanical

I. Söderback (ed.), *International Handbook of Occupational Therapy Interventions*,
DOI: 10.1007/978-0-387-75424-6_6, © Springer Science+Business Media, LLC 2010

stress), personal and psychosocial (gender, age, health habits, work style, medical conditions, anxiety, anthropomorphics, attitude, and work ethics), and work and organizational (work load, time pressures, job stress, social support, control over job tasks, role conflict, job security, social context, and supervisors' and managers' knowledge of assistive technologies and ergonomic principles; or legislation regarding work accommodations) (Cook and Polgar, 2008; Foye et al., 2002; Hamilton et al., 2005; Nieuwenhuijsen, 2004; Trujillo and Zeng, 2006; Weiss and Chan, 2008).

Many issues complicate the attribution of CTDs to computer use among individuals. Other work tasks can cause or contribute to the problem, such as the use of the telephone, filing, lifting and carrying tasks, resistive activities such as turning a stiff doorknob, and writing. Time use, rigor, vigor, and repetitive or resistive characteristics vary among individuals in relation to hobbies and leisure pursuits. Home maintenance activities such as laundry, washing dishes, and yard work are other potential contributing factors (Cook and Polgar, 2008; Hamilton et al., 2005).

Purposes

Occupational therapists (OTs) have training and skills to observe in the workplace, holistically, the ergonomic and environmental factors, the psychosocial issues, and individual characteristics. The aim is to provide a complete evaluation and intervention plan to prevent and heal CTDs that may be due to computer use. This chapter focuses on ergonomic interventions related to computer use.

Method

Candidates for the Intervention

People who have *sustained or chronic pains* due to computer use are candidates for the intervention. Examples of CTDs that have been reported related to computer use include carpal tunnel syndrome, neck strain, DeQuervain's disease, tendonitis, cubital tunnel syndrome, lateral and medial epicondylitis, Guyon's canal syndrome, radial tunnel syndrome, tenosynovitis, trigger finger, thoracic outlet syndrome, eye strain, dry eye syndrome, myofascial pain syndromes, headaches, and other general conditions such as arthralgia, sprains and strains, and back, shoulder, and neck pain (Brewer et al., 2006, Foye et al., 2002; Hamilton et al., 2005; Loy, nd; Trujillo and Zeng, 2006).

Epidemiology

Cumulative trauma disorders have been reported as prevalent in the workplace among individuals who utilize the computer extensively. Some statistics reported in the literature include the following:

- Incidence rates vary from 11 to 67 per 10,000 workers for workers in mathematics and computers, information services, and financial activities.
- Seventy percent of all occupational illnesses are musculoskeletal disorders of the upper extremity.
- The number of computer keyboard workers with CTDs is as much as 12 times that of non-keyboard users.
- The prevalence of musculoskeletal disorders has been reported to be as high as 86% among data processors.
- Over 500,000 injuries that result in days off work have been attributed to CTDs.
- Yearly costs of CTDs have been estimated at over $100 billion, which is close to 50% more than for other work-related injuries or illnesses.
- Injuries to the trunk and back are the most frequently reported, but upper-extremity musculoskeletal injuries are twice as frequent as those in the lower extremity.
- Cumulative trauma disorders are twice as common among women among workers ages 30 to 50 years (Bureau of Labor Statistics, 2007; Foye et al., 2002; Hamilton et al., 2005; Keller et al., 1998; Loy, nd; Pascarelli and Hsu, 2001; Trujillo and Zeng, 2006; Weiss and Chan, 2008; Werner, 2006).

However, some studies suggest the incidence of carpal tunnel syndrome and other CTDs among office workers is not as high as previously reported (Andersen et al., 2003; Atroshi et al., 2007; Stevens et al., 2001).

Settings

Occupational therapists typically see clients with CTDs in the workplace or in outpatient clinics in conjunction with hand or orthopedic surgeons, physical therapists, ergonomists, vocational rehabilitation specialists, case managers, or occupational health physicians or nurses.

The Role of the Occupational Therapist in Applying the Intervention

Occupational therapists are important members of the intervention team addressing CTDs among computer users. They are skilled at activity analysis. Often the problems are due to a specific activity that, if avoided, could result in elimination or reduction of symptoms. One example of this is the computer user who experiences cubital tunnel syndrome due to excessive leaning on his or her elbow on a hard surface while typing. OTs are also skilled in using interviews and observations to solve the root problem of these disorders. Restorative and adaptive approaches are used to modify the environment or to provide interventions such as rest, splinting, alteration of movement, and alteration of work schedule. The interventions seek to restore tissue integrity, allow for healing, or to prevent further injury. OTs provide education to workers, management, and caregivers regarding preventative, restorative, or adaptive measures. Finally, OTs have expertise in assistive technologies, ergonomic principles, and modifying a task or environment to maximize functional performance of occupations.

Results

Clinical Application

Interventions for Cumulative Trauma Disorders Related to Computer Use in the Workplace

Modification of the workstation can be categorized into (1) modification to eliminate factors related to posture, force, duration, intensity, positioning, or repetitive motion that may contribute to the disorder; (2) modification of schedule or work activities (including rest); (3) use of assistive devices not related to the workstation such as eyeglasses or a splint; (4) physical agent modalities, medications, surgery, or other medical interventions; (5) patient education related to the condition; and (6) behavioral interventions such as relaxation training, exercises, stress management, and interventions to improve psychosocial function in or outside the workplace (American Industrial Hygiene Association, nd; Bernaards et al., 2007; Bohr, 2000; Brewer et al., 2006; Goodman et al., 2005; Nainzadeh et al., 1999 Trujillo and Zeng, 2006).

This chapter focuses on interventions to modify the workstation and the schedule.

Modification to the Workstation

The workstation can be modified using a universal ergonomic approach, or specific CTDs can be addressed. For example, emphasis on wrist and forearm positions may be more critical in carpal tunnel syndrome. Here these options have to be prioritized due to time or cost considerations. Many resources offer guidelines for equipment and positioning using ergonomic principles. Issues on which there is a consensus include the following:

• *Proper positioning* recommendations include approximately 90 degrees of hip flexion, knee flexion, and ankle dorsiflexion with the head and neck in line with the torso and upright, and the head in slight downward tilt. There should be adequate support of the lumbar spine to facilitate normal curvature of the spine. The arms should be in line with the torso with approximately 90 degrees of elbow flexion. Feet should be resting flat on the floor or supported by a footrest. Wrists should be in neutral in all planes of motion.
• *Armrests and ergonomic chairs* should be used that allow for or encourage the above positioning guidelines and with elbow height below the "J" key, and the

horizontal location of the "J" key more than 12 cm from the edge of the desk. Chairs should adjust for seat height, seat depth, angle of seat, angle of back, height of back, amount of lumbar curve, armrest height. Chairs should be properly rated to support the weight of the worker with appropriate padding for seat and back cushions.

- *Armrests* should be properly padded and large enough to support the forearm.
- *Align the mouse* with the keyboard on a level surface and in close proximity to the keyboard (e.g., keyboard and mouse trays should accommodate left- or right-handed users).
- The *monitor* is positioned to allow 0 to 20 degrees of downward gaze at a distance that maximizes visibility for the individual user (10 to 30 inches or 25 to 75 cm from the eyes to the monitor).
- The size of the *monitor* should accommodate the visual field and take into account acuity issues.
- A padded wrist rest may be needed.
- *Glare reduction* is accomplished through lighting, glare filters, angle of the monitor, and proper shading.
- If laptops are used, detachable standard or ergonomic keyboards are recommended. Split keyboards with adjustable angles and negative slopes that reduce arm pronation and ulnar deviation are preferred for all computer use.
- *Keyboard* trays should be *adjustable* for tilt, distance from desk, and height. They should tilt in a negative direction.
- All ergonomic devices should be evaluated for adjustability to accommodate changes between persons if there are several users, or to change positions for comfort when an individual requires this.
- *Accessories* and other tasks should be ergonomically considered. Examples of this include the position and type of telephone, document holders, scanners, and printers.
- *Desk height* should be adjustable if possible. If not, clearance for knees and legs should be considered before ordering an appropriate size desk.
- *Pointing devices* should be chosen based on types and location of pain, required tasks, and physical limitations. The pointing device should match the contour of the hand, be thinner to reduce the distance between buttons, have low placement on the keyboard, and reduce the amount of shoulder abduction. Adjustments in sensitivity of the pointing device should be considered.
- Association of symptoms and duration of keyboard/mouse use differ between men (6 hours/day) and women (4 hours/day).
- *Lighting* should be adjustable for intensity, direction, and distance from work.
- *Additional environmental factors* such as temperature, ventilation, and dust should be evaluated and modified if problematic (Blatter and Bongers, 2007; Brigham Young University, 2005; Clemson University, nd; Cook et al., 2000, 2004; Cook and Polgar, 2008; Fagarasanu and Kumar, 2003; Foye et al., 2002; Goodman et al., 2005; Harvard University, nd; Keller et al., 1998; Lee and Jacobs, 2001; Loy, nd; New Jersey Department of Health and Senior Services, nd; Noack, 2005; Marcus et al., 2002; Tittiranonda et al., 1999; University of Connecticut Occupational and

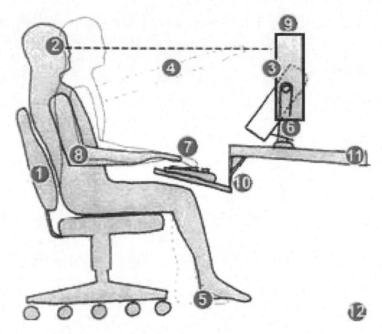

Fig. 6.1 Ergonomic guidelines for computer workstations. 1. Use a good chair with a dynamic chair back that is angled slightly to the rear. 2. The top of the monitor screen should be 2 to 3 inches above eye level. 3. There should be no glare on the screen. Use an optical glass antiglare filter where needed. 4. Sit at arms' length from the monitor, or further if the distance is comfortable and screen is readable. 5. Rest feet on the floor or on a stable footrest (move feet frequently for circulation). 6. Use a document holder, preferably in line with the computer screen. 7. Wrists should be flat and straight in relation to the forearms to use keyboard/mouse/input device. 8. Keep arms and elbows relaxed close to body. 9. Center the monitor and keyboard in front of you. 10. Use a negative tilt keyboard tray with an upper mouse platform or downward tiltable platform adjacent to keyboard. 11. Use a stable work surface and stable (no bounce) keyboard tray. 12. Take frequent short breaks (microbreaks) and stretch. (From Ergo on Demand Web site, http://www.ergoindemand.com/ergonomic-computer-workstation-guidelines.htm, with permission.).

179   Environmental Health Center, nd; University of Medicine and Dentistry of New
180   Jersey, nd; U.S. Department of Labor, nd; Weiss and Chan, 2008).

181   Figure 6.1 above demonstrates the application of the above principles.

182   **Modification of Work Activities and Scheduling**

183   Interventions designed to modify work activities and scheduling include the following:

184   • *Frequent rest breaks*, at least once an hour for continuous users and once every
185   2 hours for noncontinuous typing, and cessation or reduction of typing for a
186   specified time to allow healing.
187   • *Exercises* to stretch musculoskeletal tissues and to reduce eye strain.

- *Repositioning* of keyboard, monitor, and mouse at midday if symptoms occur in spite of desired or recommended positions (e.g., change frequently used keys and reduce key-switch force).
- *Vary activities* to intersperse typing with other tasks throughout the day.
- Analysis of all *daily activities* (including computer use activities) that require excessive force, positioning, speed, duration, or movements.
- Consider programs (wellness, smoking cessation, weight reduction, cardiovascular and endurance) that address other contributing factors.
- Consider an *alternative method* of input such as voice recognition, learning keyboard shortcuts as an alternative to mouse control, using the mouse in the nondominant extremity, or a combination of methods.
- *Modification of job* including trading activities with another worker, modification of work schedule, and changing jobs temporarily or permanently.
- Provision of *patient education* on anatomy and disease process (Brigham Young University, nd; Cook and Polgar, 2008; Delisle et al., 2004; Fagarasanu and Kumar, 2003; Goodman et al., 2005; Keller et al., 1998; Lawler et al., 1997; Lee and Jacobs, 2001; Loy, nd; New Jersey Department of Health and Senior Services, nd; U.S. Department of Labor, nd; Weiss and Chan, 2008).

A list of resources and specific ergonomic equipment is given in Table 6.1 to assist therapists with specific recommendations based on the general principles reviewed above.

Evidence to Support Various Interventions for Computer Access in the Workplace

One systematic review of the literature addresses the evidence for preventing musculoskeletal and visual symptoms among computer users (Brewer et al., 2006). The search identified over 7300 articles on this topic. Only 31 of these studies met the rigorous criteria set by these reviewers to be considered in their findings. The following evidence was reported:

- Moderate evidence that alternative pointing devices have an effect on musculoskeletal outcomes.
- Mixed evidence to support the effect of ergonomics training, alternative keyboards, rest breaks, and screen filters.
- Moderate evidence that there is no effect of rest on visual outcomes.
- Moderate evidence that rest breaks and stretching have no effect on musculoskeletal outcomes.
- Moderate levels of evidence reported no effects of workstation modifications on musculoskeletal or visual problems.
- Insufficient evidence to support the effect of stress management training, exercise training, lighting, workstation adjustment, video display terminal (VDT) glasses, or arm supports.

Table 6.1 Resources for ergonomic interventions for computer users with cumulative trauma disorders

Interventions	Company	Address	Web site	Other contact information
Guidelines for health computing; excellent checklist for ergonomics of computer workstation	OSHA; guidelines for computer workstations	U.S. Department of Labor Occupational Safety and Health Administration, 200 Constitution Avenue, Washington, DC 20210	http://www.osha.gov/SLTC/etools/computerworkstations/	1-800-321-6742
Guidelines for health computing; resources for office furniture	University of Minnesota Department of Environmental Health and Safety	University of Minnesota, W-140 Boynton Health Services, 410 Church Street SE, Minneapolis, MN 5455	http://www.dehs.umn.edu/ergo_office.htm	612-625-5422
Guidelines for health computing	HealthyComputing.com	12323 Caminito Mirada, San Diego, CA 92131	http://www.healthycomputing.com/	619-987-0246
Ergonomic keyboard, mouse, and other devices	EnableMart	EnableMart Sales Office, 4210 E. 4th Plain Blvd., Vancouver, WA 98661, USA	www.enablemart.com	888–640–1999 (Toll Free) 360–695–4133
Ergonomic keyboard, mouse, and other devices	Ergo in Demand	Ergo in Demand Inc., 4900 Industry Drive Central Point, OR 97502	http://www.ergoindemand.com/	1-800-888-6024
Ergonomic keyboard, mouse, and other devices	Ergo-Items.com	4454 N Morris blvd, Shorewood, WI 53211	http://www.ergo-items.com/	414-921-4262 fax
Ergonomic chairs, desks, and peripherals	ErgoStore Online	17319 Meadow Bottom Road, Charlotte, NC 28277	http://www.ergostoreonline.com/	1-877-971-0151

Two other review articles (Lincoln et al., 2000; Williams & Westmoreland, 1994) reported insufficient evidence to identify effective workplace rehabilitation interventions for a variety of CTDs. However, systematic evidence should be carefully interpreted.

In contrast, findings reported by OTs and that are limited to interventions for CTDs related to computer use suggest evidence supporting effectiveness of or need for these interventions:

- Eighty-two percent of musculoskeletal or visual problems were reported solved to the computer user's satisfaction 1 year following a multifaceted ergonomics program provided by occupational and physical therapists (Goodman et al., 2005).
- A holistic intervention approach, utilized by 50 workers in a computer firm, achieved a positive outcome in cost-effectiveness, decrease in lost workdays, and worker satisfaction (Lee and Jacobs, 2001).
- Seventy percent of computer users ($n = 55$) surveyed experienced symptoms related to computer use. Only 60% had been given ergonomics information regarding the computer workstation. Only 10% of respondents with access to this information reported implementing this knowledge in daily tasks (Berner and Jacobs, 2002).
- A cost-benefit analysis showed projected savings of more than $300,000 from an intervention program to reduce CTDs among computer users (Noack, 2005).
- A meta-analysis found that alternative keyboard designs decrease potentially harmful awkward postures typically assumed on a standard flat keyboard (Baker and Cidboy, 2006).
- Sixty-five of 72 female college students using laptops showed musculoskeletal complaints (Hamilton et al., 2005).
- A retrospective study of 312 workers'-compensation patients found positive correlations between a patient's eventual return to work and the OT's initial rating of the patient's rehabilitation potential as well as the patient's own initial rating of desire to return to work (Waylett-Rendall and Niemeyer, 2004).
- A mixed methodology study of 43 hand patients found the strongest correlations to reported pain intensity were the patients' physical functioning, role limitations due to emotional issues, and social functioning (Chan and Spencer, 2005).
- A qualitative case study with three participants identified psychosocial themes of depression, frustration, loss, dependence, role changes, fear and hopelessness as potential impairments to rehabilitation (Schier and Chan, 2007).

Conclusion

The literature suggests there is a high cost for and incidence of CTDs among computer users, but the relative contribution of the computer to these problems is under debate. Available lists of ergonomic principles and recommendations are remarkably consistent in addressing this problem. Many articles look at the effectiveness of interventions for computer users with CTDs, but none written by occupational therapists was considered acceptable in comprehensive and rigorous systematic review papers. A few studies written by occupational therapists were found, which specifically addressed the effectiveness of computer workstation issues.

If occupational therapists want to increase their contribution to ergonomic interventions for computer users, more research is needed to address the benefits of OT interventions that perhaps will stand the scrutiny of peer evaluation from other disciplines. Current evidence is encouraging, and suggests that these interventions are effective or at least needed.

This chapter has described best practice based on current evidence. The resources and references cited should help therapists who want to develop new programs or study the effectiveness of existing interventions. There is much more to know in this interesting and important area of practice.

References

American Industrial Hygiene Association. (n.d.). An ergonomics approach to avoiding workplace injury. http://www.aiha.org/Content/AccessInfo/consumer/AnErgonomicsApproachtoAvoiding WorkplaceInjury.htm.

Andersen, J.H., Thomsen, J.F., Overgaard, E., et al. (2003). Computer use and carpal tunnel syndrome: a 1-year follow-up study. JAMA 289(22), 2963–2969.

Atroshi, I., Gummesson, C., Ornstein, E., Johnsson, R., and Ranstam, J. (2007). Carpal tunnel syndrome and keyboard use at work. Arthritis Rheumw, 56(11), 3620–3625.

Baker, N.A., and Cidboy, E.I. (2006). The effect of three alternative keyboard designs on forearm pronation, wrist extension, and ulnar deviation: a meta-analysis. Am J Occup Ther, 60(1), 40–49.

Bernaards, C., Ariens, G., Knol, D., and Hildebrandt, V. (2007). The effectiveness of a work style intervention and a lifestyle physical activity intervention on the recovery from neck and upper limb symptoms in computer workers. Pain, 132(1–2), 142–153.

Berner, K., and Jacobs, K. (2002). The gap between exposure and implementation of computer workstation ergonomics in the workplace. Work, 19(2), 193–199.

Blatter, B., and Bongers, P. (2007). Duration of computer use and mouse use in relation to musculoskeletal disorders of the neck or upper limb. Int J Ind Ergonom, 30(4–5), 295–306.

Bohr, P.C. (2000). Efficacy of office ergonomics education. J Occup Rehabil, 10(4), 243–255.

Brewer, S., Van Eerd, D., Amick, B. III, et al. (2006). Workplace interventions to prevent musculoskeletal and visual symptoms and disorders among computer users: a systematic review. J Occup Rehabil, 16(3), 325–358.

Brigham Young University. (2005). Ergonomics safety program. http://safety.byu.edu/docs/Ergonomics SafetyProgram.pdf.

Bureau of Labor Statistics. (2007). Nonfatal occupational injuries and illnesses requiring days away from work, 2006. http://www.bls.gov/news.release/osh2.nr0.htm.

Chan, J., and Spencer, J. (2005). Contrasting perspectives on pain following hand injury. J Hand Ther, 18(4), 429–436.

Clemson University. (n.d.). Clemson University ergonomics plan. http://www.clemson.edu/ehs/ Ergonomics%20Plan.html.

Cook, A.M., and Polgar, J.M. (2008). Assistive Technologies: Principles and Practice. St. Louis: Mosby.

Cook, C., Burgess-Limerick, R., and Chang, S. (2000). The prevalence of neck and upper extremity musculoskeletal symptoms in computer mouse users. Int J Ind Ergonom, 26(3), 347–356.

Cook, C., Burgess-Limerick, R., and Papalia, S. (2004). The effect of wrist rests and forearm support during keyboard and mouse use. Int J Ind Ergonom, 33(5), 464–472.

Delisle, A., Imbeau, D., Santos, B., Plamondon, A., and Montpetit, Y. (2004). Left-handed versus right-handed computer mouse use: effect on upper-extremity posture. Appl Ergonom, 35(1), 21–28.

Fagarasanu, M., and Kumar, S. (2003). Carpal tunnel syndrome due to keyboarding and mouse tasks: a review. Int J Ind Ergonom, 31(2), 119–136.

Foye, P.M., Cianca, J.C., and Prather, H. (2002). Industrial medicine and acute musculoskeletal rehabilitation. III. Cumulative trauma disorders of the upper limb in computer users. Arch Phys Med Rehabil, 83 (Suppl 1), S12–S15.

Goodman, G., Landis, J., George, C., et al. (2005). Effectiveness of computer ergonomics interventions for an engineering company: a program evaluation. Work, 24(1), 53–62.

Hamilton, A.G., Jacobs, K., and Orsmond, G. (2005). The prevalence of computer-related musculoskeletal complaints in female college students. Work, 24(4), 387–394.

Harvard University. (nd). Computer workstation ergonomic training and evaluation program. http://www.uos.harvard.edu/ehs/training/ergo_info.html.

Keller, K., Corbett, J., and Nichols, D. (1998). Repetitive strain injury in computer keyboard users: pathomechanics and treatment principles in individual and group intervention. J Hand Ther, 11(1), 9–26.

Lawler, A.L., James, A.B., and Tomlin, G. (1997). Educational techniques used in occupational therapy treatment of cumulative trauma disorders of the elbow, wrist, and hand. Am J Occup Ther, 51(2), 113–118.

Lee, D.L., and Jacobs, K. (2001). Perspectives in occupational therapy: bridging computer ergonomics with work practice. Technol Special Interest Sect Q, 11(4), 1–4.

Lincoln, A.E., Vernick, J.S., Ogaitis, S., Smith, G.S., Mitchell, C.S., and Agnew, J. (2000). Interventions for the primary prevention of work-related carpal tunnel syndrome. Am J Prev Med, 18(1), 37–50.

Loy, B. (nd.). Accommodating people with cumulative trauma disorders. Job Accommodations Network. http://www.jan.wvu.edu/media/CTDs.html.

Marcus, M., Gerr, F., Montelh, C., et al. (2002). A prospective study of computer users. II. Postural risk factors for musculoskeletal symptoms and disorders. Am J Ind Med, 41(4), 236–249.

Nainzadeh, N., Malantic-Lin, A., Alvarez, M., and Loeser, A.C. (1999). Repetitive strain injury (cumulative trauma disorder): causes and treatment. Mt Sinai J Med, 66(3), 192–196.

New Jersey Department of Health and Senior Services. (n.d.). Cumulative trauma disorders in office workers. http://www.state.nj.us/health/eoh/peoshweb/ctdib.htm.

Nieuwenhuijsen, E.R. (2004). Health behavior change among office workers: an exploratory study to prevent repetitive strain injuries. Work, 23(3), 215–224.

Noack, J. (2005). Development of an employer-based injury-prevention program for office workers using ergonomic principles. OT Pract, 10(7), 1–8.

Pascarelli, E.F., and Hsu, Y.P. (2001). Understanding work-related upper extremity disorders: clinical findings in 485 computer users, musicians, and others. J Occup Rehabil, 11(1), 1–21.

Schier, J.S., and Chan, J. (2007). Changes in life roles after hand injury. J Hand Ther, 20(1), 57–69.

Stevens, J.C., Witt, J.C., Smith, B.E., and Weaver, A.L. (2001). The frequency of carpal tunnel syndrome in computer users at a medical facility. Neurology, 56(12), 1568–1570.

Tittiranonda, P., Rempel, D., Armstrong, T., and Burastero, S. (1999). Effect of four computer keyboards in computer users with upper extremity musculoskeletal disorders. Am J Ind Med, 35(6), 647–661.

Trujillo, L., and Zeng, X. (2006). Data entry workers perceptions and satisfaction response to the "Stop and Stretch" software program. Work, 27(2), 111–121.

University of Connecticut Occupational and Environmental Health Center. (n.d.). Cumulative trauma disorders and computer workstation problems. http://www.oehc.uchc.edu/ergo_officeergo1.asp.

University of Medicine and Dentistry New Jersey. (n.d.). Computer workstation design. http://www2.umdnj.edu/eohssweb/ergo/part_one/page01.htm.

U.S. Department of Labor. (n.d.). OSHA ergonomics solutions: computer Workstations eTool-checklist. http://www.osha.gov/SLTC/etools/computerworkstations/checklist.html.

Waylett-Rendall, J., and Niemeyer, L.O. (2004). Exploratory analysis to identify factors impacting return-to-work outcomes in cases of cumulative trauma disorder. J Hand Ther, 17(1), 50–57.

Weiss, P.T., and Chan, C.C. (2008) Computers and assistive technology. In: Jacobs, K., ed. Ergonomics for Therapists, 3rd ed. St. Louis: Mosby.

Werner, R. (2006). Evaluation of work-related carpal tunnel syndrome. J Occup Rehabil, 16(2), 207–222.

Williams, R., Westmorland, M. (1994) Occupational cumulative trauma disorders of the upper extremity. Am J Occ Ther 48(5): 411–420.

Chapter 7
Optimal Positioning: Wheelchair Seating Comfort and Pressure Mapping

May Stinson and Shelley Crawford

Pressure sores probably have existed since the dawn of our infirm species. They have been noted in unearthed Egyptian mummies, and scientific writings have addressed them since the early 1800s.

(Revis, 2005)

Abstract Pressure ulcers remain a common problem, incurring great cost to both clients and the health care system. The predominant risk factor for pressure ulcers is interface pressure, that is, the pressure exerted between the body and the seating surface. Interface pressure can be measured by pressure mapping systems, and can assist with pressure ulcer risk assessment by identifying areas of high pressure and postural abnormalities, which both increase the risk of pressure damage. Pressure mapping systems are clinically useful for assisting with cushion selection. In the clinic, the pressure-measuring mat is placed between the client and a variety of seating surfaces in turn. The seating surfaces showing high interface pressure or poor pressure distribution are eliminated. Selection is then further refined on consideration of factors such as comfort, ease of transfers, and maintenance. Pressure mapping is also a valuable tool to guide therapists in the adjustment of complex seating systems. The color-coded pressure maps provide useful biofeedback to clients, caregivers, and health professionals on the importance of weight shifts and optimal postural alignment.

Keywords Biofeedback • Healthcare • Pressure ulcers • Technology

Definition

Pressure mapping systems measure interface pressure, that is, the pressure between the body and the seating surface. Interface pressure is the predominant risk factor associated with pressure ulcers (Geyer et al., 2001). A pressure mapping system consists of an array of pressure sensors connected via an interface module box to computer software (Fig. 7.1).

I. Söderback (ed.), *International Handbook of Occupational Therapy Interventions,*
DOI: 10.1007/978-0-387-75424-6_7, © Springer Science+Business Media, LLC 2010

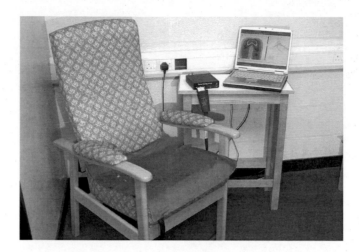

Fig. 7.1 The pressure mapping system.

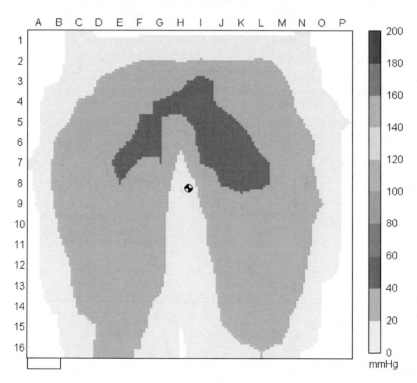

Fig. 7.2 Example of a good pressure map. There are no areas of excessively high interface pressure, and a good spread of pressure across the seating surface.

The system output is displayed numerically and visually as color-coded maps of pressure distribution. Examples are shown as "good" results, no need for interventions occur (Fig. 7.2) and "bad" results (Fig. 7.3), adaptive interventions is needed.

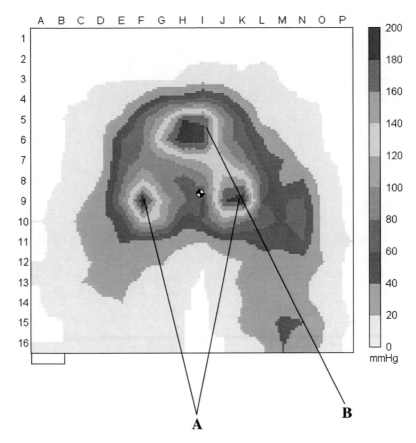

Fig. 7.3 Example of a 'poor' pressure map. There are areas of high interface pressure over the buttocks (ischial tuberosities) (A) and sacrum (B) and an uneven spread of interface pressure across the seating surface.

Pressure mapping arrays for clinical use have evolved from the early 1990s, and with advances in technology have become increasingly reliable. Designed as an objective method to measure interface pressure, they complement pen-and-paper pressure ulcer risk assessment tools, such as the Braden Scale (Bergstrom et al., 1987).

Purpose

The purpose of interface pressure mapping is to assist with the risk assessment of pressure ulcer and to educate clients, caregivers, and healthcare professionals in pressure care prevention.

Method

Candidates for Pressure Mapping

Pressure mapping can be used with children or adults at risk of pressure ulceration, particularly those with reduced mobility, poor nutrition, lack of sensation, and acute or chronic illness. Examples are people who are sitting in a wheelchair or chair for most of the daytime.

Epidemiology

Pressure ulcers remain a common problem. European prevalence rates vary from 8.3% to 22.9% (Defloor et al., 2002) and 38.1% in nursing homes (Defloor et al., 2005). The cost of pressure ulcers is immense, both to the client in terms of pain and decreased quality of life, and to health care resources in terms of financial expenditure.

Settings

Pressure mapping systems are portable and can be used in hospitals, clinics, and community settings.

The Role of the Occupational Therapist in Applying the Intervention

The role of the occupational therapist (OT) is to managing the assessment process of pressure mapping. The aim is to adapt the most appropriate wheelchair or sitting cushions and to teach clients and caregivers how to prevent pressure ulcers. This process is as follows:

- Clients are initially positioned on a firm surface, such as a mat table. This position is used for establishing a baseline of pressure distribution. Any postural abnormalities are identified.
- Clients are positioned on a selection of seating surfaces with the pressure-sensing mat placed between the buttocks and each of the surfaces in turn. Clients are requested to maintain their optimal seating position.
- The pressure maps are recorded after a consistent period of sitting time, preferably 8 minutes (Crawford et al., 2005b; Stinson et al., 2002) on each seating surface. The OT visually ranks the maps from best to worst pressure distribution. Good pressure distribution is characterized by an even spread of pressure, including

good femoral loading and no areas of excessively high pressure (Stinson et al., 2003) (Fig. 7.2).

- Bad pressure distribution (Fig. 7.3) requires inventions characterized by the selection of optimal seating surfaces from those remaining and include the consideration resulting in the client's comfort, maintenance, optimal transfers, posture, and stability (Sprigle, 2000).
- The process of testing seating positions on various surfaces (Fig. 7.4) continues until the seating surfaces showing poor pressure distribution have been eliminated.

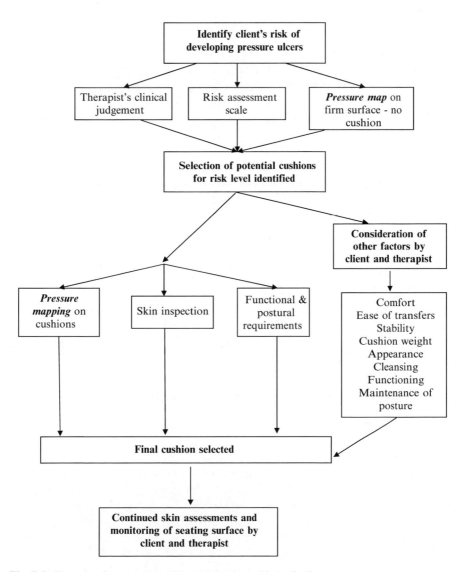

Fig. 7.4   The role of pressure mapping systems in cushion selection.

- The OT uses the results of pressure maps to educate clients, caregivers, and health professionals. This education concerns the importance of clients learning to shift weight between the buttocks, and explains what an ergonomic postural alignment entails.

Results

Clinical Application

The pressure-mapping system is used to assist clinicians and clients in eliminating unsuitable sitting surfaces aimed at preventing and healing sitting ulcers.

The results of a pressure mapping assessment demonstrate (1) sitting areas of high interface pressure, such as over the buttocks (ischial tuberosities); and (2) postural abnormalities, such as pelvic obliquity/rotation. The OT uses the results of the mapping for a comparison of seating surfaces. This procedure determines the optimal sitting surfaces for each client (Crawford et al., 2005a; Sprigle, 2000). The results are used for adapting the sitting cushions. The views of the results of the mapping system (Figs. 7.2 and 7.3) give clients, caregivers, and health professionals feedback on the differences between sitting with a risk of ulcers and sitting with the cushion and sitting position optimally adapted.

The intervention includes sessions where the clients learn the habits of optimal sitting position. The biofeedback apparatus is used by the clients for visualizing the present sitting position. Here, the OT demonstrates the benefits of shifting weight between the buttocks, and the effect of poor posture or incorrect placement of cushions. The client is informed about the importance of adjusting other components of the seating systems, such as the use or adjustment of wheelchair footplates and the use of tilt and recline functions (Stein et al., 2006). The apparatus also permits optimal cushion settings for high-risk clients, for example air-filled cushions or cushions with accessories.

How the Intervention Eases Impairments, Activity Limitations, and Participation Restrictions

Pressure mapping systems provide valuable information regarding maintenance of skin integrity (International Classification of Functioning, Disability, and Health [ICF] code b810–b849). They provide biofeedback on pelvic alignment (ICF b7201) and on the effects of changing and maintaining body position (ICF d410–d429), hence assisting clinicians in the overall management and prevention of pressure ulcers.

Evidence-Based Practice

The link between high interface pressure, as measured with pressure mapping systems, and pressure ulcer incidence has been demonstrated in randomized controlled trials. Interface pressures were significantly higher ($p < .01$) for participants who developed pressure ulcers than for those who did not (Brienza et al., 2001; Conine et al., 1994).

Numerous research studies have used pressure-mapping systems to compare pressure-reducing cushions based on interface pressure measurements (Ferrarin et al., 2000; Geyer et al., 2001; Shechtman et al., 2001; Tanimoto et al., 2000). For example, the study by Ferrarin et al. (2000) of ten wheelchair users showed that the Roho Low Profile and the Jay2 cushions had significantly lower peak pressure ($p < .05$) over the buttocks than two polyurethane gel–filled foam-based cushions had.

Discussion

Pressure-mapping systems require expertise in operation and output interpretation. Although expensive to purchase, the mapping system has potential benefits in pressure-ulcer management. Above all, the prevention of pressure ulcers is becoming increasingly valued. Further research should focus on the clinical applications of this technology with disabled clients and on the development of standard protocols for its use.

References

Bergstrom, N., Demuth, P.J., and Braden, B.J. (1987). A clinical trial of the Braden Scale for predicting pressure sore risk. Nurs Clin North Am, 22(2), 417–428.

Brienza, D.M., Karg, P.E., Geyer, M.J., Kelsey, S., and Trefler, E. (2001). The relationship between pressure ulcer incidence and buttock-seat cushion interface pressure in at-risk elderly wheelchair users. Arch Phys Med Rehabil, 82, 529–533.

Conine, T.A., Hershler, C., Daechsel, D., Peel, C., and Pearson, A. (1994). Pressure ulcer prophylaxis in elderly care patients using polyurethane foam or Jay wheelchair cushions. Int J Rehabil Res, 17, 123–137.

Crawford, S.A., Stinson, M.D., Walsh, D.M., and Porter-Armstrong, A.P. (2005b). Impact of sitting time on seat-interface pressure and on pressure mapping with multiple sclerosis patients. Arch Phys Med Rehabil, 86, 1221–1225.

Crawford, S.A., Strain, B., Gregg, B., Walsh, D.M., and Porter-Armstrong, A.P. (2005a). An investigation of the impact of the Force Sensing Array pressure mapping system on the clinical judgement of occupational therapists. Clin Rehabil, 19, 224–231.

Defloor, T., Bours, G., Clark, M., et al. (2002). EPUAP prevalence project; the project results. In: Abstracts from EPUAP Open Meeting Budapest 2002. http://www.epuap.org/reviews_1page5d.html.

Defloor, T., De Bacquer, D., and Grypdonck, M.H. (2005). The effect of various combinations of turning and pressure reducing devices on the incidence of pressure ulcers. Int J Nurs Stud, 42(1), 37–46.

Ferrarin, M., Giuseppe, A., and Pedotti, A. (2000). Comparative biomechanical evaluation of different wheelchair seat cushions. J Rehabil Res Dev, 37(3), 315–324.

Geyer, M.J., Brienza, D.M., Karg, P., Trefler, E., and Kelsey, S. (2001). A randomised controlled trial to evaluate pressure-reducing seat cushions for elderly wheelchair users. Adv Skin Wound Care, 14(3), 120–132.

Revis, D.R. (2005). Decubitus ulcers. http://emedicine.com/med/topic2709.htm.

Shechtman, O., Hanson, C.S., Garrett, D., and Dunn, P. (2001). Comparing wheelchair cushions for effectiveness of pressure relief: a pilot study. Occup Ther J Res, 21(1), 29–48.

Sprigle, S. (2000). Effects of forces and the selection of support surfaces. Topics Geriatr Rehabil, 16(2), 47–62.

Stein, F., Söderback, I., Cutler, S. K., and Larson, B. (2006). Occupational Therapy and Ergonomics. Applying Ergonomic Principles to Everyday Occupation in the Home and at Work, 1st ed. London/Philadelphia: Whurr/Wiley.

Stinson, M., Porter, A., and Eakin, P. (2002). Measuring interface pressure: A laboratory-based investigation into the effects of repositioning and sitting. Am J Occup Ther, 56(2), 185–190.

Stinson, M.D., Porter-Armstrong, A.P., and Eakin, P.A. (2003). Pressure mapping systems: reliability of pressure map interpretation. Clin Rehabil, 17, 504–511.

Tanimoto, Y., Takechi, H., Nagahata, H., and Yamamoto, H. (2000). Pressure measurement of air cushions for SCI patients. IEEE Trans Instrument Measure, 49(3), 666–670.

Chapter 8
Wheelchair Intervention: Principles and Practice

Åse Brandt and Kersti Samuelsson

> *After my wheelchair got adapted to me and my needs, it became possible for me to cook and to go out with my friends.*
>
> —Client

Abstract The purpose of wheelchair interventions is to compensate for reduced walking ability or the lack of it, which in turn supports individual performance in activity as well as participation in society. Each occupational therapist (OT) working in this field has to have high-quality competence in different products, how to adjust and adapt them, what factors affect the fitting process, and what health risks are associated with using them. A successful solution is based on a therapeutic understanding of the user, the equipment, and the environment. Even though a wheelchair primarily is an assistive device aimed at providing mobility, it is also a chair, and thus should comfortably and ergonomically seat the user while supporting effective mobility. Regular follow-ups of the prescribed wheelchair may increase the professional's knowledge and secure good clinical practice in this field, enhancing the users' occupational performance.

Keywords Activity • Assistive technology • Fitting • Mobility • Seating

Definitions

Mobility is necessary to enable a person to carry out everyday activities and to participate in society, and it has a major impact on the quality of life. For children, mobility is a prerequisite for cognitive and social development. When mobility is difficult or impossible due to mobility limitations, wheelchair interventions might enable mobility and make activities and participation possible.

I. Söderback (ed.), *International Handbook of Occupational Therapy Interventions*,
DOI: 10.1007/978-0-387-75424-6_8, © Springer Science+Business Media, LLC 2010

Types of Wheelchairs

Many different types of wheelchairs are available, classified by the International Standards Organization (ISO) 9999 International Standard on Assistive Products for Persons with Disability—Classification and Terminology as standards 12-22 and 12-23: human-driven wheelchairs and powered wheelchairs. These include wheelchairs propelled by both hands, a foot-driven type, attendant-controlled wheelchairs, scooters, and electric-motor–driven wheelchairs with powered steering (International Standards Organization, 2007). In addition, a number of brands and models are available. For example, the North American database Abledata (2008) contains nearly 1500 products, while in some low-income countries only a few products are available.

Background

The first known use of wheelchairs by people with disabilities was in the mid-1600s. The first wheelchairs were made of wood and hard to propel. In the 1930s, a new and relatively lightweight foldable wheelchair was manufactured. After World War II, light, easily maneuvered wheelchairs with a rigid frame were manufactured. The development of powered wheelchairs is much more recent. Even though the first powered wheelchair was invented in 1940, powered wheelchairs were not commonly in use until the 1960s (Cook and Hussey, 2002). In the last 10 years considerable interest in scooter models has emerged.

Purpose

The purpose of wheelchair interventions is to compensate for reduced walking ability or the lack thereof, so as to prevent activity limitations and participation restrictions.

Method

Candidates for the Intervention

The functional limitations requiring a wheelchair intervention may stem from a broad variety of diseases and may be temporary, intermittent, or permanent. Diagnoses are often diseases of the nervous system, the circulatory system, and the respiratory system, as well as injuries to the musculoskeletal system. These diseases and injuries may cause different mobility limitations, and it is the limitations that should be considered, rather than the specific medical diagnoses. Even though all age groups are represented among wheelchair users, most are older people. The reason is that mobility limitations increase with increasing age. More women than men use wheelchairs because of a higher prevalence of mobility limitations among women.

Epidemiology

The prevalence of wheelchair use depends on several factors. The main factor is the *availability of wheelchairs*, which varies from country to country and is depending on specific legislation on assistive technology services and on the socioeconomic circumstances that affect the willingness to provide for needy clients. However, the World Health Organization (WHO, 2007) estimates that about 1% of the world's population needs a wheelchair, equivalent to over 65 million people.

Settings

Wheelchair interventions are initiated within the medical service at hospitals or in municipal settings. Parts of the intervention, such as implementation, follow-up, and evaluation, often take place in the user's home.

The Role of the Occupational Therapist in Applying the Intervention

In a wheelchair fitting process, the role of the occupational therapist (OT) is to consider activity and participation in daily life and everything related to that. The wheelchair is going to be used in everyday occupations and has to fit the user with that perspective. It is of great importance that the fitting process be based on cooperation with the user and take account of his or her preferences.

Results

Clinical Application

This subsection describes the process of individually fitting a wheelchair for a client.

Overall Principles of the Wheelchair Fitting Process

Mobility is the primary aspect in wheelchair fittings, and the OT considers aspects related to the interface between the user and the wheelchair. The wheelchair is a replacement for other seating furniture, and therefore the user's seating comfort and support is a fundamental aspect that has to be taken into account. Risk factors related to wheelchair use have to be considered, such as pressure sores (see Chapter 7), back and shoulder pain, deformities, and discomfort.

Interview and evaluation with the client are fundamental to obtain an optimal wheelchair fitting. During this phase, the OT collects information about the client's occupational preferences as well as relevant environmental conditions. The Canadian Occupational Performance Measure (Law et al., 1998) might serve as a tool in this process. This information is related to the physical and cognitive prerequisites of the user. Physical capacity, joint range of motion, sensibility, body image, balance, and muscle tone are examples of aspects that should be considered before making a decision about the type and adjustment of a wheelchair.

Functional Capacity and Mobility

Propelling a manual wheelchair is hard work. Rolling resistance has to be overcome, especially outdoors. This is physically demanding, and a powered wheelchair might be a necessity. To minimize rolling resistance in a manual wheelchair, an adjustment of weight distribution might be effective. The wheels' angles are also relevant, since they may affect rolling resistance in a most significant negative way (Kauzlarich, 1999); that is, the rear wheels should be slightly cambered, which places the wheels close to the user. The users should have optimal opportunity to use their arms or legs for effective manual propulsion. The center of the shoulder joints should be over the hub of the rear wheels, and the fingertips should reach the hub for efficient push angle and joint movement (Boninger et al., 2003).

Different modes of controlling powered wheelchairs are available, such as joystick, steer, sip-and-puff, and switches. The selection of these available tools should be based on tests in the environments where the wheelchair is to be used.

A wheelchair of any type should fit the user in height, width, and depth. The seating posture is important since an upright seat position supports the cardiovascular and respiration function (Stein et al., 2006; Stewart, 1991).

Activity and Participation

A client to whom a wheelchair has been fitted needs further interventions to be able to perform activities of daily living (ADL) and to be able to participate in society. Here, the OT acts by enabling occupation, by making it possible to perform different activities in a seated position. This fitting process is dependent on the assessments together with wide knowledge about wheelchair adjustment and about potential advantages and risks.

Environment

The environment could be a hindrance as well as a support. The physical environment such as the home environment and the outdoor surroundings must be considered, and accessibility (see Chapter 6) may be required.

Complications of Using a Wheelchair

Many wheelchair users suffer from back and neck pain (Samuelsson, 2002). Deformities and a restricted range of motion together with pressure sores and discomfort are other complications associated with sitting for long periods. Wheelchair fitting and body posture are fundamental in counteracting these risks. A good range of motion in hips, knees, and pelvis enables the wheelchair user to attain a comfortable and optimal seating position. Wheelchair cushions, lumbar supports, and other equipment are helpful tools in this process.

Seating

The wheelchair user has the right to have a comfortable and appropriate sitting. The key to the seating posture is the pelvis. A close to neutral pelvic rotation and no lateral tilt supports the natural spine curvature and reduces the risk for high local under-seat pressure. Hip and knee angles affect pelvic rotation, and it is important to know and understand this relationship (Engström, 2002). Back and seat angles of the chair together with the wheelchair cushion and back support can be adjusted to provide optimal seating support. A strap-adjustable back support is preferable over a nonadjustable sling back support, because it makes it possible to "mold" the support to the individual user. A contoured seat cushion is often preferable since it supports pressure distribution and stability.

Training

It is of great importance that the client be trained in the use of the wheelchair until the necessary skills are acquired, such as managing curbs and other physical barriers. Training should be carried out both indoors and outdoors (Lois, 2004; Royston, 1995).

Follow-Up and Evaluation

A wheelchair fitting requires follow-up to be sure the chair appropriately fits the patient. A poorly fitting wheelchair can cause great harm. Investigation with a pressure mapping system (see Chapter 7) is one way to follow-up and evaluate the wheelchair fitting process. Other examples of follow-up outcome are user-estimated comfort, mobility aspects, and the user's satisfaction with the wheelchair. A simple general follow-up could include the Quebec User Evaluation of Satisfaction with Assistive Technology (QUEST) 2.0 questionnaire (Demers et al., 1997). Evaluation of the effect of wheelchair interventions requires more specific assessment tools.

How the Intervention Eases Impairments, Activity Limitations, and Participation Restrictions

Wheelchairs provide people with mobility limitations with the opportunity to perform daily occupations and to participate in social life. According to the United Nations Convention on the Rights of Persons with Disabilities, article 20, personal mobility is a fundamental human right, and the convention asks for production of and access to quality mobility devices at affordable cost (WHO, 2007).

Evidence-Based Practice

Evidence outcome of wheelchair interventions is limited, especially regarding how the client uses the wheelchair and how it facilitates the performance of occupations and social participation. One reason may be that the effects of the intervention are apparent and do not require research to prove the outcome. A recent systematic review of activity and participation outcomes of mobility device interventions did not identify any studies on manual wheelchair interventions, but two pre-post studies on powered wheelchair outcome were done (Salminen et al., submitted). One study on stroke patients' powered wheelchairs showed that the users' activity problems had been substantially reduced, and that participation in the most investigated activities increased (Petterson, 2007). Another study found that powered wheelchair interventions positively affected the users' social lives (Davies et al., 2003).

A larger body of research is available concerning evidence for mobility outcome of wheelchair interventions, even though the quality of the research and level of evidence still need to be improved. The research supports the effectiveness of wheelchair interventions (Boninger et al., 2003; Corfman et al., 2003; Hoenig et al., 2003), while attention is drawn to some of the adverse outcomes mentioned earlier in this chapter (Bottos et al., 2001; Brandt et al., 2004; Mann et al., 2004; Petterson et al., 2006).

There is no evidence of the cost-effectiveness of wheelchairs as such, but in general, assistive technology interventions have been found to be cost-effective (Gosman-Hedström et al., 2002).

Discussion

An optimal wheelchair and seating system is a human right (WHO, 2007) for people with an impaired walking ability or the lack thereof. Occupational therapists have a clear role to play in wheelchair intervention. Their professional knowledge enables them to understand clients' daily occupational needs, abilities, and contexts. The options of wheelchairs and accessories are enormous, and the importance of knowledge in all relevant details is necessary for being able to perform an optimal fitting.

Even though it often is apparent that wheelchair interventions are effective, higher quality research is required, especially regarding occupational performance outcomes.

References

Abledata. A source for assistive technology information. http://www.abledata.com.

Boninger, M.L., Dicianno, B.E., Cooper, R.A., Towers, J.D., Koontz, A.M., and Sopuza, A.L. (2003). Shoulder magnetic resonance imaging abnormalities, wheelchair propulsion, and gender. Arch Phys Med Rehabil, 84, 1615–1620.

Bottos, M., Bolcati, C., Sciuto, L., Ruggeri, C., and Feliciangeli, A. (2001). Powered wheelchairs and independence in young children with tetraplegia. Dev Med Child Neurol, 43, :769–777.

Brandt, Å., Iwarsson, S., and Ståhl, A. (2004). Older people's use of powered wheelchairs for activity and participation. J Rehabil Med, 36(2), 70–77.

Cook, A.M., and Hussey, S.M. (2002). Assistive Technologies: Principles and Practice, 2nd ed. St. Louis: Mosby.

Corfman, T.A., Cooper, R.A., Fitzgerald, S.G., and Cooper, R. (2003). Tips and falls during electric-powered wheelchair driving: effects of seatbelt use, leg rests, and driving speed. Arch Phys Med Rehabil, 84, 1797–1802.

Davies, A., De Souza, L.H., and Frank, A.O. (2003). Changes in the quality of life in severely disabled people following provision of powered indoor/outdoor chairs. Disabil Rehabil, 25(6), 286–290.

Demers, L., Weiss-Lambrou, R., and Ska, B. (1997). The Quebec User Evaluation of Satisfaction with Assistive Technology (QUEST 2.0). Webster, NY: Institute for Matching Person and Technology.

Engström, B. (2002). Ergonomic Seating. The True Challenge. Hässelby, Sweden: Posturalis.

Gosman-Hedström, G., Claesson, L., and Blomstrand, C. (2002). Assistive devices in elderly people after stroke: a longitudinal, randomized study—the Göteborg 70+ stroke study. Scand J Occup Ther, 9, 109–118.

Hoenig, H., Landerman, L.R., Shipp, K.M., and George, L. (2003). Activity restrictions among wheelchair users. J Am Geriatr Soc, 51(9), 1244–1251.

International Standards Organization. (2007). Assistive Products for Persons with Disabilities—Classification and Terminology. DS/EN ISO 9999: 2007(E). Geneva: International Organization for Standardization.

Kauzlarich, J. (1999). Wheelchair rolling resistance and tire design. In: van der Woude, L., Hopman, M., and van Kemenade, C., eds. Biomechanical Aspects of Manual Wheelchair Propulsion. The State of the Art II. Amsterdam: ISO Press.

Law, M., Baptiste, S., Carswell, A., McColl, M.A., Polatajko, H., and Pollock, N. (1998). Canadian Occupational Performance Measure, 4th ed. Toronto, ON: CAOT Publications.

Lois, K. (2004). Being in a Wheelchair. UK: Anova Books.

Mann, W.C., Llanes, C., Justiss, M.D., and Tomita, M. (2004). Frail older adults' self-report of their most important assistive device. OTJR: Occup Participation Health, 24(1), 4–12.

Petterson, I. (2007). Significance of Assistive Devices in the Daily Life of Persons with Stroke and Their Spouses [Doctoral dissertation]. Örebro, Sweden: Örebro University.

Petterson, I., Törnquist, K., and Ahlström, G. (2006). The effect of an outdoor powered wheelchair on activity and participation in users with stroke. Disabil Rehabil Assistive Technol, 1(4), 235–246.

Royston, A. (1995). Using a Wheelchair. UK: Heinemann Educational Books.

Salminen, A., Brandt, Å., Samuelsson, K., Töytäri, O., and Malmivaara, A. (Submitted). Mobility devices to promote activity and participation systematic review.

Samuelsson, K. (2002). Active Wheelchair Use in Daily Life. Considerations for Mobility and Seating [Doctoral dissertation]. Linköping/Örebro, Sweden: The Swedish Institute for Disability Research, Department of Rehabilitation Medicine, Faculty of Health Sciences, Linköping University.

Stein, F., Söderback, I., Cutler, S.K., and Larson, B. (2006). Occupational Therapy and Ergonomics. Applying Ergonomic Principles to Everyday Occupation in the Home and at the Work, 1st ed. (pp. 92–116). London/Philadelphia: Whurr/Wiley.

Stewart, C.P., Psysiological considerations in seating. Prosthet Ortho Int, 15(3), 193–198.

World Health Organization. (2007). Improving Wheelchair Provision in Developing Countries. The WHO Newsletter on Disability and Rehabilitation. http://www.who.int/disabilities/publications/newsletter/1st_Issue_Newsletter_May07.pdf. 2007, 1(1), 2.

Chapter 9
Functional Electrical Stimulation Therapy: Individualized Neuroprosthesis for Grasping and Reaching

Milos R. Popovic and B. Cathy Craven

Although conventional occupational therapy was ineffective, the client was able to grasp a soda can after four months of FES therapy.

Abstract Stroke and spinal cord injury clients experience permanent disability resulting in total or partial upper limb paralysis. The paralysis can be either unilateral (typical for stroke clients) or bilateral (typical for cervical spinal cord injury clients). Approximately 85% of people living with stroke have severe upper limb paralysis, while 45% of people living with tetraplegia have persisting upper limb motor deficits more than one year after onset. These persisting functional inabilities affect their independence in activities of daily living, thereby increasing their need for attendant care services. This chapter provides a discussion of available therapies, with a particular focus on functional electrical stimulation therapy (FES).

Keywords Grasping • Neuroprosthesis • Reaching • Stroke • Spinal cord injury

Definitions

Reaching refers to abduction or flexion of the arm with an extended elbow to shoulder height.

Grasping refers to both palmar grasp and lateral prehension. *Palmar grasp* refers to opposition of the thumb and palm followed by flexion of the thumb and fingers, and is used to hold a water bottle. *Lateral prehension* is generated by flexing the fingers to provide opposition followed by thumb flexion, and is used to hold light objects like keys or paper.

Functional electrical stimulation (FES) is provided by a group of devices, conventionally prescribed for lifetime use, in which an electrical current is applied to a muscle or group of muscles via implanted or surface electrodes to stimulate the client's paralyzed muscles to contract and perform functional or leisure activities that are not otherwise possible.

I. Söderback (ed.), *International Handbook of Occupational Therapy Interventions*,
DOI: 10.1007/978-0-387-75424-6_9, © Springer Science+Business Media, LLC 2010

In functional electrical stimulation therapy (FES-T), FES is applied intermittently for short periods of time (2 to 6 months) to elicit or augment voluntary upper limb motor function.

Purposes

Functional electrical stimulation therapy is an intervention to improve grasping and reaching in clients with stroke or spinal cord injury (SCI) and weak or paretic upper limbs.

Method

Candidates for Functional Electrical Stimulation Therapy

Acute or chronic stroke and SCI clients with upper limb impairments and an inability to voluntarily grasp or reach objects with the impaired limbs are candidates for FES-T.

Epidemiology

Implanted FES systems have conventionally been used in clients with acute tetraplegia. Surface FES systems have been used in the past as an orthotic system prescribed for long-term substitution for inadequate or absent upper limb motor function in clients with stroke or SCI. This chapter outlines the paradigm shift in using FES as a short-term therapeutic tool to improve reaching and grasping in clients with stroke or SCI and absent/inadequate upper limb function prior to FES-T.

Settings

The studies presented and discussed were conducted in tertiary stroke and SCI rehabilitation centers or university-affiliated academic institutions in Canada, the United States, and Europe.

The Role of the Occupational Therapist

Occupational therapists (OTs) are responsible for identifying clients who are candidates for FES-T, for providing FES-T, and for evaluating its effectiveness. The OT advocates for FES-T resources in the practical environment.

Results

Clinical Applications

Overview of Current Grasping and Reaching Therapies

Constraint-induced intervention (Page and Levine, 2007; Wolf et al., 2006), neuro-modulation of the motor cortex in stroke clients (Petrofsky and Phillips, 1984), robotics-assisted therapy (Nef et al., 2007), and FES-T (Popovic et al., 2005) are currently being explored as interventions to minimize upper limb impairments. Among these, the most promising is FES-T for promoting or restoring grasping and reaching.

Functional Electrical Stimulation Devices (Apparatus)

Commercially available FES systems to restore grasping based on the former FES concept of substituting for motor impairment are the Freehand system (Mulcahey et al., 2004) and the Handmaster or Bioness H200 (Alon et al., 2007). The Freehand system is an implanted system primarily used in clients with SCI, while the Bioness H200 has been used in both SCI and stroke clients.

Functional Electrical Stimulation Versus Functional Electrical Stimulation Therapy

Functional electrical stimulation devices produce muscle contractions or sequences of contractions generated by a microprocessor-controlled electric stimulator. This enables controlled stimulated sequences of functional activity such as grasping or releasing a cup. Functional electrical stimulation was previously prescribed for lifetime use throughout the day to substitute for a motor activity the client could not perform.

In contrast, FES-T refers to a group of novel therapies in which FES is applied intermittently for a short period (2 to 6 months) to elicit and or augment voluntary upper limb motor function. Electrical stimulation applied during FES-T is delivered using short electrical pulses, preferably current regulated balanced biphasic pulses that generate a sequence of action potentials of adequate amplitude in the peripheral nerves. Visible or palpable muscle contractions are elicited. FES-T is individualized for the client and can be delivered using surface, transcutaneous, percutaneous, or implanted electrodes, with surface electrodes predominating. The choice of FES versus FES-T should be based on the client's goals, prognosis, and resources.

Use of Surface Versus Percutaneous Electrodes

Surface electrodes are inexpensive and easy to apply to the skin, but they are ineffective when stimulating some peripheral nerves (i.e., those innervating the proximal

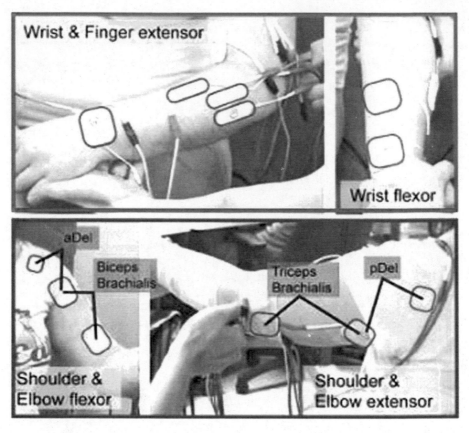

Fig. 9.1 Typical locations of the surface stimulation electrodes that are used to retrain reaching and grasping functions.

shoulder muscles). The typical locations of FES-T electrodes for grasping and reaching are shown in Fig. 9.1.

Percutaneous electrodes consist of thin wires that are inserted through the skin into the underlying muscle tissue where they remain in place up to 30 days.

Implanted electrodes are permanently implanted in the muscle or around a peripheral nerve. BION™ microstimulators (Advanced Bionics Corporation; Valencia, CA) are implanted via a hypodermic needle (Loeb, 2003); they are cylindrical in shape (2-mm diameter and 16-mm length), and are powered and controlled via radio waves from an external controller carried by the client.

Compared to surface electrodes, implanted and percutaneous electrodes have higher stimulation selectivity with much less electrical charge applied, both of which are desired characteristics. Implanted electrodes, with the exception of the BION, require lengthy surgical procedures to implant. In contrast, percutaneous electrodes are used temporarily. Implanted and percutaneous electrodes may cause local infection.

Functional Electrical Stimulation Therapy Intervention

Functional electrical stimulation therapy is typically applied using surface electrodes three to five times per week for 12 to 16 weeks with each session ranging in duration from 30 to 60 minutes.

Evidence-Based Practice

In an evidence-based practice, OTs perform standardized assessments to characterize the client's impairment and disability, identify subgroups suitable for specialized care, and assess treatment efficacy. The choice of the standardized assessment is dictated by the intent of the assessment. The Chedoke McMaster Stages of Motor Recovery (CMSMR) is an example of a valid measure with sound psychometric properties used to describe upper limb function after stroke and to help determine a prognosis. Less than 10% of stroke clients with CMSMR stages 1 or 2 recover their reaching and grasping ability (Rand et al., 1999). The reader is encouraged to become familiar with the assessments described herein for stroke and SCI clients.

The recent paradigm shift from using FES technology as an orthotic system to using it as a therapeutic tool to improve strength in clients with barely perceptible or weak voluntary upper limb motor function has resulted in improved voluntary reaching and grasping. Extensive experiments and investigations using FES-T as an intervention have been conducted by researchers around the world (Burridge et al., 2007; Gritsenko and Prochazka, 2004; Popovic et al., 2002, 2003, 2004), and by the authors' team (Popovic et al., 2005, 2006)

Surface Functional Electrical Stimulation Therapy for Stroke Clients

Many authors have experimented with surface FES-T systems over the last 5 years to restore grasping in stroke clients (Popovic et al., 2002, 2003, 2004). These studies categorize stroke clients based on their functional ability into high or low functioning groups. The high functioning group (HFG) subjects (four FES-T and four controls) (Popovic et al., 2002) could actively extend the affected wrist ≥20 degrees, and extend their metacarpophalangeal (MP) and interphalangeal (IP) joints of all digits 10 degrees prior to FES-T. The low functioning group (LFG) subjects (four FES-T and four controls (Popovic et al., 2002) could extend the paretic wrist <10 degrees, and volitionally extend the MP and IP joints of the thumb and two other digits for <10 degrees prior to FES-T.

Functional electrical stimulation therapy was applied daily for 3 consecutive weeks, up to 30 minutes per session. Controls received conventional physical therapy and OT. In the first and consecutive studies the Upper Extremity Functioning Test (UEFT) (Popovic et al., 2002) was used to assess subjects before and after FES-T. In later studies, the sample size was increased to 38 acute subjects (22 FES-T and 16 controls), and the controls were invited 12 months post-stroke to participate in the FES-T as well as the chronic clients (Popovic et al., 2003, 2004). In these later studies the UEFT, Drawing Test (DT), and the Modified Ashworth Spasticity (MAS) Scale were used to assess subject outcomes.

In all studies, acute subjects were assessed 12 months after enrollment in the study and chronic subjects up to 23 weeks after enrollment. Results of these three studies suggest that both acute and chronic stroke clients benefit from FES-T. Both the HFG and LFG benefited from FES-T, but the HFG had greater benefits and are best suited for FES-T.

Gritsenko and Prochazka (2004) used a sophisticated workstation with multiple instrumented objects typically used in activities of daily living in concert with a modified-impact cuff FES system to generate hand opening and closing. Six stroke clients (three males/three females), >12 months post stroke, participated; all had reasonable range of shoulder and elbow active range of motion, but were unable to grasp and release objects.

Functional electrical stimulation therapy was administered on 12 consecutive weekdays. The sessions were 1 hour long, during which subjects performed three tasks for 20 minutes each. Subjects were assessed on admission, on discharge, and 72 days after admission (follow-up), using the Fugl-Meyer Assessment (FMA) and Wolf Motor Function Test (WMFT) kinematics. Kinematics were assessed using the instrumented objects on the treatment and assessment days. WMFT and kinematic assessments showed improvement during treatment and on discharge, but were lower on follow-up assessment. The FMA scores did not improve. Functional electrical stimulation therapy in conjunction with an instrumented workstation was associated with improvements in hand function among hemiplegic stroke clients whose level of motor function would have precluded them from constraint-induced therapy.

Burridge et al. (2007) used an implanted FES system, the BION microstimulators, to help seven chronic (>12 months) stroke clients (four males/three females) improve voluntary hand opening and closing with CMSMR baseline stages 4 and 5. Subjects were assessed using the Action Research Arm Test (ARAT), Tracking Index (TI), and FMA assessments on admission and after 12 weeks. Functional electrical stimulation therapy was administered once or twice daily for at least 12 weeks. The ARAT, TI, and FMA showed improvements. However, the data presented were preliminary in nature, and future publications of the results are expected.

Our team (Popovic et al., 2005) is the first group to apply FES-T to restore voluntary reaching and grasping in severely impaired stroke subjects. These subjects were at CMSMR stages 1 or 2 at baseline, considerably lower than subjects in similar studies. Thirteen acute stroke subjects participated in a randomized control trial (five FES-T and eight controls) where FES-T for reaching and grasping was administered for 12 to 16 weeks, three to five times per week, 45 minutes per session. Controls received conventional PT and OT. Subjects were assessed on admission and discharge using the Functional Independence Measure (FIM), Barthel Index (BI), CMSMR, FMA, and Rehabilitation Engineering Laboratory Hand Function Test (REL test) (Popovic et al., 2005).

Statistically significant results were achieved on all tests, except FIM in favor of FES-T. FIM was not sufficiently responsive to capture improvements in arm and hand function during the study. When statistically significant results are achieved with extremely low number of participants (five FES-T and eight controls) this suggests that the administered intervention, in this case FES-T as compared to conventional PT and OT, ($p < .05$) is beneficial and merits further investigation. Our study also included detailed electrophysiologic examinations of selected subjects (article in preparation), which revealed that muscles with tone prior to the FES-T had significant tone reductions, and muscles that subjects were unable to relax or contract voluntarily prior to the intervention, were able to do so following FES-T.

Surface Functional Electrical Stimulation Therapy for Clients with Spinal Cord Injury

Our team conducted an randomized controlled trial (RCT) in which surface FES-T was applied to clients SCI as a treatment to improve grasping function (Popovic et al., 2006). Ten subjects with complete SCI (six FES-T and four controls) and 11 individuals with incomplete SCI participated (six FES-T and five controls) (Fig. 9.1). The subjects were assessed using the FIM, SCIM (Spinal Cord Independence Measure), and REL tests. Although the results to date are not statistically significant, they suggest that FES-T improves grasping in clients with motor complete or incomplete SCI as measured by the FIM, SCIM, and REL tests.

Discussion

Functional electrical stimulation therapy has the potential to improve reaching and grasping in clients with stroke and SCI.

The key factors to ensure FES-T success include (1) application early after the onset of stroke or SCI; (2) use of FES in conjunction with conventional physiotherapy or occupational therapy; (3) incorporation of customized electrical stimulation protocols, and programmable FES systems are required; (4) therapies that are delivered with the FES system; (5) repeatable yet diverse activities should be administered; and (6) FES-T administration for at least 40 minutes, three times per week is essential as this dose improves both reaching and grasping in clients with stroke and SCI.

The functional gains anticipated with FES-T are greatest in clients with acute stroke or SCI but are evident in both acute and chronic clients. This review summarizes the published benefits of FES-T among clients with stroke or SCI. The generalization of the findings are limited by small sample sizes, individualized treatment and outcome assessment protocols, diverse inclusion criteria, and the availability of FES-T equipment and OT expertise in clinical as opposed to research settings.

The OT and resource requirements associated with FES-T, although significant, have the potential to improve SCI and stroke clients' functional abilities and reduce the burden of care over their lifetime.

Acknowledgments We would like to acknowledge Karen Lepper for her assistance in preparing this chapter. The authors receive support from the Toronto Rehabilitation Institute, which receives funding under the provincial rehabilitation research program from the Ministry of Health and Long-Term Care in Ontario. We acknowledge funding from the Canadian Foundation for Innovation, Canadian Paraplegic Association Ontario, Natural Sciences and Engineering Research Council of Canada, Ontario Innovative Trust, Physicians Services Incorporated, and the Ontario Neurotrauma Foundation.

References

Alon, G., Levitt, A.F., and McCarthy, P.A. (2007). Functional electrical stimulation enhancement of upper limb functional recovery during stroke rehabilitation: a pilot study. Neurorehabil Neural Repair, 21(3), 207–215.

Burridge, J.H., Turk, R., Davis, R., et al. (2007). A clinical study using implantable microstimulators to facilitate recovery of upper limb function in hemiparesis: preliminary therapeutic outcomes. In: 12th Annual Conference of the International FES Society, pp. 82–84.

Gritsenko, V., and Prochazka, A. (2004). A functional electric stimulation-assisted exercise therapy system for hemiplegic hand function. Arch Phys Med Rehabil, 85(6), 881–885.

Loeb, G.E. (2003). Presentation highlights: bionic neurons 628 (Advanced Bionics Corporation; Valencia, CA, (BIONs™)). J Rehabil Res Dev, 39 (Suppl 6293), 5–6.

Mulcahey, M.J., Betz, R.R., Kozin, S.H., Smith, B.T., Hutchinson, D., and Lutz, C. (2004). Implantation of the freehand system during initial rehabilitation using minimally invasive techniques. Spinal Cord, 42(3), 146–155.

Nef, T., Mihelj, M., and Riener, R. (2007). Armin: a robot for patient client-cooperative arm therapy intervention. Med Biol End Comput, 45(9), 887–900.

Page, S.J., and Levine, P. (2007). Modified constraint-induced therapy intervention in clients with chronic stroke exhibiting minimal movement ability in the affected arm. Phys Ther Intervent, 87(7), 872–878.

Petrofsky, J.S., and Phillips, C.A. (1984). The use of functional electrical stimulation for rehabilitation of spinal cord injured clients. Central Nervous System Trauma, 1(1), 57–74.

Popovic, M.B., Popovic, D.B., Sinkjaer, T., Stefanovic, A., and Schwirtlich, L. (2002). Restitution of reaching and grasping promoted by functional electrical therapy. Artif Organs, 26(3), 271–275.

Popovic, M.B., Popovic, D.B., Sinkjaer, T., Stefanovic, A., and Schwirtlich, L. (2003). Clinical evaluation of functional electrical therapy in acute hemiplegic subjects. J Rehabil Res Dev, 40(5), 443–453.

Popovic, M.B., Popovic, D.B., Schwirtlich, L., and Sinkjaer, T. (2004). Functional electrical therapy (FET): Clinical trial in chronic hemiplegic subjects. Neuromodulation, 7(2), 133–140.

Popovic, M.R., Thrasher, T.A., Zivanovic, V., Takaki, J., and Hajek, V. (2005). Neuroprosthesis for retraining reaching and grasping functions in severe hemiplegic clients [article]. Neuromodulation, 8(1), 58–72.

Popovic, M.R., Thrasher, T.A., Adams, M.E., Takes, V., Zivanovic, V., and Tonack, M.I. (2006). Functional electrical therapy: retraining grasping in spinal cord injury. Spinal Cord, 44(3), 143–151.

Rand, D., Weiss, P., and Gottlieb, D. (1999). Does proprioceptive loss influence recovery of the upper limb after stroke? Neurorehabil Neural Repair, 13, 15–21.

Wolf, S.L., Winstein, C.J., Miller, J.P., et al. (2006). Effect of constraint-induced movement therapy on upper limb function 3 to 9 months after stroke: the excite randomized clinical trial. JAMA, 296(17), 2095–2104.

Chapter 10
Splints: Mobilization, Corrective Splintage, and Pressure Therapy for the Acutely Injured Hand

Josephine Man Wah Wong

> *I can touch my palm with my finger pulp again after splints and mobilization. I'd made it.*
>
> —Client

Abstract Early active and passive mobilization helps reduce edema, encourages active tendon gliding, and prevents joint stiffness after injury and operative intervention of the hands. It also enhances tensile strength of the newly repaired tendons, soft tissues, or fractured site, minimizing scar adhesion. Corrective splintage and pressure garments contribute to an effective outcome.

Keywords Corrective splintage • Injured hand • Mobilization • Pressure therapy

Background

The phases of the wound healing process are as follows:

- The *inflammatory phase* is the immediate vascular and cellular response to wounding that clears the wound of devitalized tissue, debris, and foreign materials. Edema dominates subsequent to vascular dilation. The length of this phase depends on the severity of the structures damaged and the tissue-handling approaches that follow. It usually lasts for about 5 days if no complication exists.
- The *fibroplastic phase* of repair lasts from 2 to 6 weeks, starting 3 to 5 days after the wounds occurred. This phase includes tissue granulation, collagen accumulation, and epithelialization, that is, the wound begins to heal. Here, the tensile strength of the wound grows, an increase that may last for about 3 weeks before reaching a plateau and then linearly increasing for at least 3 months further.
- *The maturation phase* begins as fibroblastic activity decreases and may last for years when the amount of collagen decreases and the wound becomes stronger (Smith, 1995).

To maximize treatment outcome, the choice of splintage should parallel the patient's tissue healing process.

Main Principles of Splintage

Splintage serves as a protective device to rest the injured finger(s) and hand in a functional and healing position. It helps relieve pain, prevents joint stiffening, and corrects joint contractures. It facilitates hand function in daily living by positioning the weakened or deformed fingers and hand optimally to facilitate occupational performance (Wong, 2002).

Main Principles of Movement Therapy Stress the Tissues of the Hand

Mobilization Through Active Motion

Mobilization through early active and passive motion aims at enhancing active tendon gliding, maintaining joint mobility, and preventing potential complications.

Early active mobilization of the hand should commence after the injured structures become stabilized. It encourages the pumping action of the muscles and the subsequent gliding of the soft tissue structures (Colditz, 1995). The aims are to decrease edematous fluid by mobilizing in an elevated position and facilitating finger-joint range of motion (Wong, 2002).

Mobilization Through Passive Motion

Passive motion is the mobilization of a joint by an external force intended to increase joint and soft tissue mobility (Maitland, 1977). It encourages tissues to reach a maximum available length within patients' pain tolerance, provided the resistance from the tissues is respected to prevent tissue damage from overstretching.

Purpose

The ultimate goal of hand therapy is to restore maximal hand function so that the client will be able to perform occupations independently.

Method

Candidates for the Interventions

People suffering from trauma that requires surgery of the hand(s) may benefit from hand therapy conducted by occupational therapists (OTs). According to the International

Classification of Functioning, Disability, and Health (ICF), the impairments relevant here concern structure of upper extremity and hand plus the function of the power of the muscles of a limb (World Health Organization, 2007).

Epidemiology

In Hong Kong, the risk of a hand injury at work occurs with odds ratios ranging from 10.5 to 26.0, as shown in a matched-pair interval analysis. The risk factors are (1) using malfunctioning tools/materials, (2) using a new work method, (3) doing an unusual work task, (4) working overtime, (5) feeling ill, and (6) being distracted and rushing (Chow et al., 2007). Another example, from the United States, of the extent of the need for hand therapy is that one fourth of workers (n = 232) who had used malfunctioning equipment or tools presented within 10 minutes with a hand injury (laceration, crush, or fracture) (Sorock et al., 2001). Hand trauma among children and in the home and during leisure time is not included in these figures.

However, there are no exact figures for how many people suffer from hand injury that may require rehabilitation, including occupational therapy, or for how many remain with a permanent disability. In the United Kingdom in 2006, the cost of hand surgery was more than £100 million (Dias and Garcia-Elias, 2006).

The Role of the Occupational Therapist

Occupational therapists (OTs) should have thorough knowledge of biologic and mechanical aspects of the injured hand, plus the clinical expertise to perform accurate clinical judgments leading to an effective splinting and movement program.

Results

Clinical Application: Mobilization of the Injured Hand

Mobilization of Repaired Tendons of the Hand

Controlled active and passive mobilization of the repaired tendons should commence within 1 week of surgery (Pettengill, 2005). Tendon excursion should be limited to a safe range but great enough to provide the stress necessary to stimulate biochemical changes that promote the healing process (Evans, 1995).

Table 10.1 presents an overview of the splintage common in rehabilitation of the injured hand.

Table 10.1 Overview of the splintage common in rehabilitation of the injured hand

Splint entitled	Splint figure	Functions of the splint
Repaired flexor tendons of the hand		
Controlled active flexor splint	Figure 10.1	A controlled active flexor tendon splint is used to allow early active mobilization of the fingers after flexor(s) repair. The active range of motion of the injured finger within the dorsal extension block splint is governed by the splint position. Passive flexion of the finger joints is allowed to maintain their suppleness.
Synergistic splint	Figure 10.2	A synergistic splint is a dynamic splint guided by wrist motion used to increase the excursion of the tendons within safe limits: from maximum wrist extension at 30 degrees to full flexion. The interphalangeal (IP) joints of fingers are passively flexed on the "place-and-hold" principle when the wrist extends to the 30-degree extension block.
Differential tendon gliding	Figure 10.3	Individual passive flexion of the IP joints enhances the isolated gliding of the flexor digitorum sublimis (FDS) and flexor digitorum profundus (FDP) in zone II.
Repaired extensor tendons of the hand		
Controlled passive extensor splint	Figure 10.4	A controlled passive extensor splint is used to allow early mobilization of the fingers after extensor repair. The injured finger is flexed actively and extended passively by the extensor assist within a controlled range. The volar flexion block is adjustable weekly.
Immediate controlled active motion splint	Figure 10.5	The immediate controlled active motion splint consists of two components. A finger extension-assist splint supports the injured finger in 20 degrees of relatively more extension than the adjacent fingers, and the finger actively extends supported by the adjacent fingers via the extension-assist splint. A wrist extension splint supports the wrist in 20 degrees of extension to relax the finger extensors.
Mobilization and passive motion of fractured fingers		
Splints for stable and nondisplaced fractures		
Buddy splint and proximal phalanx fracture resting splint	Figure 10.6	The buddy splint straps the injured finger and the adjacent finger together to facilitate the active motion of the injured finger. The night finger extension splint holds the finger and hand in a safe position to prevent potential flexion contracture developing in the IP joints and extension contracture in the metacarpophalangeal joint.

Corrective splintage

Belly gutter splint	Figure 10.7	A belly gutter splint helps correct flexion contracture of interphalangeal joints by molding a hollow space underneath the contracted joint in order to reinforce the correcting force applied by the strapping from top of the joint.
Dynamic mobilizing splint	Figure 10.8	The dynamic mobilizing splint provides low-load tensile stress via its dynamic component, trying to realign the scarred tissue.
Serial static web spreader	Figure 10.9	The serial static web spreader gradually widens the tightening first web by serial adjustment or splint remolding.
Static progressive proximal interphalangeal joint splint	Figure 10.10	The static progressive proximal interphalangeal joint splint applies passive stretching to gradually restore the passive extension and flexion range of the joint. The inelastic component of the splint is adjusted without change to its main structures.

Clinical application: Edema control

Edema control by elevation, active mobilization and pressure therapy

Pitting edema	Figure 10.11	Edema retention around the injured site, or even the whole hand after the injury. Edematous fluid is movable and soft when direct fingertip pressure is applied in the early stage.
Pressure finger tube	Figure 10.12	A pressure finger-tube with gentle circumferential pressure will help reduce local swelling over a finger. The choice of materials used depends on the severity of the swelling.
Pressure glove	Figure 10.13	A pressure glove, providing gentle and circumferential pressure, helps control swelling if all the fingers and the whole hand become swollen after injury or surgery.

Repaired Flexor Tendons of the Hand

Flexor tendon post-repair motion protocols include early-controlled forces, exerted through either passive or active motion (Strickland, 2005).

The traditional *passive way of splinting* (Kleinert et al., 1967; Lister et al., 1997) caused buckling of the repaired tendon within the synovial sheath (Horii, 1992). This way of splinting is no longer recommended.

Recent findings verify that flexor tendon rehabilitation should be based on controlled active digital motion (Lund, 2000). Here the *controlled active flexor splint* is used (Fig. 10.1).

The *synergistic splint* (Fig. 10.2), according to the Mayo Clinic protocol, is used to increase the differences (excursion) between the two digital flexors (Cooney et al., 1989; Savage, 1988). It functions at the optimal positions of the extended wrist and flexed metacarpophalanges of the hand joints to produce the least tension on a repaired flexor tendon during active digital flexion (Strickland, 2005).

Controlled *active and passive* motion should be integrated.

Passive flexion movements of the interphalangeal (IP) joints of the injured finger(s) contribute to maintaining joint mobility by influencing the edematous fluid,

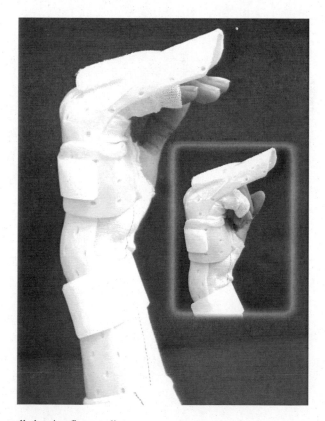

Fig. 10.1 Controlled active flexor splint.

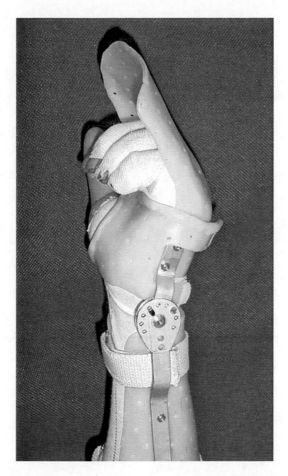

Fig. 10.2 Synergistic splint.

thus facilitating the active gliding of the tendons (Duran and Houser, 1995). Intervention in zone II flexor tendon injuries should include *differential tendon gliding exercise* to encourage isolated gliding of the two flexor tendons (Fig. 10.3).

Repaired Extensor Tendons of the Hand

The same principles are used for mobilization of the extensor tendons. *Controlled passive extension motion using a dynamic splint* seeks to prevent dense adhesions (Fig. 10.4) (Duran and Houser, 1995), and to stimulate intrinsic repair processes (Gelberman et al., 1981). The *Immediate Controlled Active Motion Extensor Tendon Program* (ICAM) gives the professional recommendations on how the pair of a wrist extension splint (wrist extended 20 to 25 degrees) and a *finger extension-assist* splint is designed to allow active digital flexion-extension. (Fig. 10.5) (Howell et al., 2005).

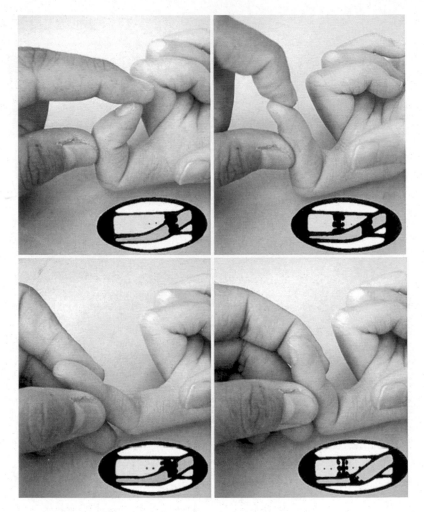

Fig. 10.3 Differential tendon-gliding splints.

Mobilization and Passive Motion of Fractured Fingers

The outcomes of managing finger fractures (especially proximal phalangeal fractures) depend on whether a stable anatomic position of the fracture is achieved and whether an *early active motion program* focusing on tendon gliding and joint mobility is conducted (Freeland et al., 2003).

Splints for Stable and Nondisplaced Fractures

Buddy taping or *splinting* (Fig. 10.6) to an adjacent uninvolved finger is sufficient to permit immediate active motion of the interphalangeal joints, enabling the extensor

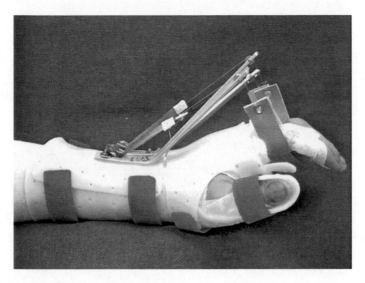

Fig. 10.4   Controlled passive extensor splint.

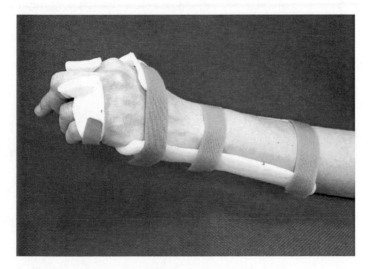

Fig. 10.5   Immediate controlled active motion splint.

mechanism to act as a tension band over the proximal phalanx. *Active motion* simultaneously compresses the fracture and stimulates periosteal callus formation, initiating the recovery of digital motion (Freeland et al., 2003). A *resting splint at night* is recommended to minimize the risk of contracture of the proximal interphalangeal (PIP) joint flexion. This splint is adapted to extend the IP joint and to keep the intrinsic tendons in a relaxed position by flexing the metacarpophalangeal (MP) joint.

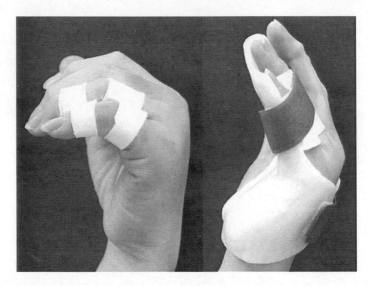

Fig. 10.6 Buddy splint and proximal Phalangial fracture resting splint.

A *dorsal block splint* is used *for displaced or open fractures* repaired with surgical stabilization. This splint is intended to relax the tensions over the fracture and is used to facilitate movement (Freeland et al., 2003).

Passive motion of fractured fingers should generally not begin before fracture callus calcification has been confirmed radiologically. Normally this occurs 10 to 21 days after the injury. Gentle passive flexion and extension of the distal IP joint can be allowed with fracture site protected (Freeland et al., 2003).

Clinical Application: Splintage

Corrective Splintage

The OT examines the fingers and the hand through his or her "end feel," that is, slow and careful stretching and tightening of soft tissue or finger joint(s). The result indicates the types of splintage to be used.

Static Splint

A *static splint* holds the finger in one specific position that applies stress to the newly repaired tissue. Its purpose is to *prevent* joint contracture and correct the new onset of joint flexion tightness (Wong, 2002).

A *belly-gutter splint* (Fig. 10.7) is intended to correct flexion tightness of the PIP joint by holding the injured finger in a safe but corrective position. The splint is positioned over the metacarpophalangeal (MCP) joints at 60 to 70 degrees of flexion and with the IP joints in full extension.

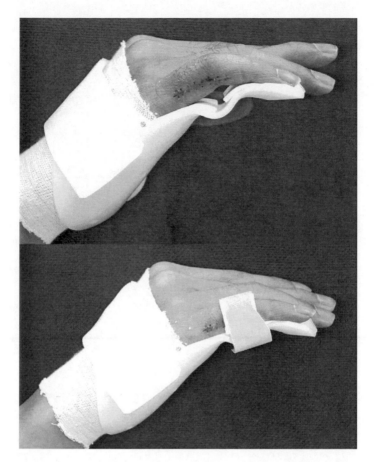

Fig. 10.7 Belly gutter splint.

Dynamic Splint

A dynamic mobilization splint (Fig. 10.8) applies a passive pulling force to a specific joint in one direction while permitting active motion in the opposite direction, using energy-storing materials such as a "Theraband," rubber band, springs, and spring wire (Wong, 2002). It applies a low-load constant and gentle force to realign the soft tissue under stress, holding tension on the joint, tendon, scar, and adhesions at the maximum tolerable limit (Flowers and LaStayo, 1994).

Serial Static Splint

Through periodic readjustment of position, the *serial static splint* (Fig. 10.9) provides serial stretching of a contracting or deforming tissue. After the tissue being stretched

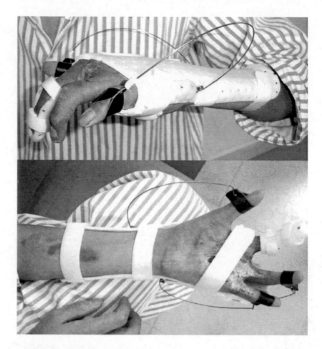

Fig. 10.8 Dynamic mobilizing splint.

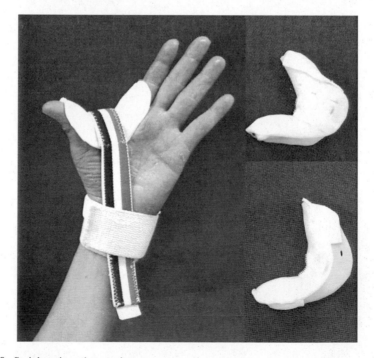

Fig. 10.9 Serial static web spreader.

it adapts to its stretching force by achieving the maximum tolerable length, the old splint is remolded or renewed in order to sustain the tissue at its maximum length again (Wong, 2002). It also functions as night resting splint, maintaining the "maximum gain" from the mobilizing splints used during the daytime. The first web spreader as shown illustrates how it regains the width of the first web space by serial adjustment.

Static Progressive Splint

Static progressive splints (Fig. 10.10) are made up of inelastic components such as hook and loop tapes, adjustable hinges, screws, or turnbuckles to apply torque to a joint statically at a position as close to end range as possible. These components allow progressive changes in joint position without changes in the structure of the splint (Schultz-Johnson, 2002). The contracted joint or shortened tissue is positioned at its maximum tolerable length by adjusting the tension of the inelastic component to reposition the tissue at a new maximum tolerable length. This type of splint is effective over stiff joints especially during the mid-to-late scar maturation stage of healing.

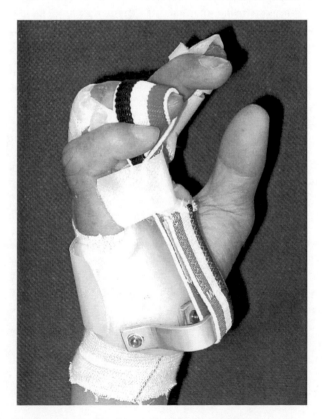

Fig. 10.10   Static progressive proximal interphalangeal joint splint.

Risks with Using Splints

All splintage has to be made with precautions to avoid excessive force from overstretching that will cause a prolonged increase in swelling retention and temperature around the stretched joint. Aggressive stress that produces more tissue damage than remodeling introduces more scarring, triggering the vicious circle of joint stiffening.

Clinical Application: Scar-Remodeling

Corrective Splintage Through Low-Load Prolonged Stress to Induce Scar-Remodeling

Dynamic or static corrective splintage is used to correct *progressive or static hand deformity* during the fibroplasia phase of healing. *Mobilizing splints* are applied to provide stress for remodeling collagen tissues, keeping the involved tissues in a prolonged state of mild tension, maximizing articular gliding and tendon excursion (Brand, 1995).

Static, serial static, or static progressive splints are used with increasing mechanical force to move the joint and tissue into the position opposite contracture.

Clinical Application: Edema Control

Edema Control Through Elevation, Active Mobilization, and Pressure Therapy

Persistent edema has detrimental effects on the intimately fitting gliding structures of the hand, causing pain, joint stiffness, and connective tissue adherence. Movable pitting edema (Fig. 10.11) usually dominates during the acute stage after the injury. It gives way when one applies direct fingertip pressure over the edematous area, though a soft feel is still noted during the "end-feel" of passive joint stretching. Fibrotic edema is found in the chronic stage of injury because of prolonged retention of edema fluid over the fingers and hand. Movable edema is replaced by fibrotic adhesion, limiting the gliding of soft tissues and finger motion. The "end-feel" from the joint passively stretched is stiff and resistive (Colditz, 1995).

Edema control by elevation, mobilization, and pressure garment (Fig. 10.12) is essential. The involved hand should be raised to above heart level to facilitate the flow of the edematous fluid from distal to proximal. Patients are encouraged to mobilize, pumping away the edema fluid, although they may experience great resistance from the extra fluid. Gentle massage, distal to proximal, will facilitate

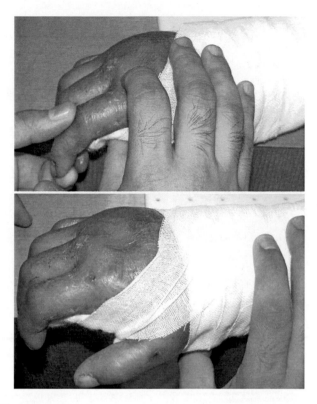

Fig. 10.11 Pitting edema.

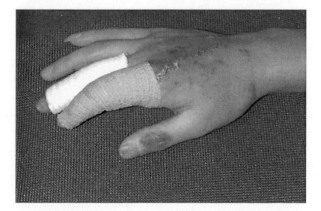

Fig. 10.12 Pressure finger tube.

blood circulation and mobility of the tissue layers. Compression with elastic bandage or pressure garment (Fig. 10.13) works when it applies gentle and constant pressure circumferentially distributed over the swollen hand (Wong, 2002).

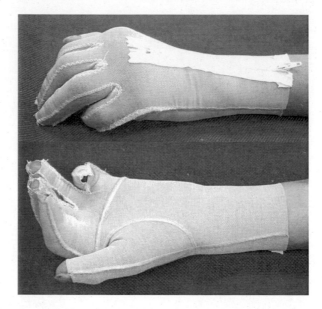

Fig. 10.13 Pressure glove.

Evidence-Based Practice

Kleinert and Duran protocols (Cetin et al., 2001) are the major guidelines for our routine flexor tendon programs for early mobilization, while programs encouraging active tendon gliding have been under investigation to enhance treatment effectiveness (Baktir et al., 1996; Brüner et al., 2003; Howell et al., 2005; Hung et al., 2005).

Discussion

Research on mobilization programs for tendon rehabilitation has been thorough and comprehensive. Further studies on the management of complications such as stiff fingers due to the splinting regime, the effectiveness of pressure therapy in swelling control, and the physical properties of materials used in treatment are needed to give us insight into the choice of evidence for hand therapy in the future.

References

Baktir, A., Türk, C.Y., Kabak, S., Sahin, V., and Karda , Y. (1996). Flexor tendon repair in zone 2 followed by early active mobilization. J Hand Surg, 21B, 624–628.
Brand, P.W. (1995). The forces of dynamic splinting: 10 questions before applying a dynamic splint to the hand. In: Hunter, J.M., Mackin, E.J., and Callahan, A.D., eds. Rehabilitation of the Hand: Surgery and Therapy, 4th ed. St. Louis, MO: Mosby.

Brüner, S., Wittemann, M., Jester, A., Blumenthal, K., and Germann, G. (2003). Dynamic splinting after extensor tendon repair in zones V to VII. J Hand Surg, 28B, 224–227.

Cetin, A., Dinçer, F., Keçik, A., and Cetin, M. (2001). Rehabilitation of flexor tendon injuries by use of a combined regimen of modified Kleinert and modified Duran techniques. Am J Phys Med Rehabil, 80, 721–728.

Chow, C.Y., Lee, H., Lau, J., and Yu, I.T. (2007). Transient risk factors for acute traumatic hand injuries: a case-crossover study in Hong Kong. Occup Environ Med, 64(1), 47–52.

Colditz, J.C. (1995). Therapist's management of the stiff hand. In: Hunter, J.M., Mackin, E.J., and Callahan, A.D., eds. Rehabilitation of the Hand: Surgery and Therapy, 4th ed. St. Louis, MO: Mosby.

Cooney, W.P., Lin, G.T., and An, K.N. (1989). Improved tendon excursion following flexor tendon repair. J Hand Ther, 2, 102–6.

Duran, R., and Houser, R. (1995). Controlled passive motion following flexor tendon repair in zones 2 and 3. In: Hunter, J.M., Mackin, E.J., and Callahan, A.D., eds. Rehabilitation of the Hand: Surgery and Therapy, 4th ed. St. Louis, MO: Mosby.

Evans, R.B. (1995). An update on extensor tendon management. In: Hunter, J.M., Mackin, E.J., and Callahan, A.D., eds. Rehabilitation of the Hand: Surgery and Therapy, 4th ed. St. Louis, MO: Mosby.

Flowers, K., and LaStayo, P. (1994). Effect of total end range time on improving passive range of motion. J Hand Ther, 7(3), 150–7.

Freeland, A.E., Hardy, M.A., and Singletary, S. (2003). Rehabilitation for proximal phalangeal fractures. J Hand Ther, 16(2), 129–142.

Gelberman, R.H., et al. (1981). The excursion and deformation of repaired flexors treated with protected early motion. J Hand Surg, 11A, 106–110.

Horii, E., Lin, G.T., and Cooney, W.P., et al. (1992). Comparative flexor tendon excursion after passive mobilization: an in vitro study. J Hand Surg [Am], 17A, 559–566.

Howell, J.W., Merritt, W.H., and Robinson, S.J. (2005). Immediate controlled active motion following zone 4-7 extensor tendon repair. J Hand Ther, 18(2), 182–190.

Hung, L.K., Pang, K.W., Yeung, P.L.C., Cheung, L., Wong, J.M.W., and Chan, P. (2005). Active mobilization after flexor tendon repair: comparison of results following injuries in zone 2 and other zones. J Orthop Surg, 13, 158–163.

Kleinert, H.E., Kutz, J.E., Ashbell, S., et al. (1967). Primary repair of lacerated flexor tendons in no man's land. J Bone Joint Surg, 49A, 577–578.

Lister, G.D., Kleinert, H.E., Kutz, J.E., et al. (1997). Primary flexor tendon repair followed by immediate controlled mobilization. J Hand Surg [Am], 2, 441–451.

Lund, A.T. (2000). Flexor tendon rehabilitation: a basic guide. Oper Tech Plast Reconstruct Surg, 7(1), 20–24.

Maitland, G.D. (1977). Peripheral Manipulation. London: Butterworth.

Pettengill, K.M. (2005). The evolution of early mobilization of the repaired flexor tendon. J Hand Ther, 18(2), 157–168.

Savage, R. (1988). The influence of wrist position on the minimum force required for active movement of the interphalangeal joints. J Hand Surg [Br], 13, 262–268.

Schultz-Johnson, K. (2002). Static progressive splinting. J Hand Ther, 15(2), 163–178.

Smith, K.L. (1995). Wound care for the hand patient. In: Hunter, J.M., Mackin, E.J., and Callahan, A.D., eds. Rehabilitation of the Hand: Surgery and Therapy, 4th ed. St. Louis, MO: Mosby.

Sorock, G.S., Lombardi, D.A., Hauser, R.B., Eisen, E.A., Herrick, R.F., and Mittleman, M.A. (2001). A case-crossover study of occupational traumatic hand injury: methods and initial findings. Am J Ind Med, 39(2), 171–179.

Strickland, J.W. (2005). Biologic basis for hand and upper extremity splinting. In: Fess, E.E., Fettle, K.S., Philips, C.A., and Janson, J.B., eds. Hand and Upper Extremity Splinting: Principles and Methods. New York: Elsevier, Mosby.

Wong, J.M.W. (2002). Management of stiff hand: an occupational therapist perspective. Hand Surg, 7(2), 261–269.

World Health Organization. (2007). ICF Introduction. http://www.who.int/classifications/icf/site/index.cfm.

Chapter 11
Splinting: Positioning, Edema, and Scar Management Due to Burn Injury

Megan Simons

After burn injury, the ultimate goal is to assist an individual to achieve optimal function and independence.

Abstract To achieve optimal function and independence, an individual relies on the combined use of a number of treatment modalities available to therapists (Simons et al., 2003). This chapter provides an overview of (1) classification and epidemiology of burn injury; and (2) intervention modalities that aim to minimize impairment to body structures and body functions after burn injury, by using positioning and splinting, and edema and scar management.

Keywords Burns, Contracture • Cicatrix hypertrophic • Edema • Rehabilitation

Purposes

Health professionals have been treating clients with burns for two millennia. Medical advances over the past three decades have resulted in declining mortality and shorter periods of hospitalization when burns are treated in a specialist burn unit. From this time, it was also realized that morbidity was reduced if occupational therapists, physical therapists, dieticians, psychologists, and social workers became an integral part of burns care (Herndon and Blakeney, 2007; Janzekovic, 1970).

Method

Candidates for the Intervention

People with wounds caused by burn injury should be referred for occupational therapy. The severity of a burn injury is determined according to the surface area affected and depth of the burn. The total body surface area (TBSA) affected is

I. Söderback (ed.), *International Handbook of Occupational Therapy Interventions*,
DOI: 10.1007/978-0-387-75424-6_11, © Springer Science + Business Media, LLC 2010

reported as a percentage (%TBSA), which ranges from <1% to 100%. The depth of the burn wound relates to the layers of skin that have been affected. Skin is considered to have two layers: the epidermis and dermis (Sheridan and Thompkins, 2007). The dermal layer is further classified as papillary dermis (upper layer) and reticular dermis (lower layer). Traditionally burns were classified as first, second, or third degree, depending on whether the burn was superficial, partial thickness, or full thickness. Fourth-degree burns involve underlying tissues such as muscle and fascia. However, since 2001, the main classification system used throughout the world is superficial, superficial partial, deep partial, or full thickness (Shakespeare, 2001).

Superficial burns involve only the epidermis. Although painful, healing usually occurs within 1 week without any residual scarring (Bessey, 2007).

Superficial partial-thickness burns involve only papillary dermis and epidermis. Burns of this depth are expected to heal in 1 to 2 weeks and should not result in visible changes to the skin beyond 6 months (Bessey, 2007).

Deep dermal partial-thickness burns involve epidermis and dermis to reticular dermis. It is usually expected that burns of this depth would take longer than 3 weeks to heal, and skin grafting is recommended to promote early wound closure and to reduce the degree of residual scarring (Bessey, 2007).

Full-thickness burns entail involvement of the whole thickness of the skin and possibly subcutaneous tissue. Skin grafting is essential since there is little potential for spontaneous healing (Greenhalgh, 2007).

To obtain the objective of optimal function and independence, treatment modalities to minimize the risk of impairment to body structures and body functions must be commenced upon admission after the burn injury. If wounds are considered partial or full thickness in depth on a flexor surface of the body (e.g., cubital fossa, popliteal fossa), the client is at significant risk of long-term functional impairment. If a burn heals spontaneously (i.e., without the need for skin grafting) with complete skin coverage of the affected area within 2 weeks, it will do so without a hypertrophic (red, raised, rigid) scar or functional impairment, but can result in long-term pigment changes. If healing takes more than 3 weeks, hypertrophic scarring inevitably results and can lead to functional impairment (Greenhalgh, 2007). As a general rule, the depth of the burn is usually underestimated at initial presentation (Sheridan, 2002), and the burn is rarely of uniform thickness (Johnson, 1994).

Epidemiology of Patients with Burns

The majority of burns are caused by scalding, fire, or hot surfaces (Forjuoh, 2006). Worldwide, burns in the under-5 age group account for a quarter to a half of all burn injuries treated in burn centers (Ansari-Lari and Askarian, 2003; Komolafe et al., 2003; Laloe, 2002). The majority of burns to young children occur as accidents in the home environment (Ansari-Lari and Askarian, 2003; Hemeda et al., 2003;

Laloe, 2002; Van Niekerk et al., 2004), while adult burns occur in the home, work-place, and outdoors in approximately equal proportions (Forjuoh, 2006). Most regions report scalds as causing the majority of burns to young children and the elderly (Al-Shehri, 2004; Ansari-Lari and Askarian, 2003; Belba and Belba, 2004; Dewar et al., 2004; Forjuoh, 2006; Tarim et al., 2005; Van Niekerk et al., 2004). Flammable liquid burns are common from cooking accidents in developing countries and in adolescent and young adult boys experimenting with petrol and other accelerants (Henderson et al., 2003). Burns from house fires or clothing ignition generally produce the most severe and lethal injuries (Forjuoh, 2006). Low socio-economic status of the family and low educational level of the mother are the main demographic factors associated with a high risk of childhood burn injury (Ahuja and Bhattacharya, 2004; Van Niekerk et al., 2004). Nonaccidental burn injury (i.e., abuse) is present in a higher proportion of families with a single parent, a younger mother, a low income, or an unemployed parent (Brown et al., 1997).

Settings

The overall care of clients with burns depends on the depth and extent of the injury, their age, the degree of wound healing, the presence of infection, and the psycho-social status of the client and family. Therefore, a multidisciplinary team is required to ensure that every aspect of the client's physical, psychological, and social needs is met during hospitalization and following discharge. Complex social issues often affect the delivery of a client's care, and therefore require skilled personnel to manage adjustment to hospitalization (Phillips and Rumsey, 2008). Often, for reasons of managed care or distance, clients with burns are referred to their local service providers for regular follow-up upon discharge, with less frequent reviews by the specialist burns unit. Therapists working outside a specialist burns center are encouraged to consult closely with their colleagues within the specialist units for advice and support in burn client therapy management (Simons et al., 2003).

The Role of the Occupational Therapist in Applying the Intervention

The occupational therapist (OT) is an integral part of a multidisciplinary burn team. The OT will be involved from the time of admission to the hospital to assess and treat impairment to body structures and function (e.g., contractures and scarring), as well as facilitating clients' ability to participate in meaningful occupation throughout their recovery to scar maturation and beyond.

Results

Clinical Application

This section describes three interventions provided by occupational therapists in burn care: splinting and positioning, edema management, and scar management.

Splinting and Positioning

Appropriate splinting and positioning, whereby tissues are maintained in an elongated state, are fundamental to the prevention of contractures, compression neuropathies, and decubitus ulcers following burn injury (Spires et al., 2007). Skin requires sustained mechanical stretch to facilitate alignment and lengthening of collagen and other fibers (Richard and Ward, 2005). The splinting protocols commenced by Willis (1969) continue as the basis for therapeutic intervention today.

Contractures, that is, the inability to perform full range of motion (ROM), result from factors such as limb positioning, duration of immobilization, and muscle, soft tissue, and bone pathology, placing the person with a burn injury at risk of secondary medical and functional deficits (Fig. 11.1) (Schneider et al., 2006). Joints overlaid by deep partial-thickness or full-thickness burns are at high risk for developing contracture. Contractures are a common problem following burn injury, and have been reported in up to 42% of patients receiving burn care (Esselman et al., 2006). The shoulder, elbow, and hand are most commonly affected (Schneider et al., 2006).

Minimizing contractures generally involves positioning of the actual joint. Positioning promotes extension and abduction (Fig. 11.2). Specific injuries require an individualized approach (Richard and Staley, 1994). A splinting or positioning device may be required for the prevention of ankle contractures during prolonged bed rest and also when exposed tendons require protection (Spires et al., 2007).

Splinting of the burned area may be undertaken using a range of media (foam, thermoplastics, neoprene) (Richard and Staley, 1994). The time needed for use of both pre- and postsurgical splinting depends on factors such as the client's age, the length of time since burn injury, and the severity of the deformity (Esselman et al., 2006). Prolonged *static splinting* is required following skin grafting procedures, but therapy should be started within 2 to 3 weeks with the splint removed for each session. Six weeks after the surgery, night splinting alone should be sufficient and may need to be continued for 1 or 2 years (Schwarz, 2007). If full ROM is not maintained, a program of stretching is recommended. A *positioning and splinting schedule* is developed for each client by the OT in collaboration with the burn team. Once the acute phase is over, occupational and physical therapists monitor and modify exercises and splints to maintain functionality until the reconstructive phase begins. At that time, prosthetic and orthotic devices and splints focus on rehabilitating the patient, with an emphasis on activities of daily living (Latenser and Kowal-Vern, 2002; Richard and Staley, 1994).

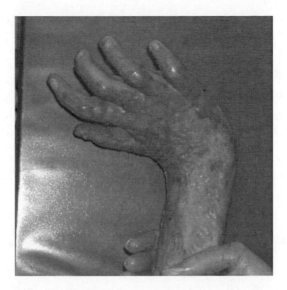

Fig. 11.1 Contractures to wrist and fingers because of hypertrophic scarring.

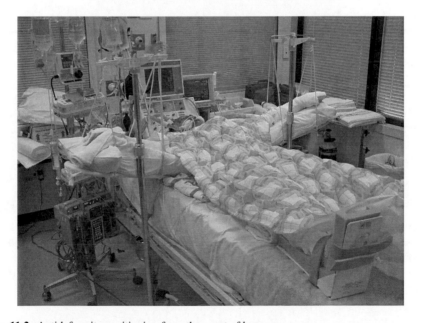

Fig. 11.2 Antideformity positioning from the onset of burn care.

Considerations for Treatment

The centripetal movement of skin peripheral to the wound is thought to increase tension in surrounding tissue, which decreases tissue reserves and makes the tissue that remains less responsive to elongation. The deleterious effects of these natural biologic occurrences are further compounded when extremities are not positioned appropriately (Richard et al., 1996). When contracture is present, a sustained force to tissue will produce tissue elongation and a subsequent plastic change in length, resulting in improved range of movement. Treatment intensity is determined by scar blanching (the clinical sign that the tissue's yield point is approaching) and tolerable pain (Spires et al., 2007). Gentle, prolonged stretch to healing tissue at its longest tolerable length for at least 6 to 8 hours per day is most effective (Chapman, 2007). The joint needs to be moved slowly and repeatedly to its end range several times before applying a prolonged stretch, which is maintained until the tissue blanches (Spires et al., 2007).

Splints must be "user-friendly," as poorly applied splints can cause nerve injury, loss of skin grafts, and worsening of a burn wound. An effective splint avoids pressure over bony prominences and is compatible with wound dressings and topical medications. Splints fabricated of re-mouldable materials can be modified, as the client's needs change. Factors to consider when prescribing a splint include the area of the body injured, extent and type of injury, the functional goal being addressed, and patient cooperation (Spires et al., 2007).

Evidence-Based Practice

There is much evidence, predominantly level IV studies (Edlund et al., 2004), which demonstrates that splinting is common practice, frequently used at the time of admission to the burn unit, for full-thickness burns and after grafting (Esselman et al., 2006). When compared with a multimodal approach (massage, exercises, pressure), those treated with progressive treatment, including static or dynamic splints and serial casting, required significantly fewer days to correct the contractures (Richard et al., 2000).

Edema Management

Edema is an interstitial protein-rich substance that forms a gel-like consistency and impedes vascular clearance. The superficial lymphatic plexus resides within the dermal–epidermal junction; therefore, deep partial-thickness and full-thickness burns can cause impairment to the superficial or deep lymphatic system. Edema arises from the lymph vascular safety system being exceeded, or lymph transport capacity being compromised (Hettrick et al., 2004).

On admission to the hospital, the severely burned client requires fluid resuscitation, which increases edema in the extravascular space that can limit joint motion (Latenser and Kowal-Vern, 2002; Spires et al., 2007). Edema develops within 8 to 12 hours after burn injury and peaks at approximately 36 hours. Failure to reduce edema in the first 48 to 72 hours can result in a fixed deformity (Richard and Staley, 1994).

Edema management is especially important with hand burns due to the dependent position of the hand (Esselman et al., 2006). Lymphedema, that is, chronic edema that is sustained for more than 3 months, is a rarely reported complication associated with burn injuries. Risk factors for lymphedema development include circumferential extremity involvement and fascial excision (Hettrick et al., 2004).

Considerations for Treatment

In the acute phase, *edema reduction* is pursued by elevation of the extremities above heart level. Elevating the hand and arm is accomplished using splints, bedside troughs, or similar devices (Richard and Staley, 1994). Web spacers (i.e., strips of foam/dressing product/molds) can be placed between digits to prevent fluid collection and edema formation (Latenser and Kowal-Vern, 2002) and elasticized bandages are used to decrease edema (Esselman et al., 2006). Exercise of the burned body parts helps to maintain joint mobility and muscle function (Latenser and Kowal-Vern, 2002). If the patient is alert and able to participate, a program of active and active-assisted exercise is appropriate. In obtunded or critically ill patients, passive range-of-motion exercises that emphasis the outermost wrinkle of the joints are prescribed to reduce contractures and functional loss.

Immediately following autografting, active and passive exercises are not performed on the limb. Depending on the type of graft, the condition of the graft wound, and the judgment of the surgeon, no exercise is performed for approximately 3 days on mesh grafts and 5 days for sheet grafts. Heterografts, synthetic dressings, escharotomies, and surgical debridements are not contraindications to exercise (Spires et al., 2007).

Wrapping burned extremities with elastic bandages when the patient is sitting or ambulating contributes to a decrease in edema and is used to avoid venous pooling, which can lead to graft sloughing (Spires et al., 2007). Should lymphedema be present, it can be managed with specific manual techniques, special bandaging and compression wraps, and remedial exercise (Hettrick et al., 2004).

The OT, in conjunction with the physiotherapist, is generally responsible for providing a positioning program, as well as either a passive or active exercise program from the day of admission until patients are fully mobilized and exercising (Latenser and Kowal-Vern, 2002). The OT enables clients to complete their daily functional tasks independently. Using assessment tools with demonstrated reliability the OT looks for (1) the presence of edema or lymphedema, such as the "figure of 8 method" (Maihafer et al., 2003; Pellecchia, 2003); (2) deepening of skin folds; and (3) absence of visible venous alterations and Stemmer's sign (Hettrick et al., 2004).

Education and communication among all burn team members, clients, and caregivers are necessary if an effective positioning and exercise program is to be successful (Richard and Staley, 1994).

Evidence-Based Practice

To date, evaluations of edema management techniques are predominantly based on case reports (Esselman et al., 2006). Further research would benefit from a scrutiny of the methods in both adult and pediatric populations, as well as focusing on the relationship between impairments to body structures and functions, and participation in a broad range of activities post-burn injury.

Scar Management

Hypertrophic scarring is caused by proliferation of dermal tissue following skin injury (Aarabi et al., 2007). Scar is considered immature if it is red, raised or rigid, and mature when it is nonvascular, flat, pliable, and soft. Approximately 1 to 3 months after healing of deep partial-thickness or full-thickness burns, hypertrophic scarring typically appears and may create a wide range of cosmetic and functional problems. The inflexibility of the scar may limit motion of the joint or soft tissue (Spires et al., 2007).

Scar management interventions include compression and the use of silicone. The use of pressure as a major treatment modality for scar suppression commenced in the early 1970s, following observed improvements of scarring with the use of a pressure garment (Macintyre and Baird, 2006). The use of silicone gel sheeting started in 1981, with treatment of burn scars (Perkins et al., 1983). The first silicone applications (elastomers) were individually made as a pressure device or pad to solve concavity problems under pressure garments (Malick and Carr, 1980).

The purpose of scar management is to prevent the development of impairments of body structures and functions from scarring, edema, or musculoskeletal changes, and to remediate or compensate for musculoskeletal or neurologic deficits. The estimated prevalence of hypertrophic scarring varies due to many factors but is reported as high, ranging from 32% to 67% in individuals with severe burn injury (Bombaro et al., 2003; Esselman et al., 2006). Wounds that need more than 10 to 14 days to heal are at risk of developing hypertrophic scarring and are therefore treated prophylactically (Chapman, 2007).

Considerations for Treatment

Pressure garments are typically introduced as soon as the patient is able to tolerate pressure (Fig. 11.3). The use of pressure in the pregrafting or healing stages has been advocated by some authors to prepare the wound bed and assist graft retention. Compression to healed wounds can prevent raised scarring if applied early and can accelerate scar maturation (Chapman, 2007; Van den Kerckhove et al., 2005). Garments are to be worn continuously for at least 23 hours, removed only for hygiene purposes and laundering. Pressure is continued until scar maturation has occurred, which generally takes up to 6 to 18 months, and in exceptional cases up to 5 years (Chapman, 2007; Macintyre and Baird, 2006). Commonly a silicone Silastic sheet, gel sheet, or pad is used in combination with a pressure garment. Inflatable silicone inserts are available in which the pressure on the scar can be adjusted using a pump (Van den Kerckhove et al., 2001).

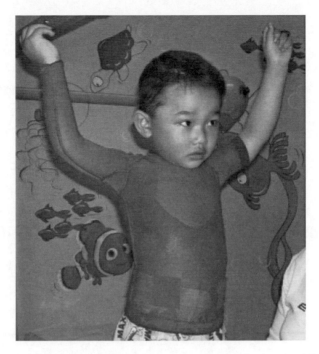

Fig. 11.3 Custom-made pressure garments are measured and fitted when the child's skin is able to withstand pressure and edema has resolved.

Garments should extend at least 5 cm (2 inches) beyond the margins of the scar(s) in order to apply an even pressure. Where it is difficult to provide pressure, such as at the web spaces between fingers, additional inserts of silicone or moldable materials are required to ensure an intimate fit (Spires et al., 2007). Silicone gel sheeting is ideally applied up to 24 hours per day from when epithelialization (i.e., healing) has occurred until the scar matures. The recommended initial duration of the treatment is 12 hours/day, particularly when it is used in combination with pressure, on children or in warm weather or climates. Strict guidelines are necessary for cleaning and disinfecting both the product and the skin. Gel sheeting may be stabilized at the edges with tape to prevent slippage and displacement during body movement (Van den Kerckhove et al., 2001).

The OT prescribes a pre-fabricated pressure garment. The fit of the garment is assessed regularly, and adjustments are made or new garments are supplied to ensure that adequate pressure is maintained (Macintyre and Baird, 2006). A reduction in the pressure of the garment is more significant over the first month of wear for garments that provide pressure >20 mm Hg (Van den Kerckhove et al., 2005). It is generally recommended that the garment be replaced every 2 to 3 months (Esselman et al., 2006).

Complications from compressive garments have been reported as wound breakdown, skeletal deformation, growth retardation, and obstructive sleep apnea

(Bourget et al., 2007; Rappoport et al., 2008). Complications from silicone gel sheeting (rash, ulcer, erythema, and pruritus) have been reported by some authors in over 50% of cases (Rayatt et al., 2006). While these complications are more common in children and when the gel is kept in place with pressure garments or adhesive tape, they usually resolve when the therapy is stopped temporarily or with hygiene measures (Van den Kerckhove et al., 2001).

Evidence-Based Practice

Hypertrophic scarring is collagen arranged in random orientation with whorls and nodules. Mechanical pressure facilitates the alignment of collagen fibers in a more parallel, normal orientation (Spires et al., 2007). Additionally, it is widely believed that pressure controls collagen synthesis by limiting the supply of blood, oxygen, and nutrients to the scar tissue, and reduces collagen production to the levels found in normal scar tissue more rapidly than the natural maturation process by replacing the pressure exerted by the destroyed skin on underlying tissues. A common belief is that the application of pressure alleviates the itchiness and pain associated with active hypertrophic scarring (Macintyre and Baird, 2006). Silicones are entirely synthetic polymers generally based on a dimethyl siloxane monomer and contain a repeating unit of structure. They have a silica-derived backbone and organic groups such as SiOC chains attach directly to a silicon atom via silicon carbon bonds (Van den Kerckhove et al., 2001). The working mechanism of silicone is unclear but the effects may be mediated through the pressure therapy principle (optimizing pressure) and hydration of the scar, due to a diminished water vapor loss through the silicone pad. It is thought that hydration should also benefit joint motion when used over a burn wound contracture due to diminished mechanical stress on the tissue (i.e., less tension or traction in the wound) (Van den Kerckhove et al., 2001). Little scientific evidence regarding the clinical effectiveness of pressure therapy has been reported, but a large body of dermatologic/histologic, clinical, and anecdotal or case-study evidence supports its use (Macintyre and Baird, 2006). When objective measures of scar thickness and erythema were considered with patients randomized to high-pressure/low-pressure groups, it was reported that garments must deliver a pressure of at least 15 mm Hg to accelerate scar maturation (Van den Kerckhove et al., 2005). Studies that randomized patients to pressure/no pressure or to high-pressure/low-pressure treatment and used a subjective measure (number of days pressure therapy required) reported no difference between the two groups (Chang et al., 1995).

Trials evaluating silicone gel sheeting as treatment for scarring are of poor quality and highly susceptible to bias. Weak evidence exists of a benefit of silicone gel sheeting as a prevention of abnormal scarring in high-risk individuals. When compared to no treatment, silicone gel sheeting reduced the incidence of hypertrophic scarring in people prone to scarring (relative risk [RR] 0.46, 95% confidence interval [CI] 0.21–0.98) and improved scar elasticity (RR 8.60, 95% CI 2.55–29.02)

(O'Brien and Pandit, 2006). Silicone gel sheeting has also been reported to effectively reduce thickness, pain, itchiness, and pliability of severe hypertrophic scarring in a Chinese population ($n = 45$). Objective measures of pigmentation and scar thickness and subjective measures of scar appearance, pain and itchiness, were used (Li-Tsang et al., 2006).

Additional studies to understand the prevalence and risk factors for the development of hypertrophic scarring are required. It is currently not known how pressures exerted on the surface of the body are diffused into the underlying tissue (Macintyre and Baird, 2006), nor is there clear scientific evidence that pressure therapy is effective for the treatment of hypertrophic scarring or what the optimal pressure to be applied is (Esselman et al., 2006). Further randomized trials are needed in this area.

References

Aarabi, S., Longaker, M.T., and Gurtner, G.C. (2007). Hypertrophic scar formation following burns and trauma: new approaches to treatment. PLoS Med, 4(9), e234.

Ahuja, R.B., and Bhattacharya, S. (2004). Burns in the developing world and burn disasters. BMJ, 329(7463), 447–449.

Al-Shehri, M. (2004). The pattern of paediatric burn injuries in Southwestern, Saudi Arabia. West Afr J Med, 23(4), 294–299.

Ansari-Lari, M., and Askarian, M. (2003). Epidemiology of burns presenting to an emergency department in Shiraz, South Iran. Burns, 29(6), 579–581.

Belba, M.K., and Belba, G.P. (2004). Review of statistical data about severe burn patients treated during 2001 and evidence of septic cases in Albania. Burns, 30(8), 813–819.

Bessey, P.Q. (2007). Wound care. In: Herndon, D.N., ed. Total Burn Care, 3rd ed. (pp. 127–135). Edinburgh: Elsevier Saunders.

Bombaro, K.M., Engrav, L.H., Carrougher, G.J., et al. (2003). What is the prevalence of hypertrophic scarring following burns. Burns, 29(4), 299–302.

Bourget, A., Dolmagian, J., Lapierre, G., and Egerszegi, E.P. (2007). Effects of compressive vests on pulmonary function of infants with thoracic burn scars. Burns, 34(5):707-12.

Brown, D.L., Greenhalgh, D.G., DeSerna, C.M., et al. (1997). Outcome and socioeconomic aspects of suspected child abuse scald burns [abstract]. J Burn Care Rehabil, 18(1, Part 3), S167.

Chang, P., Laubenthal, K.N., Lewis, R.W. II, Rosenquist, M.D., Lindley-Smith, P., and Kealey, G.P. (1995). Prospective, randomized study of the efficacy of pressure garment therapy in patients with burns. J Burn Care Rehabil, 16(5), 473–475.

Chapman, T.T. (2007). Burn scar and contracture management. J Trauma, 62(6 Suppl), S8.

Dewar, D.J., Magson, C.L., Fraser, J.F., Crighton, L., and Kimble, R.M. (2004). Hot beverage scalds in Australian children. J Burn Care Rehabil, 25(3), 224–227.

Edlund, W., Gronseth, G., and Yuen, S., , eds. (2004). American Academy of Neurology Clinical Practice Guideline Process Manual. St. Paul, MN: American Academy of Neurology.

Esselman, P.C., Thombs, B.D., Magyar-Russell, G., and Fauerbach, J.A. (2006). Burn rehabilitation: state of the science. Am J Phys Med Rehabil, 85(4), 383–413.

Forjuoh, S.N. (2006). Burns in low- and middle-income countries: a review of available literature on descriptive epidemiology, risk factors, treatment, and prevention. Burns, 32(5), 529–537.

Greenhalgh, D.G. (2007). Wound healing. In: Herndon, D.N., ed. Total Burn Care, 3rd ed. (pp. 578–595). Edinburgh: Elsevier Saunders.

Hemeda, M., Maher, A., and Mabrouk, A. (2003). Epidemiology of burns admitted to Ain Shams University Burns Unit, Cairo, Egypt. Burns, 29(4), 353–358.

Henderson, P., Mc Conville, H., Hohlriegel, N., Fraser, J.F., and Kimble, R.M. (2003). Flammable liquid burns in children. Burns, 29(4), 349–352.

Herndon, D.N., and Blakeney, P.E. (2007). Teamwork for total burn care: achievements, directions, and hopes. In: Herndon, D.N., ed. Total Burn Care, 3rd ed. (pp. 9–13). Edinburgh: Elsevier Saunders.

Hettrick, H., Nof, L., Ward, S., and Ecthernach, J. (2004). Incidence and prevalence of lymphedema in patients following burn injury: a five-year retrospective and three-month prospective study. Lymphat Res Biol, 2(1), 11–24.

Janzekovic, Z. (1970). A new concept in the early excision and immediate grafting of burns. J Trauma, 10(12), 1103–1108.

Johnson, C. (1994). Pathologic manifestations of burn injury. In: Richard, R.L., and Staley, M.J., eds. Burn Care and Rehabilitation: Principles and Practice (pp. 29–48). Philadelphia: FA Davis.

Komolafe, O.O., James, J., Makoka, M., and Kalongeolera, L. (2003). Epidemiology and mortality of burns at the Queen Elizabeth Central Hospital Blantyre, Malawi. Cent Afr J Med, 49(11–12), 130–134.

Laloe, V. (2002). Epidemiology and mortality of burns in a general hospital of Eastern Sri Lanka. Burns, 28(8), 778–781.

Latenser, B.A., and Kowal-Vern, A. (2002). Paediatric burn rehabilitation. Pediatr Rehabil, 5(1), 3–10.

Li-Tsang, C.W., Lau, J.C., Choi, J., Chan, C.C., and Jianan, L. (2006). A prospective randomized clinical trial to investigate the effect of silicone gel sheeting (Cica-Care) on post-traumatic hypertrophic scar among the Chinese population. Burns, 32(6), 678–683.

Macintyre, L., and Baird, M. (2006). Pressure garments for use in the treatment of hypertrophic scars—a review of the problems associated with their use. Burns, 32(1), 10–15.

Maihafer, G.C., Llewellyn, M.A., Pillar, W.J., Jr., Scott, K.L., Marino, D.M., and Bond, R.M. (2003). A comparison of the figure-of-eight method and water volumetry in measurement of hand and wrist size. J Hand Ther, 16(4), 305–310.

Malick, M., and Carr, J. (1980). Flexible elastomer molds in burn scar control. Am J Occup Ther, 34(9), 603–608.

O'Brien, L., and Pandit, A. (2006). Silicon gel sheeting for preventing and treating hypertrophic and keloid scars. Cochrane Database Syst Rev (1), CD003826.

Pellecchia, G.L. (2003). Figure-of-eight method of measuring hand size: reliability and concurrent validity. J Hand Ther, 16(4), 300–304.

Perkins, K., Davey, R.B., and Wallis, K. (1983). Silicone gel: a new treatment for burn scars and contractures. Burns, 9(3), 201–204.

Phillips, C., and Rumsey, N. (2008). Considerations for the provision of psychosocial services for families following paediatric burn injury—a quantitative study. Burns, 34(1), 56–62.

Rappoport, K., Muller, R., and Flores-Mir, C. (2008). Dental and skeletal changes during pressure garment use in facial burns: a systematic review. Burns, 34(1), 18–23.

Rayatt, S., Subramaniyan, V., and Smith, G. (2006). Audit of reactions to topical silicon used in the management of hypertrophic scars. Burns, 32(5), 653–654.

Richard, R., and Staley, M. (1994). Burn Care and Rehabilitation: Principles and Practice. Philadelphia: F.A. Davis.

Richard, R., and Ward, R.S. (2005). Splinting strategies and controversies. J Burn Care Rehabil, 26(5), 392–396.

Richard, R., Steinlage, R., Staley, M., and Keck, T. (1996). Mathematic model to estimate change in burn scar length required for joint range of motion. J Burn Care Rehabil, 17(5), 436–443; discussion 435.

Richard, R., Miller, S., Staley, M., and Johnson, R.M. (2000). Multimodal versus progressive treatment techniques to correct burn scar contractures. J Burn Care Rehabil, 21(6), 506–512.

Schneider, J.C., Holavanahalli, R., Helm, P., Goldstein, R., and Kowalske, K. (2006). Contractures in burn injury: defining the problem. J Burn Care Res, 27(4), 508–514.

Schwarz, R.J. (2007). Management of postburn contractures of the upper extremity. J Burn Care Res, 28(2), 212–219.

Shakespeare, P.G. (2001). Standards and quality in burn treatment. Burns, 27(8), 791–792.

Sheridan, R.L. (2002). Burns. Crit Care Med, 30(11 Suppl), S500–S514.

Sheridan, R.L., and Thompkins, R.G. (2007). Alternative wound coverings. In: Herndon, D.N., ed. Total Burn Care, 3rd ed. (pp. 239–245). Edinburgh: Elsevier Saunders.

Simons, M., King, S., and Edgar, D. (2003). Occupational therapy and physiotherapy for the patient with burns: principles and management guidelines. J Burn Care Rehabil, 24(5), 323–335; discussion 322.

Spires, M.C., Kelly, B.M., and Pangilinan, P.H., Jr. (2007). Rehabilitation methods for the burn injured individual. Phys Med Rehabil Clin North Am, 18(4), 925–948, viii.

Tarim, A., Nursal, T.Z., Yildirim, S., Noyan, T., Moray, G., and Haberal, M. (2005). Epidemiology of pediatric burn injuries in southern Turkey. J Burn Care Rehabil, 26(4), 327–330.

Van den Kerckhove, E., Stappaerts, K., Boeckx, W., et al. (2001). Silicones in the rehabilitation of burns: a review and overview. Burns, 27(3), 205–214.

Van den Kerckhove, E., Stappaerts, K., Fieuws, S., et al. (2005). The assessment of erythema and thickness on burn related scars during pressure garment therapy as a preventive measure for hypertrophic scarring. Burns, 31(6), 696–702.

Van Niekerk, A., Rode, H., and Laflamme, L. (2004). Incidence and patterns of childhood burn injuries in the Western Cape, South Africa. Burns, 30(4), 341–347.

Willis, B. (1969). The use of orthoplast isoprene splints in the treatment of the acutely burned child: preliminary report. Am J Occup Ther, 23(1), 57–61.

Chapter 12
Assistive Devices for Children with Disabilities

Sigrid Østensjø

Assistive devices widen the gate to everyday activities for children with various impairments.

Abstract Intervention for children with disabilities should be anchored in an activity-based approach and use everyday life as a source of children's learning opportunities. A wide range of assistive devices is available to support everyday activities in children with different types of problems in functioning. Providing these children with assistive technology can be an important intervention strategy for improving functional abilities, improving caregiving, and encouraging participation in everyday activities. Further research is needed to enhance our knowledge of how assistive devices can benefit children and their families to help to guide clinicians in day-to-day practice.

Keywords Activities of daily living • Caregiver • Disabled children • Play and playthings • Rehabilitation • Self-help devices

Theoretical Framework and Definitions

Traditionally, intervention for children with disabilities was based on impairment-oriented models, with the child as the only focus of intervention, denying the influence of the environment on development and functioning. More recently, interventions have emerged that emphasize the interaction among child, tasks, and environmental factors. Today, the best practice is based on an activity-based approach and on everyday life as sources of children's learning opportunities (Dunst and Raab, 2004; Valvano, 2004).

Every day a child eats, grooms, dresses, maintains continence, changes positions, moves around, understands requests, communicates basic needs, solves problems, and plays and interacts with peers. Performances of these daily activities are supported by wide ranges of assistive devices.

I. Söderback (ed.), *International Handbook of Occupational Therapy Interventions*,
DOI: 10.1007/978-0-387-75424-6_12, © Springer Science+Business Media, LLC 2010

An assistive device is commonly defined as "any item, piece of equipment, or product system, whether acquired commercially, modified, or customized, that is used to increase, maintain, or improve the functional capabilities of individuals with disabilities" (Definitions and Rule of the Assistive Technology Act of 1998).

The assistive devices used are either simple, such as adapted spoons and switch-adapted battery-operated toys, or complex, such as augmentative communication aids and powered mobility equipment.

The Purposes of Assistive Devices

In a family-centered approach to pediatric rehabilitation, assistive devices may be effective in the following ways: (1) supporting the child's functional independence, defined as the ability to perform essential tasks of mobility, self-care, and social function (Msall et al., 2001); (2) increasing the child's participation in everyday activities (Haley et al., 1992), and (3) lightening the day-to-day caregiver burden (Floyd and Gallagher, 1997).

Method

Candidates for Assistive Technology

Assistive devices are provided for children with different types of impairments causing activity limitations. Children with cerebral palsy (CP) (International Classification of Diseases [ICD 10] G80) are highly frequent users of assistive devices due to severe limitations in mobility, self-care, and social functions, such as communication and play (Korpela et al., 1993; Østensjø et al., 2005).

Role of Physical and Occupational Therapist Applying the Intervention

Using a family-centered approach, physical and occupational therapists work together with the child and the family during the different stages of the provision process: assistive technology assessment, setting goals for the provision process, selection and application of devices, and teaching the child and the family how to use them. This assessment and intervention process is dynamic and ongoing, changing in response to the needs of the child and the family.

Results

Clinical Applications

Decision-Making to Foster Use of Assistive Devices

Over the past decade, physical and occupational therapists have embraced the concept of outcome-driven clinical decision-making as a framework when designing intervention plans for children with disabilities (Campbell, 1999). In outcome-driven models of intervention, compensatory strategies, such as assistive devices, receive equal priority with other interventions in achieving consumer-based activity and participation goals.

Family-centered assistive technology is based on incorporating a parent and professionals in a partnership for making decisions about the selection and use of assistive devices. More specifically, parents are closely involved in the assessment and intervention processes. The decisions should increase the likelihood of functional use of the technology in the child's natural environment (Judge, 2002).

Use of Assistive Devices

Systematic documentation of the use of assistive devices to support everyday activities among children with disabilities is scarce. Østensjø et al. (2005) reported that nine of ten children with CP (age range 2 to 7.5 years) used assistive devices for mobility, self-care, and social functions when devices were supplied free to the family. Eighty percent of the devices belonged to children with severe limitations in gross motor function (Gross Motor Function Classification System, level IV and V; Palisano et al., 1997). However, the numbers of devices in use varied much within the same severity level. Most of the devices were used for indoor and outdoor mobility, transferring into and out of an automobile, eating, and playing. Many of the functionally nonspeaking children did not use available alternative or augmentative communication assistive devices, such as sign language, pictures and pictograms, and dialogue units.

Nonuse of devices provided among children is reported from 0 to 23%, depending on the type of device (McGrath et al., 1985; Østensjø et al., 2005).

Several obstacles to the effective integration of assistive devices into the child's everyday life were identified. Examples from the child's perspective are (1) the appropriateness of the device, (2) time constraints, (3) housing accessibility, (4) availability of transportation to get the assistive devices, and (5) insufficient training of users (Østensjø et al., 2005). Professional obstacles were (1) limited assistive-technology competence among therapists and teachers, (2) negative attitudes toward assistive devices, (3) inadequate assessment and implementation, and (4) difficulties in managing the equipment (Copley and Ziviani, 2004).

The high costs of many assistive devices and lack of available funds were frequently mentioned in the literature as an obstacle to using necessary assistive devices (Long et al., 2003).

Effect of Assistive Devices on Child and Caregiver Function

A review of 54 prospective studies concerning the effect of assistive devices on child and caregiver function found that the studies assessed effects of alternative and augmentative communication and powered mobility; devices used for play were not included in the review (Henderson et al., 2008). Among these studies, 51 focused on the outcomes of the child's performance and involvement in communication, computer use in school, mobility, and eating and nutrition. Only 11 studies incorporated caregiver outcomes. The conclusion was that the use of assistive devices had positive influences on the children's and the caregiver's situation. However, most of the studies had a low level of evidence.

In a cross-sectional study, Østensjø et al. (2005) assessed the influence of assistive devices on mobility, self-care, and social function among preschool children with CP. The devices influenced mobility: parents reported that children with some abilities in sitting and limited self-mobility increased their independence in moving around with the use of walking systems, powered mobility, and adapted tricycles, while seating systems, pushchairs, manual and powered wheelchairs, and suitable vans made care easier. Among children with the severest limitations in gross motor function, the parents judged that the assistive devices had benefits for the functional independence of the child.

The Effect of Assistive Devices on Self-Care

Four of five parents reported no or minor effect on the child's performance. However, three of four judged that the modification facilitated the care of the child, at least moderately. Adapted seating, eating utensils, and nonskid mats enhanced independence in eating and drinking, while seating systems, height-adjustable bathtubs, and shower and changing tables facilitated care of children unable to sit by themselves.

Effect of Assistive Devices on Social Function

Communication Aids

The parents judged the benefits of using assistive devices for communication as much less useful. The reason might be the complexities of activities such as communication and playing. Moreover, half of the communication aids provided were used in kindergarten and school, and not at home. This indicates that parent–child communication was mainly achieved by natural methods, such as vocalization, signs, and gestures. Communication with aids requires new skills of caregivers, plus positive attitudes toward the devices (Fallon et al., 2001; Parette et al., 2000).

Influence of Assistive Devices on Children's Play

Play is a fundamental aspect of a child's development and learning. It encompasses engagement in purposeful activities with objects or toys alone or in with others (Besio, 2002; Brodin, 1999). Parents of children with disabilities have an active role in helping the child to play (Brodin, 1999; Østensjø et al., 2005). Few studies have assessed the influence of assistive technology on playing. Østensjø et al. (2005) found that one of five parents of preschoolers with CP experienced that various sitting furniture and adapted toys and games enhanced the child's playing, and the parents' participation in the play situation. In a study of toddlers with severe sensory, motor, and cognitive impairments, three of four children learned to use switches to control adapted toys and other devices through basic technology intervention (Sullivan and Lewis, 2000).

Evidence-Based Practice: The Effectiveness of Assistive Devices

Studies addressing outcomes of assistive devices have provided evidence of improving the functional abilities, participation, and care within everyday activities of young children with disabilities. However, the significance of the studies may remain an open question because of the poor validity of the studies (Henderson et al., 2008).

Problems of the effective use of assistive devices seem to arise from an interaction of factors associated with the child's type of impairment; parents' and professionals' attitudes toward assistive devices; characteristics of the technology; design of the environment; and services, systems, and processes that currently guide the provision of assistive technology (Copley and Ziviani, 2004; Long et al., 2003; Østensjø et al., 2005).

Discussion

It is recommended that service delivery of assistive technology be integrated into an outcome-driven and family-centered model. The use of standardized assessments is requested for the investigation of how assistive devices facilitate and affect children's and their caregivers' everyday functioning in their actual living environment.

References

Besio, S. (2002). An Italian research project to study the play of children with motor disabilities; the first year of the activity. Disabil Rehabil, 24, 72–79.

Brodin, J. (1999). Play in children with multiple disabilities: play with toys—a review. Int J Disabil Dev Educ, 46, 25–34.

Campbell, S. (1999). Models for decision-making in pediatric neurologic physical therapy. In: Campbell, S., ed. Decision-Making in Pediatric Neurologic Physical Therapy (pp. 1–22). New York: Churchill Livingstone.

Copley, J., and Ziviani, J. (2004). Barriers to use of assistive technology for children with multiple disabilities. Occup Ther Int, 11, 229–243.

Dunst, C.J., and Raab, M. (2004). Parents' and practitioners' perspectives of young children's everyday learning environments. Psychol Rep, 93, 251–256.

Fallon, K.A., Light, J.C., and Page T.K. (2001). Enhancing vocabulary selection for preschoolers who require augmentative and alternative communication. Am J Speech-Lang Pathol, 10, 181–195.

Floyd, F.J., and Gallagher, E.M. (1997). Parental stress, care demands, and use of supportive services for school-aged children with disabilities and behavior problems. Fam Rel, 46, 359–371.

Haley, S.M., Coster, W.J., Ludlow, L.H., Haltiwanger, J.T., and Andrellos, P.J. (1992). Pediatric Evaluation of Disability Inventory (PEDI). Development, Standardization and Administration Manual. Boston: Boston University.

Henderson, S., Skelton, H., and Rosenbaum, P. (2008). Assistive devices for children with functional impairments: impact on child and caregiver function. Dev Med Child Neurol, 50, 89–98.

Judge, S. (2002). Family-centered assistive technology assessment and intervention practices for early intervention. Infants Young Child, 15, 60–68.

Korpela, R.A., Säppanen, R.-V., and Koivikko, M. (1993). Rehabilitation service evaluation: a follow up of the extent of use of technical aids for disabled children. Disabil Rehabil, 15, 143–140.

Long, T., Huang, L., Woodbridge, M., Woolverton, M., and Minkel, J. (2003). Integrating assistive technology into an outcome-driven model of service delivery. Infants Young Child, 16, 272–283.

McGrath, P.J., Goodman, J.T., Cunningham, S.J., MacDonald, B.-J., Nichols, T.A., and Unruch, A. (1985). Assistive devices: utilization by children. Arch Phys Med Rehabil, 66, 430–432.

Msall, M.E., Tremont, M.R., and Ottenbacher, K.J. (2001) Functional assessment of preschool children: Optimizing development and family supports in early intervention. Infants Young Child, 14, 46–66.

Østensjø, S., Carlberg, E.B., and Vøllestad, N.K. (2003). Everyday functioning in young children with cerebral palsy: functional skills, caregiver assistance and modifications of the environment. Dev Med Child Neurol, 45, 603–612.

Østensjø, S., Carlberg, E.B., and Vøllestad, N.K. (2005). The use and impact of assistive devices and other environmental modifications on everyday activities and care in young children with cerebral palsy. Disabil Rehabil, 27, 849–861.

Palisano, R., Rosenbaum, P., Walter, S., Russell D., Wood, E., and Galuppi, B. (1997). Development and reliability of a system to classify gross motor function in children with cerebral palsy. Dev Med Child Neurol, 39, 214–223.

Parette, H.P., Jr., Brotherson, M.J., and Huer, M.B. (2000). Giving families a voice in augmentative and alternative communication decision-making. Educ Train Mental Retardation Dev Disabil, 35, 177–190.

Sullivan, M., and Lewis, M. (2000). Assistive technology for the very young: creating a responsive environment. Infants Young Children, 12, 34–52.

US Government. Accessibility & Workforce Division, in the U.S. General Services Administration's Office of Government-wide Policy. Assistive Technology Act of 1998. S.2432. Sec. 3. Definitions and rule. 105–394, HYPERLINK "http://www.section508.gov/docs/AT1998.html Retrieved 5/3 2009 http://www.section508.gov/docs/AT1998.html Retrieved 5/3 2009.

Valvano, J. (2004). Activity-focused motor interventions for children with neurological conditions. Physical and Occupational Therapy in Pediatrics, 24, 79–107.

Chapter 13
Low Vision Intervention: Decision-Making for Acquiring and Integrating Assistive Technology

Al Copolillo

> *The occupational therapist and optometrist were very helpful and introduced me to a lot of technology. The OT had a pretty good grasp of the technology and was fairly abreast of what was available. I take my hat off to her.*
>
> —Client

Abstract Occupational-therapy intervention can enable strong, independent decision-making primarily related to assistive device acquisition and use for clients with *low vision*. In developed nations, occupational therapists provide interventions for older adults with acquired vision impairments more frequently than for any other population. Therefore, the information here will be applicable mostly to that age group. This chapter explores two main topics: (1) the decision-making process involved in acquiring and integrating low-vision assistive technology for clients with low vision, and (2) the types of assistive technologies available to clients with low vision.

Keywords Assistive technology • Low vision.

Definition of Assistive Low-Vision Technology

Low-vision assistive technology is any item, piece of equipment, or product system, whether acquired commercially, modified, or customized, that is used to increase, maintain, or improve the functional visual capabilities of an individual with a disability (adapted from the general definition of the U.S. Assistive Technology Act of 2004).

Categories of low-vision assistive devices are as follows:

- *Hand-held magnifier:* portable magnifier designed to be carried by the user.
- *Stand magnifier:* magnifier placed over the material to be viewed; designed primarily for reading, in a stationary situation, usually while the user is sitting at a table.

I. Söderback (ed.), *International Handbook of Occupational Therapy Interventions*,   147
DOI: 10.1007/978-0-387-75424-6_13, © Springer Science+Business Media, LLC 2010

- *Closed-circuit television* (CCTV): a video magnifier; items to be viewed are placed under a camera, and magnified images are projected onto a television screen for easier viewing.
- *Controlled area lighting:* high-intensity, glare-controlled light for reading and detail work.
- *Screen magnification and voice output readers:* accessories or software available to assist with computer use.
- *Activities of daily living (ADL)/instrumental activities of daily living (IADL) adaptive devices:* a variety of low-vision devices used throughout the home and community to enhance visibility, reduce risk of injury, or enable use of other senses to compensate for vision loss.

Background

Persons with vision impairment require substantial assistance to acquire low-vision assistive devices and integrate them into their daily routines. Since visual input is so essential to searching for and examining the wide range of assistive technologies one might choose, the vision impairment itself poses a considerable barrier to accessing the technologies. Persons with vision impairment must often rely on others for this process, especially in cases of severe vision loss. The information they receive comes from a variety of sources of varying degrees of reliability. Occupational therapy from skilled low-vision specialists that simplifies access to assistive technology is, therefore, greatly appreciated, and often life-changing for persons with low vision and blindness. However, for this population, improving access meets only part of the need. Other important components of successful intervention include assisting the low-vision client to choose the right technology by experimenting with a variety of devices; customizing use through exploration of specific device characteristics; moving from controlled, therapist-guided device acquisition and use to independence in the natural environment; and adjusting to lifestyle changes imposed by vision impairment.

Purpose

The main purpose of using low-vision assistive technology (AT) is to optimize usable vision and compensate for vision loss. Persons with low vision use assistive technology mainly for reading and writing. Therefore, ADLs requiring these skills, such as reading medicine bottles or recipes, paying bills, and reading mail are often improved with AT. Reducing the risk of injury is another main purpose for the use of AT. For example, simple devices that improve depth perception and contrast on stairs or reduce the potential for spilling hot liquids are frequently used.

Method

Candidates for the Intervention

Major causes of blindness worldwide are cataract, glaucoma, and age-related macular degeneration. The most prevalent diseases leading to blindness and low vision in developed nations are macular degeneration, diabetic retinopathy, and glaucoma. Occupational therapists (OTs) provide services to clients with these diagnoses but also design interventions for people with vision loss from stroke, traumatic brain injury, and multiple sclerosis.

Epidemiology: World Statistics on Vision Impairment

World Health Organization data from 2002 set the worldwide prevalence of vision impairment in excess of 161 million people, of whom 37 million were blind (Resnikoff et al., 2004). The prevalence of blindness in developed countries is typically less than 0.3%, but increases to greater than 1% in the least developed countries.

Cataract, typically remediated through ocular surgery in developed countries, is the leading cause of blindness and low vision in developing countries and globally, due to increased incidence plus the limited availability of surgery (Resnikoff et al., 2004). Throughout the world, the prevalence of visual impairment is substantially greater for people with diabetes (Center for Disease Control and Prevention, 2004).

Settings

Service Provision Process

Low-vision rehabilitation services are provided in a variety of health system contexts and by health professionals with a wide range of training backgrounds, including low-vision specialists, vision rehabilitation teachers, orientation/mobility specialists, and OTs. Among the specialists in low-vision rehabilitation, OTs typically obtain training through continuing education and post-degree programs and courses (Copolillo et al., 2007). Throughout the world, there is a vast shortage of low-vision health care practitioners trained to provide rehabilitation services (American Foundation for the Blind, 1999). This represents a barrier to adequate care of persons with vision impairment and reduces the potential for obtaining and using devices in a timely and effective manner.

When low-vision rehabilitation services are available, referral by ophthalmologists and other physicians is limited and often delayed (Crews, 2000). Patients who may have benefited from rehabilitation early in the disease process frequently become aware of such programs only after their vision impairments have become severe. Anecdotal evidence from practitioners indicates that intervention early in a progressive eye disease process can be highly beneficial because it is easier to learn to use adapted strategies, apply methods for finding AT, and make appropriate environmental adaptations when available vision is at its highest. As low vision approaches blindness in progressive eye diseases, the challenges to learning and initiating adaptive strategies for the first time become substantially greater and decrease the potential for success.

Types of Low-Vision Services

Low-vision rehabilitation services are provided in both group and individual therapeutic venues. Health-promotion and self-management programs are effective methods for teaching persons with low vision and blindness about available assistive technologies and their application. Group interactions provide opportunities for individuals to make decisions about what devices to acquire and how to integrate them into their lives (Brody et al., 2002, 2005; Ivanoff et al., 2002).

Within some health care systems, occupational therapy practitioners primarily intervene with clients with low vision on a one-to-one basis. Patients are seen in low-vision rehabilitation programs, typically with a two-person rehabilitation team consisting of either an ophthalmologist or optometrist and an OT. Additional professional services may be provided regularly by psychologists, nurses, or orientation/mobility specialists, but services from these professionals are more frequently acquired through referral from the low-vision rehabilitation team.

In a low-vision rehabilitation program, the physician conducts detailed eye examinations and interviews patients to determine the extent of their disability. The physician prescribes optics and identifies appropriate magnification and lighting needs. The OT collects specific information about the client's performance of basic ADL and IADL, work skills, and recreation and leisure activities, thus taking the basic results of the physician's vision testing and identifying the impact of the vision loss on performance of daily activities. The OT's evaluation leads to interventions that assist the client in performing desired activities by further identifying the functional extent of usable vision and teaching the client to make the best use of it (Warren, 1995; Warren et al., 2006).

The Role of the Occupational Therapist

Occupational-therapy practitioners working in low-vision rehabilitation collaborate with their clients to develop multifaceted interventions. Identification and use of all available vision and compensation for vision loss are the primary objectives. Activities that rely particularly on reading skills and mobility are frequently at the core of the intervention. Therefore, technologies that improve the ability to read, increase safety and ease of mobility, improve performance of IADL, and, on a lesser scale, basic ADL are identified and explored in the rehabilitation process.

Results

Clinical Application

Making Decisions About Use of Assistive Technology

As part of the process of acquiring new skills in rehabilitation, the client is assisted in finding the most useful assistive technologies and environmental adaptations for performance of desired activities. The client and therapist work together to perfect the use of the devices and adaptations, primarily through practice in multiple settings and under various conditions. Through exposure to a variety of technology resources, including the Internet and local, national, and international vision associations, the client learns a process of accessing, acquiring, and integrating needed technologies. Clients learn to judge the usability of technology by questioning its application in multiple settings, comparing costs, and seeking or requesting trial use before finally deciding to accept devices for longer-term or permanent use.

Decision-making is a special form of problem solving in which, from a variety of potential solutions, the client identifies the most satisfying outcome (Yates and Patalano, 1999). This requires the OT to compare and contrast possibilities and weigh benefits against obstacles. This complex procedure depends on the client's individual problem-solving strategies. How the problem is defined, life experience, familiarity with the problem, and the impact of the environment all contribute to decision-making (Berg et al., 1998).

Assistive Technologies for Low Vision

A wide variety of assistive technology devices are commercially available to the client with low vision. Low-vision rehabilitation programs often keep devices on site to allow clients to find ones that best fit their needs and practice using them before purchasing or accepting them for ongoing use.

Magnification and Controlled-Area Lighting

The most appropriate and useful technologies for persons with low vision provide the right combination of magnification, controlled-area lighting, and proper contrast for optimizing usable vision. Finding the right magnifiers and lighting options, therefore, are two of the main responsibilities of the OT practitioner working with persons with low vision. There is a wide range of magnifiers available, typically divided into *stand* and *hand-held* varieties. Stand magnifiers are used on a flat surface. The user learns to place the magnifier over the item to be read or examined and to look through it at an optimal distance and position from it. Stand magnifiers can have lighting attached and can include glare filters. Examples of how a stand magnifier might be used include reading a newspaper, book, or letter while seated at a desk or table. Hand-held magnifiers are designed for the user to carry; their usefulness is in being portable. They are often smaller and lighter than stand magnifiers. The key to their use lies in learning to distance the magnifier correctly from the object to be observed and then to place the head and eyes in the optimal position and at the correct distance from the magnifier. This varies according to the level of magnification of the magnifier and the size of the object. Examples of the use of hand-held magnifiers are reading labels on items in a grocery store, price tags on clothing, dosage on prescription medicine bottles, or menus in a restaurant. High-intensity lighting or filtered lighting to reduce glare are often built into magnifiers or used in combination with them. Figure 13.1 shows both stand and hand-held magnifiers and accompanying lighting systems that improve functional vision.

Closed-Circuit Television

Magnification, lighting, and contrast are also the main features on closed-circuit television (CCTV), which many people with vision impairment regard as a life-changing device (Copolillo and Teitelman, 2005). The user places an item on a platform below the magnifier; the item is enlarged to a set magnification and projected onto a television screen directly in front of the user (Fig. 13.2). For many, the cost of these items is an inhibiting factor, especially in health care systems where assistive technology is not reimbursed, as is the case for most health insurance in the United States.

Personal Computers and Computer Software

Personal computers (PCs) and the Internet have become popular for people with mild-to-moderate visual acuity problems. Many software systems purchased with PCs have built-in disability resources that can be turned on by the user, allowing for such adaptations as changes in background and print, and icon color and size. Other software, such as ZoomText, Jaws, and Kurzweil, are commercially available. These screen-magnification voices output readers provide some variety of contrast adjustment, and audible text, all features that may be appealing to persons with vision impairments.

Adaptive Devices

There is a wide variety of devices designed to compensate for vision loss while simplifying daily routines and improving safety (Fig. 13.3). Extra-large universal

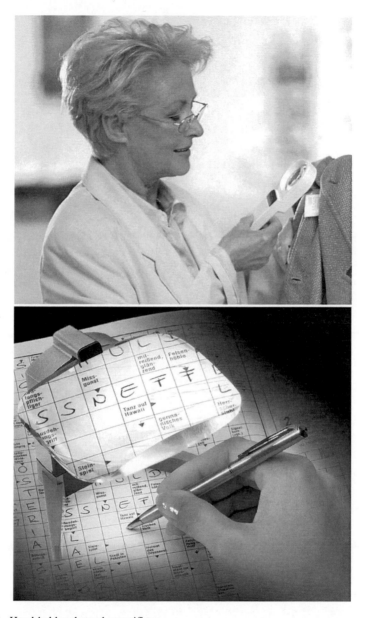

Fig. 13.1 Hand-held and stand magnifiers.

remote controls, extra-large calendars, large-print books, watches with magnifying lenses, and liquid-level indicators are among the many items that can be purchased. As more people acquire vision impairments, Internet resources for online shopping have become more sophisticated and accessible to the low-vision community. OT practitioners should strive to stay up-to-date on these resources so that they can teach clients how to navigate through them and make needed viewing adjustments.

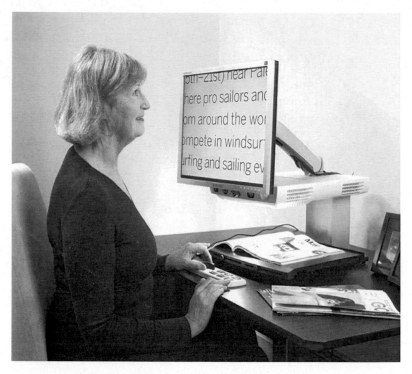

Fig. 13.2 Closed-circuit television.

Some online Web sites offer opportunities for contacting vendors and for consumers to receive electronic alerts when new equipment becomes available. OTs knowledgeable about such features will be more helpful to their clients.

How Low-Vision Rehabilitation Enables Independence

Low vision creates major disruptions in family life, employment, and social interaction, and often leads to functional dependence and depression (Horowitz and Reinhardt, 1998). While assistive technology improves function and decreases problems with mood and depression (Raasch et al., 1997), older adults unfamiliar with the devices and how to acquire them may experience difficulty in deciding about their initial and ongoing use.

Obstacles to the Use of Assistive Technology

Cost has been identified as the primary barrier to acquiring all assistive technology, including low-vision devices (LaPlante et al., 1992). Limited knowledge of the

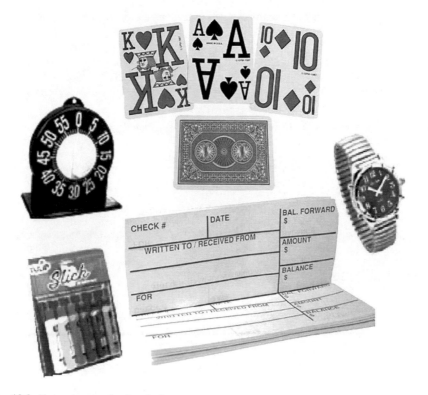

Fig. 13.3 Examples on adaptive devices.

varieties and types of device available also contributes substantially to either never acquiring devices or delaying acquisition (Leonard, 2002; Mann et al., 1993). Once solutions to these barriers are found, older adults face other concerns in the process of making decisions. For example, with self-images altered from disability, older adults often ask how assistive devices might change others' perceptions of them and their own sense of roles, responsibilities, and status in their families and communities (Copolillo, 2001; Gitlin et al., 1998).

Questions about one's capability of using a device arise, and older adults react to them by examining whether they are young and healthy enough to manage, sometimes concluding they are too old and too sick (D'Allura et al., 1995). Older adults' perceptions that device use is not yet warranted can also delay the decision to search for, acquire, and integrate a device (Copolillo, 2001). Some studies indicate that stigma and a potential for marginalization are considered when deciding when and under what circumstances to use devices (Copolillo, 2001; Fine and Asch, 1988; Mann and Tomita, 1998; Zola, 1985).

In addition to the negative attitudes toward low-vision devices, other problems that may affect device use include increased dissatisfaction with the devices as vision worsens (Mann et al., 1993), and quality and quantity of training in their use.

Poor ability to transfer what has been learned in a training environment to the
community can also hamper ongoing device use (D'Allura et al., 1995).

References

American Foundation for the Blind. (1999). National Aging and Vision Network Work Group,
March 6–7, 1999, report from the Josephine L. Taylor Leadership Institute: Chapter 2,
Advocacy Efforts. http://www.afb.org/section.asp?Documentid = 609.
Berg, C.A., Strough, J., Calderone, K.S., Sansone, C., and Weir, C. (1998). The role of problem
definitions in understanding age and context effects on strategies for solving everyday problems.
Psychology and Aging, 13(1), 29–44.
Brody, B.L., Roch-Levecq, A.C., Gamst, A.C., Maclean, K., Kaplan, R.M., and Brown, S.I.
(2002). Self-management of age-related macular degeneration and quality of life: a rand-
omized controlled trial. *Archives of Ophthalmology*, 120(11), 1477–1483.
Brody, B.L., Roch-Levecq, A.C., Thomas, R.G., Kaplan, R.M., and Brown, S.I. (2005). Self-
management of age-related macular degeneration at the 6-month follow-up: A randomized
controlled trial. *Arch Ophthalmol*, 123 (1), 46–53.
Centers for Disease Control and Prevention. (2004). Prevalence of visual impairment and selected
eye diseases among persons aged >50 years with and without diabetes—United States, 2002.
MMWR (Morbidity and Mortality Weekly Report), 53(45), 1069–1071.
Copolillo, A., and Teitelman, J.L. (2005). Acquisition and integration of low vision assistive
devices: understanding the decision-making process of older adults with low vision. *Am J
Occup Ther*, 59(3), 305–313.
Copolillo, A., Warren, M., and Teitelman, J.L. (2007). Results from a survey of occupational
therapy practitioners in low vision rehabilitation. *Occup Ther Health Care*, 21(4), 19–37.
Copolillo, A.E. (2001). Use of mobility devices: the decision-making process of nine African-
American older adults. *Occup Ther J Res*, 21(3), 185–200.
Crews, J.E. (2000). Patterns of activity limitation among older people who experience vision
impairment. In: Stuen, C., Arditi, A., Horowitz, A., Lang, M.A., Rosenthal, B., and Seidman,
K.R., eds. Vision Rehabilitation: Assessment, Intervention and Outcomes (pp. 754–757).
Exton, PA: Swets and Zeitinger.
D'Allura, T., McInerney, R., and Horowitz, A. (1995). An evaluation of low vision services. *J Vis
Impair Blindness*, 89(6), 487–493.
Fine, S.M., and Asch, A. (1988). Disability beyond stigma: social interaction, discrimination, and
activism. *J Social Issues*, 44, 3–21.
Gitlin, L.N., Luborsky, M.R., and Schemm, R.L. (1998). Emerging concerns of older stroke
patients about assistive device use. *Gerontologist*, 38, 169–180.
Horowitz, A., and Reinhardt, J.P. (1998). Development of the adaptation to age-related vision loss
scale. *J Vis Impair Blindness*, 92(1), 30–41.
Ivanoff, S.D., Sonn, U., and Svensson, E. (2002). A health education program for elderly persons
with visual impairments and perceived security in the performance of daily occupations: A
randomized study. *Am J Occup Ther*, 56, 322–330.
LaPlante, M.P., Hendershot, G.E., and Moss, A.J. (1992). Assistive Technology Devices and
Home Accessibility Features: Prevalence, Payment, Need, and Trends. Advance Data from
Vital and Health Statistics; No. 217. Hyattsville, MD: National Center for Health Statistics.
Leonard, R. (2002). Statistics on Vision Impairment: A Resource Manual, 5th ed. New York:
Arlene R. Gordon Research Institute of Lighthouse International.
Mann, W.C., Hurren, D., Karuza, J., and Bentley, D.W. (1993). Needs of home-based older visu-
ally impaired persons for assistive devices. *J Vis Impair Blindness*, 87, 106–110.
Mann, W.C., and Tomita, M. (1998). Perspectives on assistive devices among elderly persons with
disabilities. *Technol Disabil*, 8, 119–148.

Raasch, T.W., Leat, S.J., Kleinstein, R.N., Bullimore, M.A., and Cutter, G.R. (1997). Evaluating the value of low-vision services. *J Am Optom Assoc*, 68 (5), 287–295.

Resnikoff, S., Pascolini, D., Etya'ale, D., et al. (2004). Global data on visual impairment in the year 2002. *Bull WHO*, 82(11), 844–851.

Relton, J. Policy Issues. (2005). The Assistive Technology Act of 2004. AFB ACCESSWORLD ®. Technology and People Who Are Blind or Visually Impaired. (6)1. http://www.afb.org/afbpress/pub.asp?DocID=aw060109.

Warren, M. (1995). Providing low vision rehabilitation services with occupational therapy and ophthalmology. *Am J Occup Ther*, 49, 877–883.

Warren, M., Bettenhausen, D., Kaldenberg, J.M., Sokol-McKay, D.A., and Weisser-Pike, O.M. (2006). Low-vision rehabilitation: A reflection on specialized practice. *OT Pract*, 11(5), 19–23.

Yates, J.F., and Patalano, A.L. (1999). Decision making and aging. In: Park, D.C., Morrell, R.W., and Shifren, K., eds. Processing of Medical Information in Aging Patients: Cognitive and Human Factors Perspectives (pp. 31–54). Mahwah, NJ: Lawrence Erlbaum.

Zola, I.K. (1985). Depictions of disability—metaphor, message, and medium in the media: a research and political agenda. *Soc Sci J*, 22(4), 5–17.

Chapter 14
Universal Design: Principles and Practice for People with Disabilities

Nancy Rickerson

Application of universal design principles improves environmental access for people with disabilities.

Abstract People with disabilities are dependent on or function best with adaptations to environments, which enable them to function optimally and perform daily activities. However, many of these adaptations would not be necessary if universal design was applied to environments as a standard. Outlined in seven principles, universal design may be applied to environments to improve everyday functioning. In so doing, universal design improves access for people with and without disabilities (Bowe, 2000; Burgstahler, 2001; McGuire et al., 2001).

Examples for application of universal design in occupational therapy environments and sessions are described. These principles may be used to maximize client access and intervention outcomes. Applications of universal design principles are consistent with occupational therapy values and assists OTs in meeting the therapeutic needs and potential of all our clients regardless of their disabilities or learning differences (Bowe, 2000; Burgstahler, 2001).

Keywords Access • Adaptation • Occupation • Universal design • Usability.

Definitions

Universal design is "the design of products and environments to be usable by all people, to the greatest extent possible, without the need for adaptation or specialized design" (North Carolina State University, the Center for Universal Design, 2008).

Occupation is any purposeful, meaningful, and productive activity that is occupying people's time. This means that whether a person is grocery shopping, working at a computer, or gardening, each is engaged in occupation (Christiansen and Baum, 1997). Such occupation may be functionally enhanced with the use of universal design.

I. Söderback (ed.), *International Handbook of Occupational Therapy Interventions*,
DOI: 10.1007/978-0-387-75424-6_14, © Springer Science+Business Media, LLC 2010

Background

People with disabilities are dependent on or function best with adaptations to environments, which enable them to function optimally and perform daily activities. However, many of these adaptations would not be necessary if universal design was applied to environments as a standard.

Universal design embodies multiple means of improving every day functioning. In so doing, universal design improves access for people with and without disabilities (Bowe, 2000; Burgstahler, 2001; McGuire et al., 2001).

For example, people using wheelchairs, as well as these carrying packages and pushing shopping carts, appreciate automatic doors. In addition, curb cuts, ramps, lights on movement sensors, and adjustable tables and chairs provide maximum access and usability to all people depending on their situation and need. Products of universal design have improved access for people with a wide range of disabilities (Burgstahler, 2001; McGuire et al., 2001).

Application of the principles of universal design are consistent with occupational therapy values of client-centered care, the concepts of which include provision of flexible approaches, person-centered service and communication, and encouragement of active involvement in tasks in relationship to personal and environmental needs (Law et al., 2002).

While concepts of universal design are familiar to occupational therapists (OTs), universal design is too seldom incorporated in the occupational therapy interventions regarding assessment and planning of environmental adaptations. Therefore, when applied to occupational therapy intervention as standard, clients may need fewer specific adaptations.

Purpose

The purpose is to improve the understanding of (1) the principles of universal design by OTs, (2) how these principles may be applied in occupational therapy interventions aimed at enhancing disabled people's usability of their surrounding environments.

Results

The Role of the Occupational Therapist

The occupational therapist's ultimate role is to assist disabled people in achieving the optimal level of occupational functional performance in self-care, work, and leisure activities. Clinical applications of universal design require the OT's understanding of (1) the seven universal design principles; (2) their advantages for clinical use; and (3) how they should be applied in order to structure the clients' intervention sessions, and to enhance functional advantage through use of additional and specific accommodations among people with disabilities.

Clinical Application

There are seven universal design principles that, when applied, reduce the client's physical, sensory, and cognitive barriers that are imposed on the therapeutic environment. Specifically, interventions are provided in environments and methods that adapt for physical, sensory, and cognitive impairments for the vast majority of clients; thus, the need for specific accommodations for the client may be reduced.

The seven principles guiding the design of the client's environmental structures are as follows:

Equitable Use

Equitable use means that the "design is useful and marketable to people with diverse abilities" (North Carolina State University, the Center for Universal Design, 2008). This requires that the design provides equality, privacy, security, and safety; avoids segregating or stigmatizing; and is appealing and available to all users.

Applying the principle of equitable use in occupational therapy intervention environments is easily accomplished when considering the environment and provision of information through means that will meet the needs of the majority of individuals, irrespective of their disability. For example, intervention environments in wheelchair-accessible private rooms provide ample private physical space with soundproofing to allow for cognitive focus in a quiet, nondistracting environment for an individual with a traumatic brain injury who may have both physical and cognitive impairments. In a different intervention session, a nondistracting intervention-friendly environment with enough physical space allows for a person who transports himself in a wheelchair and also needs portable oxygen apparatus to perform activities of daily living (ADLs) or to learn energy conservation.

Flexibility in Use

Flexibility in use means that the "design accommodates a wide range of individual preferences and abilities" (North Carolina State University, the Center for Universal Design, 2008). The design requires that the users be free to make their choice in the performance method that is most appropriate for their functioning. The design should facilitate accuracy and precision, accommodate to right- or left-handed access and use, and be possible to adapt to the user's pace.

The flexibility principle may be applied; thus, the OTs use pictorial instructions for home exercise and energy conservation programs instead of written ones.

This is suitable, for example, to clients suffering from a decreased ability to understand spoken language. Here, multiple sensorial modes of presentation serve to enhance the learning process by providing information understandable to all individuals regardless of their learning style. Another example of flexibility design is the use of a pair of scissors, which is designed for use with either hand.

Simple and Intuitive Use

Simple and intuitive use is the "the design that is easy to understand, regardless of the user's experience, knowledge, language skills, or current concentration level" (Canadian Association of Occupational Therapists, 1990). The design should not be complex, and should give prompting and feedback during use of the object. The instructions for use should be stated in various ways in a wide range of languages, and should meet the users' expectations and intuition (North Carolina State University, the Center for Universal Design, 2008).

Application of the simple and intuitive principle means that standard and familiar structures and formats should be used. Equipment should be straightforward to use and understand. For instance, microwaves placed in the kitchen of the occupational therapy department should require a simple two-step standard operation. Use of equipment is verbally described by therapists and additionally displayed in large, bold, clear print and demonstrated with pictures. The key is to be intuitive and usable for the majority of individuals using the object or equipment.

Perceptible Information

Perceptible information is the design that "communicates necessary information effectively to the user, regardless of ambient conditions or the user's sensory abilities" (North Carolina State University, the Center for Universal Design, 2008).

Perceptible information should be usable by people with sensory limitations. Ensuring perceptible information during instruction means that information is provided in a variety of modes (pictorial, verbal, tactile) to address varied sensory abilities. For example, visual information is provided through a variety of means, such as written handouts with pictorials or on screens where the letter font is easily increased. The design should allow legibility of essential information; that is, a great contrast between the information and the surroundings is required. Auditory information is provided through auditory sources such as oral explanation, or audiotape, or CD to allow for repetition of information. Kinesthetic information is provided through compatibility with a variety of techniques or devices such as experiential exercise or by hands-on guidance. The aim is to guide the client to use the correct technique and improve motor memory learning for performing various activities. Providing perceptible information in a variety of formats ensures the highest level of comprehension and learning for all individuals regardless of ability or disability.

Tolerance for Error

"The design minimizes hazards and the adverse consequences of accidental or unintended actions" (North Carolina State University, the Center for Universal Design, 2008). It is required that the elements of objects are safely designed so that there are warnings for minimizing hazards and errors.

The most clear-cut example of applying this principle in occupational therapy interventions is the OTs' tolerance for human variance and mistakes. Far too often OTs claim that clients "fail to comply" with exercise programs or with activities of daily living (ADL) intervention expectations, but they do not consider clients' personal factors or life events. Being tolerant of errors indicates that OTs allow for and understand human variance in cognitive ability, learning style, and the interference of other life factors when clients are learning programs and new routines. The need for and practice of nonjudgmental repetition and retraining is understood and expected in standard procedures. When educating clients, applying the principle of tolerance of error entails asking: "Where did the training fail?" This approach examines the effectiveness of our interventions and allows for client variation in understanding and response, rather than to assume that the client merely failed.

Low Physical Effort

Low physical effort means the "design can be used efficiently and comfortably and with a minimum of fatigue" (North Carolina State University, the Center for Universal Design, 2008). This implies that the design should minimize sustained physical effort and use minimal operating forces, and the performances should be done in a neutral position.

Application of this principle of universal design requires that no excessive energy output be required. Energy conservation techniques are accessible by all. For example, an automatic door entry to the clinic allows for wheelchair, walker, and cane users to access it with little effort. In addition, the clinic space is fully accessible by wheelchair and has both wide aisles and linoleum for ease of mobility.

Size and Space for Approach and Use

A size and space suitable for approach and use means that the "appropriate size and space is provided for approach, reach, manipulation, and use regardless of the user's size, posture, or mobility" (North Carolina State University, the Center for Universal Design, 2008).

Using this principle requires that the objects used for standing and seating allow a clear line of sight and ability to reach other components. The design should accommodate variations in hand and grip size and the environmental space for the use of assistive devices, or personal assistance should be enough.

Universal design requires that clinic spaces be of appropriate size for access. Tables, computer stations, and chairs should be adjustable in height to allow ease of use. Equipment is likewise placed on adjustable-height tables for ease of use by all.

Intervention and mat tables are electronically adjustable for ease of use by staff with a variety of client physical needs. Environmental considerations include, yet are not limited to, adequate space allotted for wheelchair mobility and positioning of objects (e.g., phones, desks, tables, equipment, and supplies) in the physical environment to facilitate access. In addition, items on shelves are placed in easy reach from a seated or wheelchair position. Workstations are ergonomically designed with adjustable chairs, tables, keyboard trays, and monitor stands.

Benefits of Universal Design

Use of universal design has many advantages. It requires less specific adaptation for individuals with disabilities. Individuals with *orthopedic or neurologic impairments* who use wheelchairs find structures and equipment in proximity and easy to use. Individuals with *low vision* are able to perceive information within their functional range of sight when large print and high contrast in written materials are provided as standard practice. Individuals with *impaired hearing* are able to better hear and understand therapist's instructions when distracting background noise is eliminated. Individuals with *cognitive deficits* learn more readily when repetition and multisensory information is routinely provided. In addition to these functional benefits, additional accommodations for individuals may be avoided, thus providing a cost savings for therapy departments. For instance, ergonomic workstations decrease repetitive work injuries and the need for specific environmental adaptations per individual.

Accommodations in Addition to Universal Design

Despite the many advantages of the application of universal design principles, some individuals with disabilities will still require accommodations. Examples are (1) a deaf client who needs a sign language interpreter, (2) a client who is an upper extremity amputee and needs a one-handed keyboard, and (3) a blind client who needs a Braille system for written communication.

Discussion

The advantage of universal design is that it enables client function and therapeutic benefit regardless of ability, thus decreasing the need for specific accommodations. Universal design reflects OTs' ethical values of regarding each person as unique and worthy of individual experiences within the larger societal spectrum, and assists in meeting the therapeutic needs and potential of all clients regardless of their disabilities or learning differences (Bowe, 2000; Burgstahler, 2001).

Application of the seven principles of universal design in occupational therapy adaptive interventions holds the potential of being an effective method of ensuring that all clients have full access to the interventions without disadvantage. Research is needed to both quantitatively and qualitatively determine specific benefits of universal design for clients with a variety of disabilities, and in a variety of therapeutic settings.

References

Bowe, F.G. (2000). Universal Design in Education. Westport, CT: Bergin and Garvey.
Burgstahler, S. (2001). Universal Design of Instruction. Seattle: DO-IT, University of Washington.
Canadian Association of Occupational Therapists. (1990). Position paper on the role of occupational therapy in adult physical dysfunction. Can J Occup Ther, 57(5), suppl 1–8.
Christiansen, C., and Baum, C., eds. (1997). Person-environment occupational performance. A conceptual model for practice. In: Occupational Therapy. Enabling Function and Well-Being, 2nd ed. Thorofare, NJ: Slack.
Law, M., Gaum, C.M., and Baptiste (2002). Occupation-Based Practice: Fostering Performance and Participation. Thorofare, NJ: Slack.
McGuire, J., Scott, S., and Shaw (2001). Principles of Universal Design for Instruction. Storrs, CT: Center on Postsecondary Education and Disability.
North Carolina State University, the Center for Universal Design D-492, 2008. The Principles of Universal Design. http://www.design.ncsu.edu/cud/about_ud/udprinciples.htm.

Chapter 15
The Design of Artisans' Hand Tools: Users' Perceived Comfort and Discomfort

Lottie F.M. Kuijt-Evers

Using the new masonry trowel, the bricklayer was not suffering from pain anymore during his work.

Abstract Is artisans' comfort in using hand tools a necessity or a luxury? Ergonomically well-designed hand tools, which provide comfort to the user, decrease the risk of occupational health problems and increase the job performance. Therefore, it is not a luxury, but rather a necessity that hand tools be designed with a focus on comfort, and that artisans make themselves informed about the use of ergonomically well-designed hand tools.

Keywords Artisans • Comfort • Complaints • Discomfort • Hand tools • Performance

Background

A hand tool is a device for doing a particular job. It can be freely manipulated and is held by a person. Hand tools, such as hammers, pliers, scalpels, and knives, are used very frequently by many people in daily life and in their work.

The use of hand tools is very often accompanied by discomfort. Feelings of discomfort can reduce job satisfaction and cause musculoskeletal problems in the long term. Therefore, it is important that people work with well-designed hand tools. Occupational therapists (OTs) and ergonomics consultants should be able to recognize well-designed hand tools in order to advise their clients.

Method

Candidates for the Intervention

Candidates for interventions are professional groups that work with hand tools for long periods of time during the day, such as surgeons, carpenters, assembly workers, hairdressers, cooks, and gardeners.

I. Söderback (ed.), *International Handbook of Occupational Therapy Interventions*,
DOI: 10.1007/978-0-387-75424-6_15, © Springer Science+Business Media, LLC 2010

Epidemiology

Although the relationship between hand tool design and musculoskeletal disorders was directly obtained from the study of Tichauer (1978, cited in Chaffin et al. (1999), other studies have indicated poor hand tool design as a risk factor of musculoskeletal disorders (Chaffin et al., 1999; Mital and Kilbom, 1992). Moreover, some studies show that less discomfort was experienced by using appropriately designed hand tools (Chang et al., 1999; Dempsey et al., 2002; Kilbom et al., 1993). This is important, as discomfort can lead to musculoskeletal problems in the long term (Hamberg-van Reenen et al., 2008).

Risk Factors for Occupational Hand and Arm Injuries

Besides the risk on injuries due to accidents, other risk factors can cause discomfort and physical complaints:

* Awkward postures and movements of hands, wrists, and arms
* High-force exertions (working with the tool on material) or low static force supply (holding a tool above shoulder height)
* Highly repetitive movements or force exertions
* High precision requirements (e.g., use of dental instruments)
* Vibrations and high impact
* Local friction or pressure on the skin of the hand

The risk of physical complaints increases the more times a day workers are exposed to the physical load and as the frequency of use rises. Appropriate hand tool design can contribute to a reduction of the risk factors such as awkward postures or high-force exertions. However, the tasks that have to be performed and the context in which a hand tool is used also affect the way it is used, the risk of physical complaints, and the feelings of discomfort and comfort. For example, in pruning a grapevine using pruning shears, the shears can be very well designed, but the wrist position and body posture are mostly determined by the direction and the height of the branches that have to be cut.

Results

Hand Tool Evaluation Studies

Studies in a laboratory setting as well is in the field are conducted in order to compare different kinds of hand tools with the risk factors for musculoskeletal disorders. Objective as well as subjective measurements are used to determine the risk factors of using hand tools.

Objective measurements are used to measure body postures, force exertion, and pressure on the hand. Several objective measurements can be used:

- Awkward postures and movements of wrist and forearm can be measured by (electro-)goniometrics (Fig. 15.1).
- Force exertion can be measured directly:
    - In the hand–tool interface by a glove with force sensors
    - By built-in force sensors in the handgrip (McGorry, 2001).
- Force exertion can be measured indirectly:
    - Measuring the external reaction forces on the tool and calculating the wrist load moment value
    - Measuring electromyography (EMG) especially during static force exertions (Fig. 15.2) (Hoozemans and van Dieën, 2003).
- Pressure distribution on the hand surface can be recorded using a hand mat with pressure sensors (Fig. 15.3).

Subjective measurements (e.g., questionnaires) are valuable in measuring discomfort or comfort in using hand tools. The most common subjective method to assess

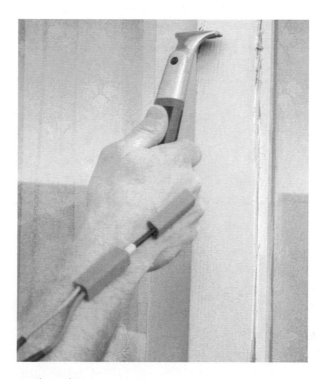

Fig. 15.1 Electrogoniometrics.

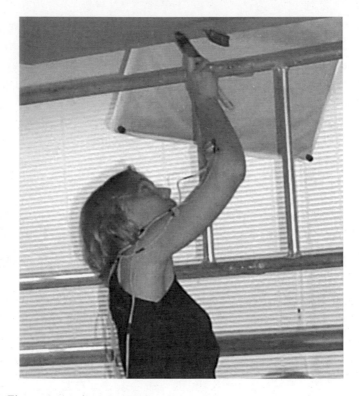

Fig. 15.2 Electromyograph measurements.

discomfort is using a body map or a detailed hand map (Fig. 15.4) (Corlett and Bishop, 1976). For each region, the feelings of discomfort are rated on a scale from no discomfort to extreme discomfort.

The workers' perception of comfort in using hand tools is assessed with the Comfort Questionnaire for Hand Tools (CQH) (Kuijt-Evers et al., 2007). This questionnaire uses phrases, such as "fits the hand," "causes pressure," "nice-feeling handgrip") that describe the needs of artisans regarding comfort in using hand tools. The CQH can be used for several purposes:

• Investigate the most important comfort aspects for a specific type of hand tool
• Find starting points for hand tool design improvement
• Compare the comfort of different kinds of the same type of hand tool

Clinical Application

Hand tool evaluations and design studies lead to design guidelines. Some general guidelines for hand tool design are as follows:

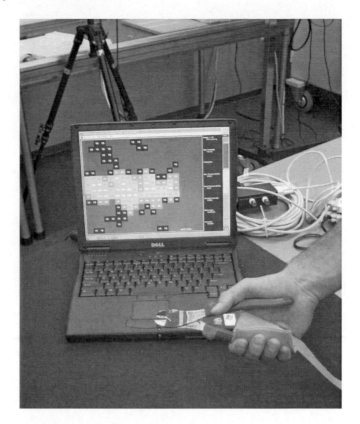

Fig. 15.3 Pressure distribution measurement.

Criteria for Optimal Design of Hand Tools

Handgrip Length

The optimum handgrip length depends of the type of grip that is used. When a power grip is used (such as for a masonry trowel), the handgrip length should be longer than the size of the user's hand to avoid points of excessive pressure on the palm (Aptel et al., 2002). To arrive at this dimension, the handbreadth at the metacarpal phalange is often used (Das et al., 2005). In the literature, lengths of 110 to 135 mm are recommended depending on the population and glove use.

Handgrip Diameter

In the literature, different handgrip diameters for use in a power grip are recommended, ranging from 30 to 50 mm. From an ergonomics viewpoint, it is apparent that one size of handgrip will not accommodate or satisfy the entire working population, male and female. Therefore, ergonomists recommend small, medium, and

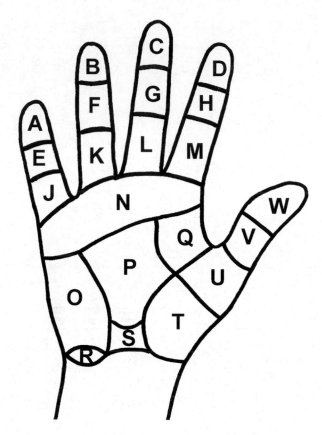

Fig. 15.4 Hand map. Drawing by L.F.M. Kuijt-Evers. Published in Kuijt-Evers L,F,M., Comfort in Using Hand Tools; Theory, Design and Evaluation. 2006. TNO Kwaliteit van Leven, Hoofddorp, proefschrift. Published with permission.

large handgrip diameters of 30, 35, and 40 mm, respectively (Das et al. 2005; Kuijt-Evers and Eikhout, 2006).

Handgrip Shape

The dimensions of the handgrip cross section should vary over the length of the handgrip, as this (1) reduces the movement of the tool forward and backward, (2) accommodates the shape of the hand, (3) permits greater force to be exerted along the tool axis due to a better bearing surface, and (4) acts as a shield if placed at the front (Konz, 1995).

A rectangular or an oval cross section allows tactile orientation of the tool. However, if the handgrip is used in different orientations (e.g., it is rotated in the hand during use), a circular cross section is preferred, to avoid pressure on the hands.

Furthermore, the handgrip should have a smooth surface, without (sharp) edges or finger holes. The connection between two parts (e.g., soft and hard material) should be smooth, as should the shape of the handgrip.

Handgrip Material

The handgrip material is important in regard to surface friction properties and the ability to grasp and manipulate the tool. Frictional characteristics vary with the pressure exerted by the hand, the smoothness and porosity of the surface, and the type of contamination (sweat increases the coefficient of friction, and oil reduces it) (Bobjer et al., 1993; Bucholz et al., 1988).

Rubber, compressible plastic, or wood are better handgrip materials than are hard plastic or metal. Compressive materials tend to dampen vibration and allow better distribution of pressure, reducing feelings of fatigue and hand tenderness (Fellows and Freivalds, 1991).

Balance and Mass of the Tool

The tool weight should be balanced around the grip axis to minimize the wrist load moment value. The maximal acceptable mass of the tool depends on the task, the direction of force exertion, the frequency of use, and the total task duration during a day. Sometimes the mass of a tool supports the task, as the gravity force is in the same direction as the force exertion of the user, such as drilling a hole in vertical direction or using a circular saw. In other situations, the optimal tool weight is about 1 kg with a maximum of 1.5 kg for one-hand use. When tools are used with two hands, the maximum recommended weight is 3 kg.

Work Side of the Tool

The work side of the tool (e.g., the blade of the saw) is especially important. It determines the functionality of the tool. A study on handsaws showed that if the functionality of the handsaw is lacking (due to a blunt saw blade or a too flexible blade), the performance is reduced 50%, the carpenters works less accurately, and the discomfort level increases.

Users' Perceived Comfort of Using Hand Tools

As comfort is a personal experience and a reaction to the environment, a product can never be comfortable in and of itself. It becomes comfortable (or not) in its use (Vink et al., 2005). Comfort is affected by the interaction between the user, the hand tool, and the task in an environment. Figure 15.5 illustrates these interactions.

Tool–Task Interaction

The primary goal of using a hand tool is to perform a task, for example, to cut a wooden beam or to fix elements together. The interaction between the task and the

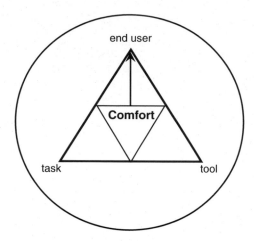

Fig. 15.5 Illustration of the interactions between the user, the hand tool, and the task, as illustrated by the triangle within the environment (illustrated by the large circle). Drawing by L.F.M. Kuijt-Evers. Publiced: Kuijt-Evers, L.F.M. Comfort in Using Hand Tools; Theory, Design and Evaluation. 2006. TNO Kwaliteit van Leven, Hoofddorp, proefschrift. Published with permission.

hand tool is mostly determined by the work side of the tool. This part of the tool is also the part that is very important for the functionality of the tool. If the end-user cannot fulfill the task in an appropriate way, due to the hand tool, then the hand tool can never be comfortable to work with. The functionality of the tool is one of the most important factors in comfort in using hand tools. It is the basis of good hand tool design and an integral part of the task–tool–user triad.

Interaction Between User and Tool

The physical interaction between the hand tool and the hand, along with functionality, is the most important predictor of comfort in using hand tools. For designers, it is important to know how the physical interaction can be optimized by proper handgrip design, and it is important for OTs to recognize good or bad handgrip designs. Adverse body effects (or the absence of adverse body effects) are the second important predictor of comfort in using hand tools, which include numbness and lack of tactile feeling in the hand, inflamed skin of the hand, and pressure on the hand.

Interaction Between User and Task

The way in which the hand-tool user performs his task is related to his experience. There are differences in comfort experience between professionals and layman. This may be explained by the fact that professionals very often have preferences for a particular type of tool and have better physical capabilities to perform the job. Feelings of discomfort will be less if the user is better trained for the job.

Hand Tool–Specific Comfort Factors

We described how the interaction among the tool, the task, and the user in the environment affects the feeling of comfort. To optimize comfort, one should know the factors that determine comfort in using hand tools. These factors include the task intensity (movement frequency and force exertion) and the force direction (perpendicular or parallel to the handgrip surface) (Kuijt-Evers et al., 2007). The flow chart in Fig. 15.6 shows which aspects should be taken into account, depending on the task characteristics.

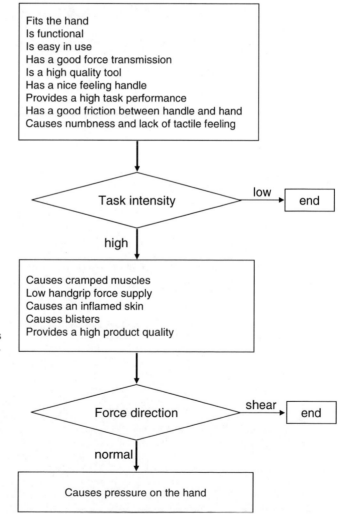

Fig. 15.6 Flow chart to support designers and researchers to focus on the appropriate comfort descriptors in hand tool design. Drawing by L.F.M. Kuijt-Evers. Publiced: Kuijt-Evers, L.F.M. Comfort in Using Hand Tools; Theory, Design and Evaluation. 2006. TNO Kwaliteit van Leven, Hoofddorp, proefschrift. Published with permission.

To recap, the main factors related to comfort in using hand tools are the functionality of the tool, the physical interaction with the tool, and the adverse body effects (on the skin and on soft tissues). The importance of the comfort factors differs among different kinds of hand tools (as shown by the flow chart) (Fig. 15.6).

Discussion

For OTs, it is important to recommend to their clients well-designed tools that avoid discomfort, as discomfort can lead to musculoskeletal disorders in the long term. Furthermore, the occurrence of discomfort can result in productivity loss and days on sick leave. On the other hand, a well-designed hand tool in itself cannot prevent discomfort (or provide comfort). The feelings of comfort and discomfort and the physical load also depend on the task that is performed, the capacities of the user, and the environment in which the task is performed. Therefore, it is not sufficient to look at the tool out of context; rather, all tool–task–user interactions in the working environment should always be taken into account.

References

Aptel, M., Claudon, L., and Marsot, J. (2002). Integration of ergonomics into hand tool design: principle and presentation of an example. Int J Occup Safety Ergonom, 8, 107–115.
Bobjer, O., Johansson, S.E., and Piguet, S. (1993). Friction between hand and handle: effects of oil and lard on textured and non-textured surfaces. Appl Ergonom, 24, 190–202.
Bucholz, B., Frederick, L.J., and Armstrong, T.J. (1988). An investigation of human palmer skin friction and the effects of materials, pinch force and moisture. Ergonomics, 31, 317–325.
Chaffin, D.B., Andersson, G.B., and Martin, J.M. (1999). Occupational Biomechanics. New York: Wiley.
Chang, S.R., Park, S., and Freivalds, A. (1999). Ergonomic evaluation of the effects of handle types on garden tools. Int J Ind Ergonom, 24, 99–105.
Corlett, E.N., and Bishop, R.P. (1976). A technique for assessing postural discomfort. Ergonomics, 19, 175–182.
Das, B., Jongkol, P., and Ngui, S. (2005). Snap-on-handles for a non-powered hacksaw: an ergonomics evaluation, redesign and testing. Ergonomics, 48, 78–97.
Dempsey, P.G., McGorry, R.W., Leamon, T.B., and O'Brien, N.V. (2002). Bending the tool and the effect on human performance: further investigation of a simulated wire-twisting task. AIHA J, 63, 586–593.
Fellows, G.L., and Freivalds, A. (1991). Ergonomics evaluation of a foam rubber grip for tool handles. Appl Ergonom, 22, 225–230.
Hamberg-van Reenen, H.H., van der Beek, A.J., Blatter, B.M., van der Grinten, M.P., Mechelen, W., and Bongers, P.M. (2008). Does musculoskeletal discomfort at work predict future musculoskeletal pain? Ergonomics, 51, 637–648.
Hoozemans, J.M., and van Dieën, J.H. (2003). Prediction of handgrip forces using surface EMG of forearm muscles. J Electromyogr Kinesiol, 15, 358–366.
Kilbom, Å., Mäkäräinen, M., Sperling, L., Kadefors, R., and Liedberg, L. (1993). Tool design, user characteristics and performance: a case study on plate-shears. Appl Ergonom, 24, 221–230.

Konz, S. (1995). Work Design: Industrial Ergonomics, 4th ed. Arizona: Publishing Horizons.

Kuijt-Evers, L.F.M., and Eikhout, S.M. (2006). Development process of a new masoner's trowel. In: Pikaar,R.N.,Koningsveld, E.A.P., Settels, P.J.M., eds. Meeting Diversity in Ergonomics: Proceedings IEA2006 Congress. Oxford: Elsevier, CD-ROM: art0571.

Kuijt-Evers, L.F.M., Groenesteijn, L., de Looze, M.P., and Vink, P. (2004). Identifying factors of comfort in using hand tools. Appl Ergonom, 35, 453–458.

Kuijt-Evers, L.F.M., Vink, P., and de Looze, M.P. (2007). Comfort predictors for different kinds of hand tools: Differences and similarities. Int J Ind Ergonom, 37, 73–84.

McGorry, R.W. (2001). A system for measurement of grip forces and applied moments during hand tool use. Appl Ergonom, 32, 271–280.

Mital, A., and Kilbom, Å. (1992). Design, selection and use of hand tools to alleviate trauma of the upper extremities. II. The scientific basis (knowledge base) for the guide. Int J Ind Ergonom, 10, 7–21.

Vink, P., Overbeeke, C.J., and Desmet, P.M.A. (2005). Comfort experience. In: Vink, P., ed. Comfort and Design: Principles and Good Practice. (pp.1–12)Boca Raton, FL: CRC.

Chapter 16
Temporal Adaptation for Individuals Living with Serious Mental Illness in the Community

Terry Krupa, Megan Edgelow, and Debbie Radloff-Gabriel

I found the intervention helpful because it allowed me to monitor my activity, and thus I could see my progress. I am happier being productive and useful; I am proud of my improvements and the better use of my time.

—Client

Abstract This chapter provides a brief description of an intervention designed to address the time use and activity patterns of individuals with serious mental illness, living in the community, with a view to improving their quality of life and promoting recovery through occupation. The intervention uses (1) a client-centered practice approach, (2) evidence-based behavioral activation, and (3) education techniques to effect change. Initial pilot testing of the intervention established its clinical acceptability, relevance, and utility, and suggested positive changes in the amount of time spent in activities other than sleep. More research is needed to determine its effectiveness in influencing other time use patterns.

Keywords Activities of daily living • Mental disorder • Quality of life.

Definitions and Background

Occupational therapy interventions that focus on temporal adaptation address human activity patterns with a view to improving personal health, well-being, and social participation. These interventions are based on the notion that the human impact of social roles and activities cannot be understood separately from the way in which time is allocated to these activities (Bird and Fremont, 1991).

Theoretical perspectives on temporal adaptation explain the complex relationship among human activity patterns, time allocation, and health. These perspectives focus on how time is allocated to self-care, productivity, leisure, and rest, and organized with attention to sleep–wake cycles; the balance of rest with exertion; the balance of free and obligatory activities; social and cultural expectations with regard to activity participation; opportunities for participation in personally and

I. Söderback (ed.), *International Handbook of Occupational Therapy Interventions*,
DOI: 10.1007/978-0-387-75424-6_16, © Springer Science+Business Media, LLC 2010

community valued activities; and the shifts in human activity patterns across the life span (Eklund et al., in press).

A broad range of health and community adjustment outcomes have been associated with temporal adaptation, including improvements in personal satisfaction and a sense of meaning, quality of life, adjustment to illness and disability, maintaining biologic rhythms, and better community integration (Eklund et al., in press). Information about the time use patterns of the general population is derived from studies conducted in several countries, often in the context of a national censuses; this allows for comparisons of activity patterns between populations.

In occupational therapy there has been a particular interest in the time use and activity patterns of people living with disability and other health related circumstances (see, for example, Pentland et al., 1998; Söderback, 1999).

Purpose

The primary purpose of this intervention is to modify daily activity patterns so that individuals will experience improvements in a range of outcomes associated with health, well-being, and community participation. The intervention is developed in the form of a clinician/client workbook titled, *Action Over Inertia: Reconnecting with Activity to Promote Health and Well-Being* (Krupa et al., 2007).

Method

Candidates for the Intervention

The *Action Over Inertia* workbook has been developed for adults with serious mental illness who are living in the community. Specifically it has been designed for those individuals (for example, those with a diagnosis of schizophrenia or major affective disorder) who experience (1) significant occupational disengagement as reflected in a lack of investment in and emotional detachment from activities, and (2) significant occupational alienation reflected in a lack of involvement in activities emerging from forces of social and cultural exclusion or stigma (Krupa et al., in press).

Epidemiology

Serious mental illness includes a group of mental disorders that are characterized by diagnosis (specifically schizophrenia and major affective disorders), significant disability, and long-standing duration (Schinnar et al., 1990). While the prevalence of mental illness in the adult population is quite high, estimated in the range of 10% to 20%, the prevalence of *serious* mental illness is much lower, at about 2% to 5% (U.S. Department of Health and Human Services, 1999; World Health Organization, 2001).

Recent studies have demonstrated that disrupted time use patterns are common among people with serious mental illness. Their activity patterns are characterized by underoccupation, day-night reversal, fewer hours in productivity activities, and an inordinate amount of time spent in passive and isolated activity (Bejerholm and Eklund, 2004; Farnworth, 2003; Krupa et al., 2003; Leufstadius et al., 2006; Minato and Zemke, 2004). The reasons for these activity patterns are complex, but factors include disruptions in the experience of activity associated with impairments of mental illness; very high levels of unemployment and subsequent difficulties organizing the day around productivity; high levels of stigma and discrimination that lead to exclusion from social roles and activities and inequity in access to health and social services; high levels of poverty; and limited experiences and networks connecting people to community roles and activities.

Settings

The *Action Over Inertia* workbook has been designed for use within assertive community mental health outreach services that aim to facilitate the social recovery of individuals with serious mental illness. The relevance of the intervention is determined by individual clients and service providers in a collaborative manner, and is guided by the evaluation of significant disruptions in activity patterns (Tables 16.1 and 16.2).

Table 16.1   Determining relevance of the intervention: activity patterns

The individual may find the intervention beneficial if they meet three or more of the following criteria:	Check √
The person's daily activities demonstrate an imbalance among self-care, productivity, and leisure.	
The person spends a large amount of time without defined activity on a day-to-day basis.	
Much of the individual's day is spent in passive activities or rest.	
There is a lack of organized routine/structure to the person's daily activity.	
The person's daily activities limit his/her contact with others.	
The person's daily activities limit his/her access to a range of community environments.	
The person cannot define activities/occupations that are meaningful or of personal interest.	
The person experiences distress, or is easily overwhelmed in activity.	
The person's involvement in activity is impacted by a limited experience of enjoyment.	

Table 16.2 Determining relevance of the intervention: realizing the benefits of activities

If six or fewer are checked, then this may be a helpful intervention for the individual
Client engages in activities that provide the opportunity for…   √
Skill and/or knowledge development
Making a contribution to society
Gaining physical health benefits
The enjoyment of beautiful things
Self-expression and creativity
A range of social interactions
Meeting personal goals and experiencing accomplishment
Expressing personal values
Earning a personal income
Giving to others, such as family and friends

Result

Clinical Application

- The *Action Over Inertia* workbook is intended to be used in partnership between the occupational therapist (OT) and the client.
- It begins by engaging individuals with serious mental illness, either individually or within a group treatment setting, in *collecting information on their actual time use* over the course of a few typical days. Time logs (Fig. 16.1) are used to keep track of activities engaged in, the location of these activities, social contacts during these activities, and the personal experiences of these activities.
- This is followed by a process of guided reflection on time-use patterns, including time-use dimensions. For example, the therapist and client discuss the time use patterns with respect to balance, level of occupational engagement, passive and active participation, structure and routines, meaningfulness and personal values, satisfaction, social interactions and access to community environments.
- Clients are also provided with *education* about the relationship between serious mental illness, activity involvement, and time use as well as information about the potential health and citizenship benefits of activities.
- The client is then engaged in *structured exercises* of planning for change with regard to *time use* and activity *involvement*. In addition to *long-term activity planning* that directly addresses the supports and resources required to overcome activity challenges, clients are encouraged to identify a few "quick and simple activity fixes" to gain momentum.

My Current Time Use Log _____

Client's name: _____

Therapist's name: _____

Date: _____

In the chart below, fill in how you have recently spent a typical **weekday**.

Time	Activity	Where?	Anyone else present?	How did you experience activity?
7 am				
7:30 am				
8:00 am				
8:30 am				
9.00 am				
9:30 am				

Time log continues for a complete 24 hour cycle

Fig. 16.1 Time use log.

• Finally, changes in activity patterns and actual time use are monitored and plans refined accordingly. The therapist is encouraged to use motivational and teaching techniques to facilitate the client's commitment to the process of change.

The Role of the Occupational Therapist

The intervention is based on an occupational view of health and recovery from serious mental illness and is thus grounded in the domain of occupational therapy. It can be implemented by other members of the health care team, and supported by peer specialists, but it is advised that an OT be involved in overseeing the training, supervision, and evaluation of the intervention within the service.

How the Intervention Eases Impairments, Activity Limitations, and Participation Restrictions

Activity involvement is presented as a public health concern and as an important determinant of health in recovery from serious mental illness. The intervention directly addresses temporal activity patterns as the focus for change. It uses educational and behavioral activation techniques, consistent with evidence-based practices in community mental health and recovery (Cuijpers et al., 2007; Mueser et al., 2003) to empower people with serious mental illness to develop the knowledge and support they need to engage in activity patterns that are personally and socially meaningful and associated with physical and mental health.

Evidence-Based Practice

To date, the evidence for occupational therapy interventions focused on time use and temporal activity patterns in mental health practice has largely been anecdotal (see, for example, Kielhofner et al., 2002). The construction of a psychometrically sound and sensitive measurement of occupational engagement, the Profiles of Occupational Engagement in Persons with Schizophrenia (POES) (Bejerholm et al., 2006) has advanced both clinical applications and research in the area.

The *Action Over Inertia* workbook is new and only now undergoing research. A pilot study, using the randomized controlled trial method, demonstrated a positive change: specifically, the reduction in the amount of time spent sleeping for individuals with serious mental illness who received this intervention over 12 weeks. There was no significant change in other dimensions of time use patterns. Qualitative feedback from OTs and clients indicated that the intervention was considered useful and well structured. The 3-month time frame of the pilot study was considered too brief to lead to major changes in activity patterns (Edgelow, 2008).

Discussion

Occupational therapists may need to advocate for the implementation of this intervention within community-based treatment teams where biomedical treatment, housing support, and crisis management are prioritized. Demonstrating how changes in temporal adaptation are related to community stability and integration for people with mental illness may be an important aspect of these advocacy efforts.

The intervention itself is lengthy, perhaps requiring several months for meaningful change. Of course, this limitation needs to be evaluated with consideration of the likelihood that clients receiving the intervention have experienced a lengthy period of profound occupational alienation and disengagement. While the intervention itself does not evaluate any particular forms of activity, therapists should keep in mind the extent to which involvement in productivity, and specifically education and employment, is considered integral to successful community integration and socioeconomic recovery from mental illness (Waghorn and Lloyd, 2005).

References

Bejerholm, U., and Eklund, M. (2004). Time-use and occupational performance among persons with schizophrenia. Occup Ther Mental Health, 20(1), 27–47.

Bejerholm, U., Hansson, L., and Eklund, M. (2006). Profiles of occupational engagement in people with schizophrenia (POES): the development of a new instrument based on time-use diaries. Br J Occup Ther, 29(2), 58–69.

Bird, C. E., and Fremont, A.M. (1991). Gender, time use and health. J Health Social Behav, 32(2), 114–129.

Cuijpers, P., van Straten, A., and Warmerdam, L. (2007). Behavioral activation treatment of depression: a meta-analysis. Clin Psychol Rev, 27, 318–326.

Edgelow, M. (2008). Effectiveness of an Occupational Therapy Time Use Intervention for People with Serious Mental Illness. Unpublished master's thesis, Queen's University, Kingston, ON.

Eklund, M., Leufstadius, C., and Bejerholm, U. (2009). Time use among people with psychiatric disabilities: implications for practice. Psychiatr Rehabil J. 32(3), 177–191

Farnworth, L. (2003). Time-use, tempo and temporality: Occupational therapy's core business or someone else's business. Aust Occup Ther J, 50, 116–126.

Kielhofner, G., Forsyth, K., Federico, J., et al. (2002). Self-report Assessments. In: Kielhofner, G., ed. Model of Human Occupation, 3rd ed. Baltimore, MD: Lippincott Williams & Wilkins.

Krupa, T., Edgelow, M., Chen, S., et al. (2007). Action Over Inertia: A Focused Intervention for Reconnecting Individuals with Serious Mental Illness with Activity to Promote Health and Well-Being. Kingston, ON: Queen's University.

Krupa, T., Fossey, E., Anthony, W., Brown, T., and Pitts, D. (2009). "Doing daily life" as means to health, personal growth and empowerment: occupational therapy, psychiatric rehabilitation and recovery. Psychiatr Rehabil J. 32(3), 155–161.

Krupa, T., McLean, H., Eastabrook, S., Bonham, A., and Baksh, L. (2003). Daily time use as a measure of community adjustment for persons served by assertive community treatment teams. Am J Occup Ther, 57, 558–565.

Leufstadius, C., Erlandsson, L., and Eklund, M. (2006). Time use and daily activities in people with persistent mental illness. Occup Ther Int, 13(3), 123–141.

Minato, M. and Zemke, R. (2004). Time use of people with schizophrenia living in the community. Occup Ther Int. 11(3), 177–191.

Mueser, K.T., Torrey, W. C., Lynde, D., Singer, P., and Drake, R.E. (2003). Implementing evidence-based practices for people with severe mental illness. Behav Mod, 27(3), 387–411.

Pentland, W., Harvey, A., and Walker, J.T. (1998). The relationship between time use, health and well-being in men with spinal cord injury. J Occup Sci, 5(1), 14–25.

Schinnar, A., Rothbard, A., Kanter, R., and Jung, S. (1990). An empirical literature review of definitions of severe and persistent mental illness. Am J Psychiatry, 147(12), 1602–1608.

Soderback, I. (1999). Validation of the theory: satisfaction with time-delimited daily occupations. Work, 12(2), 165–174.

U.S. Department of Health and Human Services. (1999). Mental Health: A Report of the Surgeon General—Executive Summary. Rockville, MD: U.S. Department of Health and Human Services, Substance Abuse and Mental Health Services Administration. http://www.surgeongeneral. gov/library/mentalhealth/summary.html.

Waghorn, G., and Lloyd, C. (2005). The employment of people with mental illness. Aust J Advancement Mental Health, 4(2), Supplement, 1–19.

World Health Organization (WHO). (2001). Mental Health: New Understanding, New Hope. Geneva: World Health Organization.

Part III
Interventions: The Occupational Therapist Teaches and the Client Learns

Chapter 17
Teaching Interventions: Overview

Ingrid Söderback

Abstract This chapter provides an overview of the chapters of this handbook that exemplify the occupational therapist's role as a teacher of the client. This teaching addresses cognitive, neuromusculoskeletal, and movement-related and sensory functioning plus psychosocial and work-related participation. Natural and intermediary learning are introduced, and the latter is illustrated by the case of Jane. The therapeutic learning process is described. Therapeutic educational theory approaches, such as behavioral and cognitive programs for active learning applied in clinical practice, are summarized. The various teaching facilitators or therapeutic media, such as dialogue techniques, strategies, and mediated learning related to therapeutic teaching, are presented and exemplified with clinical use.

Keywords Cognitive • Movement-related • Neuromusculoskeletal • Participation • Psychosocial • Sensory functioning • Teaching • Teaching facilitators • Traumatic brain injury • Work-related.

Teaching Interventions

Natural Learning

For most people, learning continues throughout their life, and mostly with no involvement of a teacher. Natural learning arises from human beings' biologic instinct: people meet new, unknown, and unpredictable situations and new challenges when performing occupations in their daily life (Schwartz, 1991).

Intermediary Learning

Most people with a permanent disability need intermediary learning with professional teaching that is one of the OTs roles (Fig. 17.1). This kind of educational participation in teaching interventions occurs intermittently during one's lifetime or initially after a disability has arisen.

I. Söderback (ed.), *International Handbook of Occupational Therapy Interventions*,
DOI: 10.1007/978-0-387-75424-6_17, © Springer Science+Business Media, LLC 2010

The occupational therapist

teaches

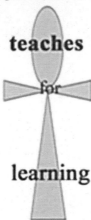

learning

Fig. 17.1 The figure shows the OT's role in teaching the occupational therapy interventions aimed at facilitate the client's learning or relearning of occupational performances of daily living tasks. The figure is a stylized Ankh-sign.

These teaching interventions are symptom-oriented and aim at *maintaining*, *improving,* or *restoring* functioning (i.e., are directed to various body functions and structures) or disabilities (i.e., are directed to impairments, activity limitations, or participation restrictions, according to the International Classification of Functioning Disability and Health [ICF] [World Health Organization, 2008]). Thus, interventions are adapted to match the client's symptoms with the task to be performed.

The diagnoses and disabilities of the clients who may be candidates for symptom-oriented teaching interventions were shown in Table 2.1 in Chapter 2, and are exemplified in the case of Jane (see below). Here the teaching and learning process constitutes a base for the interventions aimed at preventing ill-health and supporting wellness (see Chapter 5).

The Case of Jane

Jane was 54 years old and was divorced several years ago. She was a highly qualified woman in her career, and the mother of four adult children. She lived alone in an apartment. During a day at the beach 3 months ago, together with some women friends, Jane became unconscious and fell flat on her face. She was taken to a neurologic hospital for acute care. Jane underwent surgery for a cerebral hemorrhage caused by an aneurysmal rupture. Jane recovered, and now has no motor impairment, and when talking with her no specific cognitive impairment is obvious. Before discharge from the rehabilitation hospital, Jane was to spend at least two weekends at home to ascertain whether she needed assistance from the community care services.

On a Monday morning on the rehabilitation clinic ward, Jane returned after her first home leave weekend. I was there to investigate another client's need for assistance with eating. I noticed that Jane was eating a huge amount of food, as though she was famished! I realized something must be wrong.

Later that day, Jane came to the training kitchen to take the Intellectual Housework Assessment (IHA) (Soderback, 1988b). Jane was asked to cook lunch, including baking bread rolls and making potato soup. (Remember that Jane had spent years cooking for her four children.)

I had set out all the ingredients and utensils on the kitchen counter. To begin with cooking the stock, Jane would need to measure half a litre of water and open two small packets of stock cubes. Jane read the recipe aloud and talked to herself about what she had to do. She picked up the stock cubes, one in each hand and stood there, but did nothing for several minutes. I asked, "What should you do with the stock packets?" Jane answered that that they should be opened and the contents put into the pot, but she did nothing until I took one of the packets and demonstrated what to do.

This observation during the IHA assessment showed that Jane had a mental impairment, that is, disturbances of higher cortical functions. These disturbances can occur with a lesion to the frontal region of the brain. Clients' behavior is characterized by "no sign of disturbance of movement, gnosis, praxis, and speech; nevertheless, … their complex psychological activity was grossly impaired …. They are unable to produce stable plans and became inactive and aspontaneous" (Luria, 1980).

This cognitive dysfunction might also explain Jane's behavior at breakfast on the ward. When I asked her, she admitted that she had not eaten a full meal for the 4 days she was at home! I realized that Jane needed an occupational therapy program to *relearn* how to initiate and perform all her housework tasks independently (Soderback, 1988c, 1991).

Thus, for Jane and clients with similar problems, occupational-therapy interventions become an ongoing learning process.

The Therapeutic Teaching Process

The occupational therapy teaching intervention approach is a dynamic and continuing process in applying the open-system theory (Levine, 1991; von Bertalanffy, 1968). This dynamic process is distinguished by the interaction among the OT, the clients' performances of occupations (tasks/activities), and the environmental context.

A fundamental component is the *therapeutic instructions* the OT uses to provide the client with cues for task performance (Sabari, 2001). These instructions are intended to result in the client's doing of the tasks.

The teaching process are mediated by various tasks and activities, such as grooming, dressing, cooking, cleaning, playing games, reading, calculating, performing simulated tasks or work tasks, or handicrafts (Ludwig, 1993; Soderback, 1988c). (For meditated learning, see below).

The Occupational Therapist's Role

The OT as the teacher is a *traveling companion*, not the doer. He or she *guides, coaches*, and *facilitates* the client's occupational performance. In this way, the client is taught to initiate the performance of tasks that are adapted to the actual context. A favorable outcome helps the client acquire new, more adaptive, and effective knowledge.

Learning

These interventions are accomplished through *learning*, defined as "a process of acquiring, knowledge, skills, attitudes, from studies, instructions, experience" (Institute of Education Sciences, 2008). It is a set of cognitive processes adapted to the client's present environmental circumstances (Schwartz, 1991). The outcome of learning is "a change in an individual's capacity to respond to the environment and is associated with practice or experience" (Abreu and Hinojosa, 1992). Learning contributes to defining ourselves, to living in social groupings, and to saving our vital energy. The latter occurs because a task does not need to be learned anew every time one wants to do it. Instead, the new information and experience is assimilated to existing cognitive schemas, or represents an accommodation and revision of existing brain schemata. The results are evident in the person's behavior.

Theoretical Approach to Therapeutic Teaching

Therapeutic teaching focuses on the educational approaches the OT uses. The application is based on OTs' use of their professional and pedagogical knowledge, including activity analysis/synthesis, and disability and disease information (see Chapter 2).

The following factors are crucial for designing a client's therapeutic teaching process: (1) a realistic intervention goal for the client, (2) prognosis of the medical diagnosis or disease, (3) disability status, (4) present condition, and (5) present capacity for learning (Niestadt, 1998). The combination of these factors contributes to the OT's choice of appropriate therapeutic teaching, that is, a *behavioral* or a *cognitive* theoretical approach, or combinations of these, used to conduct the interventions (Schwartz, 1991).

The Behavioral Educational Approach

In a *behavioral* approach, an antecedent stimulus (S) induces a behavioral response (R). Here the OT acts as an *instructor* (S). He or she gives sequentially one instruction for each component of the task. For example, "(1) Take the pot. (2) Hold it under the tap. (3) Turn on the tap. (4) Half-fill the pot with water." The client acts (R) according to each of the instructions.

This is a *training* approach. The OT is responsible for how the task should be performed. The client is expected to memorize this prescribed solution, which, it is hoped, will be repeated next time. The prerequisites are that the task is prepared and performed in exactly the same manner, situation, and environment (Sabari, 2001).

Participating Clients

The behavioral educational approach is relevant to clients with neurologic degenerative diseases (e.g., Alzheimer's disease, people with severe cognitive disabilities), and those with static prognoses. They have lost their ability to learn, or have very restricted ability to store and recall information (Hadas and Katz, 1992). The approach is also relevant to clients who have given up their will to perform daily tasks or are not allowed by relatives to perform, tasks that they in fact should be able to do (Soderback and Lilja, 1995). These clients need another person to do the tasks for them. At best, they are able to perform one or two components of a task, though successful performance requires use of very simplified instructions.

One clinical application of behavioral teaching is *habit training*. The intervention consists of having the client daily and habitually repeat the task or routine. Practicing these daily routines is expected to "contribute to healing among clients living with severe mental illness" (Reed, 1998).

Teaching Facilitators

The behavioral educational approach includes *reinforcement strategies* for how to apply *instructions* to clients suffering from dementia. The teaching uses a specified form of problem-solving (Gitlin et al., 2005; also see Chapter 18), or a model for home interventions (Graff, 2008; also see Chapter 19) developed to support daily activities.

When giving the instructions, the OT chooses the most suitable hierarchy level depending on the client's present level of learning capacity. A top-to-bottom approach in connection with analysis of the task's degree of difficulty is used to determine what hierarchy level is effective (Allen, 1985; Allen et al., 1992). When the most appropriate level is used, it will initiate the client's action to complete the task. This hierarchy of instructions includes the following:

- *Guided movement.* The OT needs to do the same action, which the client is expected to perform. For example, it might entail putting a comb in the client's hand. The OT may keep her hand above the client's hand and follow the client's movement. When successful, this gives the client a feeling of competence.
- *Simplified demonstrations for imitation.* The simplified demonstration approach was effective in the case of Jane. The OT demonstrated how to open one of the packets of stock cubes. Then Jane followed the OT's movements and was able

to imitate the action. This simplified demonstration initiated Jane's action, and she was able to complete the task.

- *Visual signs.* In the case of Jane, the OT had prepared the session by having put all the ingredients and utensils on the kitchen counter. Their visibility prompted the initiation of action, which may have helped Jane to start the procedure of boiling the stock. However, this level proved too difficult for Jane's current capacity for transferring of learning.
- *Verbal instructions* are used in both behavioral and cognitive therapeutic teaching. These instructions have to be modified by *quantity* (how much should be said), *complexity* (the construction of the language, such as clarity, consistency, logical sequence), and *moderation* (the loudness of the voice). The OT tried to instruct Jane verbally, but this instruction level was too difficult for Jane to follow.

It might be concluded that instructions to Jane should mainly include demonstrations intended for imitation, gradually increasing visual signs and then verbal instructions (Schwartz, 1991).

The Cognitive Educational Approach: The Dialogue Technique Approach

The Client's Role

The *cognitive* educational approach requires the client's *active participation* during the information processes. Preferably, the client should develop an effective way of performing the tasks. The effect of this approach is *learning,* which results in the client's *acquisition of assimilated or accommodated, retained knowledge,* applicable in a variety of situations and environments. In other words, the learned knowledge might be *generalizable* (Sabari, 2001).

Learning originates in the cognitive process that is of value for the client when manage unexpected situations, to become a member of society, for developing personal identity and internal adaptations (see Chapter 3). Moreover, through the learning process the client might increase awareness of the consequences of the disability (Schwartz, 1991).

During the *cognitive* educational process, the client is the prime actor, in whom active memory and reflective brain processes are in play. Here, the genesis of learning acquisition lies in the schemata of conceptions stored in the brain and that are possible to recall. When new knowledge is added to these schemata, either assimilation or accommodation occurs.

Greatly simplified, in *assimilation processes,* new information is added to existing schemata, and in *accommodation,* the organization of existing schemata is altered (Schwartz, 1991). The latter process is probably the most used in occupational therapy among adult clients with recent remedial diseases or disabilities and where the sessions seek to promote the client's *relearning* how to perform daily occupations.

The Occupational Therapist's Role

Here the OT acts as "the agent who plans and structures" occupational performance "in such a way as to effect beneficial changes for the client" (Schwartz, 1991); that is, the therapist acts as a *coach,* using various teaching facilitators (see below) to promote the client's learning process.

The term *teaching facilitator* is associated with the term *learning strategy,* meaning that the OT uses various teaching techniques during the learning process. These techniques (1) assist the client in overcoming occupational obstacles; (b) help the client to focus, be motivated, pay attention, and persist with, and accomplish daily occupations that present difficulties, and not give up; and (3) promote the most rational principles for improving problem-solving (Katz, 1992; Schwartz, 1991).

Teaching Facilitators

In the cognitive educational approach, the following teaching facilitators are used with people suffering from brain damage (see Chapters 20 to 22). However, they apply also to active learning programs (see Chapters 24 to 28).

Dialogue Technique

Dialogue technique is one of the most important facilitators in the cognitive educational approach. The client is expected to be the prime mover in the communication process. Dialogue takes place between (1) the client and the task performance, and (2) the OT, the client, and the task performance. The latter form contains speech, facial expressions, gestures, body language, and action, which constitute a base for developing the *strategies* (see below) used to complete tasks. The fundamental principle of the dialogue technique is how the OT designs the questions that direct the client's action.

As an example of how to apply the dialogue technique, a 4-year-old girl and I were peeling and cutting up potatoes together. The potatoes had to be divided into at least four pieces to fit into a ricer. The girl cut the oval potatoes in half. Then she placed the oval side on the cutting board, so that when she started to cut, the potato slipped away. For me, the easiest way to instruct her would have been to pick up the potato and place it flat-side down (the behavioral educational approach).

> Instead, I asked, "Why do you think the potato slipped away?" She responded, "It thinks it was fun." I asked, "Do you want every potato to slip away like that?" "No." "Then what is the best way to put the potato on the cutting board?" She immediately placed the flat part of the potato down on the board, saying to it: "Now you should not play. I want to eat you!"

Here, I was teaching by using the dialogue technique that had become ingrained in me. Moreover, I am convinced that the girl had assimilated new knowledge into her current repertoire. This situation corresponds to many occasions that will be applied in the cognitive teaching of people with mental, motor, or sensory impairments.

Strategies

Strategies are "organized plans or sets of rules that guide action in variety of situations" (Sabari, 2001). The clients use strategies, that is, behaviors and thoughts, that differ from those they have used earlier (Schwartz, 1991) (see Chapter 22). A variety of strategies are used to facilitate the learning process:

- *Associations and imagination* prompt the client to create ideas containing connections between two elements. For example, associations may accompany relearning of logical functions, such as sequential performance of an task. This application is addressed in Chapter 21 for clients suffering from brain damage (Liu et al., 2004). The goal is that the client relearns to plan and execute daily living tasks.
- *Self-speech–induced facilitation* is used to assist simple movements such as reaching for and lifting a glass, in clients with Parkinson's disease (Maitra et al., 2006; also see Chapter 32) and in stroke patients (Kwakkel et al., 2004).
- *Prompting* occurs when the OT or the client initiates a task performance with a perceptual modality not normally used. The prompt should at best result in the client automatically completing the task.

Here is an example of using strategies with prompting as the teaching facilitator: A woman was suffering from verbal amnesia, and thus had difficulty naming objects. This impairment caused a serious speech disturbance. In the learning situation, the OT used pictures of objects. The client's speech was prompted by writing the first letter of the word on the palm of her left hand—a sensory modality. Using this prompting strategy decreased the client's frustration and was helpful. After a few learning sessions, she used this prompting on her own (Soderback, 1991; Stein et al., 2006).

- *Feed-forward and feedback* is the form of dialogue that occurs *between the client and the task* to be performed. The client's usual habits are confronted with new ways of performing occupations, which may results in completion of the task.
- *Feed-forward* refers to a problem-solving process where dialogue-technique instructions are used. The aim is to prevent clients from doing tasks in ways that run the risk of mistakes or damage.
  - Example: a client is to learn to move from his bed to his wheelchair by himself. The client might be asked in beforehand to explain how to position the wheelchair, adjust the height of the bed, and how to carry out the transfer before the task is actually undertaken.
- *Feedback* is the client's response to his or her performance of an action or task. Such responses make the client aware of success or failure and are a way of changing occupational behavior.

- The teaching process is facilitated by using *intrinsic or extrinsic feedback* (Sabari, 2001).

  - *Intrinsic feedback* concerns the client's learning through designing instructions based on the use of a single *perceptual input modality* or combinations. The modalities are verbal/auditory; visual includes the use of drawings, signs, and physical touch; visuospatial orientation includes movement guidance, tasting, smelling, or combinations thereof (Hadas and Katz, 1992). The choice of appropriate modalities may be decisive for the client's success in performing daily occupations (Hadas and Katz, 1992; Simon, 1993). Investigation of the client's learning style may reveal what combination of perceptual modalities is most effective (Schwartz, 1991).

Examples:

(a) A blind person uses his or her tactile sense and hearing ability to compensate for visual loss.
(b) The OT teaches clients suffering from intellectual dysfunctions to use the most effective combinations of perceptual input modalities, which may enable them to complete a task. For example, for clients with difficulties in perceiving correct spatial orientation (visuospatial dysgnosia), the information input may be strengthened by adding tactile, motor, and verbal perceptual inputs.
(c) In contrast, for clients with information-storing impairments (memory dysfunction), the information process may be strengthened by using as many perceptual modalities as possible, including encoding aids like imagination or categorization of information (Soderback, 1981, 1988c, 1991).

  - *Extrinsic feedback* concerns learning that occurs as reactions to perceptual input from the environment (Sabari, 2001). The client's experienced result arising from completion of a task may affect the client's accommodated or assimilated knowledge (Guiffrida, 1998). Numerous pedagogic aids may be used to bring about extrinsic feedback, such as films, lectures, diaries, biofeedback, and performance of critical tasks. Here, it is important to use a task that motivates the client to act in a realistic context (Schwartz, 1991).

- Examples of extrinsic feedback:

  - Four clients with right-hemisphere stroke and deficits in spatial orientation to the left of their body (unilateral neglect) participated in Intellectual Housework Training (Soderback, 1988a, 1991). Videorecordings were used to document the clients' actions. The films were shown to every client. Watching the video involved mirrored views; that is, the client perceived his neglected behavior in his right field of vision (with normal perception). The views gave the client feedback about his or her neglect behavior through viewing how she or he placed cakes on a baking plate (Soderback et al., 1992).

- Lifestyle interventions use feedback from monitoring, and review of dialogues and diaries is used among clients suffering from anxiety disorders (Lambert et al., 2007; also see Chapter 27).
- Electronic equipment for biofeedback is used for making the client aware of a negative internal process that is causing ill-health. Electric signals show the client's degree of muscle tension, blood pressure, heart rate, and skin temperature. The measurement results are used for feedback that gives the client an opportunity to gain voluntary control over processes or functions (Bain, 1993). Biofeedback is often a part of stress management, where progressive relaxation, relaxation responses, meditation, yoga, t'ai-chi, and music therapy accompany the intervention. The aim is to reduce hyperarousal of the sympathetic nervous system (Stein, 2002).
- Electronic equipment is also used for electrical stimulation of paretic muscles (Stein and Roose, 2000, see Chapter 9).

Mediated Learning

Mediated learning is based on the OT's analysis and synthesis of a *selected activity* (see Chapter 2, page 13) that offers the client meaning and purpose. *Activity analysis* is the OT's way to identify the sequential steps that constitute the task, that is, the performance components. This analysis is used for moderating a task's degree of difficulty by changing the number of components to be done and the time required for completion. *Activity synthesis* is a process for integrating performance components with the client's symptom(s). It has applications in mental, neuromuscular, or sensory biologic theories and depends on the client's present developmental level. The OT's teaching is based on his or her broadly medical, psychological, sociological knowledge (Hadas and Katz, 1992; Lamport et al., 1989; Soderback, 1988c). The results of a training session depend on whether the client understands the rationale, the goal, and what is to be learned (Ludwig, 1993; Soderback, 1988c). This educational approach is advocated by Govender and Kalra (2007).

Programs for Active Learning

The specific intervention programs exemplified below are distinguished by the messages they convey for the management of various illnesses. Often clients are taught in small groups (see, for example, the description of psychoeducational groups in Chapter 24) for a set of lessons. These include theoretical information about the disorder and its consequences for performance of daily activities as well as help with practical application to daily life activities. The educational approach is varied, but ordinary lessons comparable to adult education are used, and extrinsic feedback is expected to improve the client's knowledge and behavior. Ideally, active learning is applied, where the client is effectively engaged in understanding and suggesting solutions to impediments to perform daily activities (Johannessen, 2000; Stein et al., 2006).

Energy Conservation Course

Energy conservation teaching focuses on occupational performance methods that require the client to use as little energy as possible. The aims are to make the client aware of how much energy is required to do the task (Matuska et al., 2007; also see Chapter 23). Energy conservation intervention is used among clients' suffering from neuromuscular impairments that cause fatigue, such as multiple sclerosis, muscular dystrophy, cancer, diagnoses with symptoms of exhaustion.

Psychoeducational and Social-Skills Training

Psychoeducational and social-skills training may be appropriate for clients with chronic mental ill-health (Buchain et al., 2003; also see Chapter 26). Clients participate in simulated or real-life learning sessions, such as role playing, management of money and medication, and leisure activities. Teaching situations aimed at gradual improvement and control of interpersonal behavior such as anger (Cowls and Hale, 2005; also see Chapter 24) or substance-use disorders (see Chapter 28). *Reinforcement,* including assertive responses, nonverbal behavior such as voice volume adjustment or speech duration, or conversional questions, is used. The OT acts as moderator giving feedback on the client's behavior (Crist, 1993; Lieberman et al., 1993). This approach is used among clients with acute schizophrenia (Chan et al., 2007; also see Chapter 25) to improve insight into their disorder and promote health.

Neuromusculoskeletal and Movement-Related Learning

Neuromusculoskeletal and movement-related educational programs are based on neurophysiologic theory applied to activity performance in daily life. The aim is to reorganize motor function systems, and the programs are intended for clients suffering from brain damage or spinal-cord injury (Warren, 1991).

Traditionally, the Rood (Royeen et al., 2001) and the Brunstrom (Pedretti, 2001) approaches, Proprioceptive Neuromuscular Facilitation (Pope-Davis, 2001), or neurodevelopmental treatment, such as the Bobath approach (Terms, 2001), are used. However, the database search underlying the selection of interventions represented in this handbook identified no new scientific articles concerning occupational therapy that meet the stipulated search criterion and is therefore not further represented here.

The following newly originated neuromuscular reeducational interventions presented in the Handbook represent approaches to remediation of neuromuscular motor dysfunction:

- *Immersive or nonimmersive technology* is used to identify effective training strategies applied to virtual reality (Henderson et al., 2007; also see Chapter 29).
- In *constraint-induced movement therapy* (CIMT), the client may wear a restraining mitten on the less involved, more active hand/arm for 90% of waking time. He or she participates in movement-learning sessions (Bowman et al., 2006; also see Chapter 30) with performance of real daily living tasks (Sterr et al., 2006; Stevenson and Thalman, 2007; also see Chapter 31). The approach is grounded in learning theory, and on findings on the brain's adaptive capacities through the neural networks. [The OTs work contains] coaching, cheerleading, reminding, changing, and contemplating" (Boylstein et al., 2005).
- *Musculoskeletal preventive and remediation educational programs* are exemplified in this handbook by the *Looking After Your Joint Program* for people with moderate to severe rheumatoid arthritis (Hammond, 2004; also see Chapter 33). An extensive intervention program aimed at improving joint stiffness caused by a hand injury includes integrative and problem-focused teaching in combination with an external adaptive process where active and passive low-load stress mobilization and corrective splinting occur (Man Wah Wong, 2002; also see Chapter 10).

Sensory Functional Training

Sensory functional training programs are directed at children with congenital impairments and at clients suffering from neuromusculoskeletal pain.

- *Sensory integration therapy* is used with children with cerebral paresis or mental retardation. This age-developmental–mediated learning focuses on control of sensory input for stimulation of the child's somatosensory and vestibular sensations that bring about pleasurable, playful, and accomplished functional movement-based activities (Stein and Roose, 2000; Walker, 1993). Sensory integration (Ayres, 1979) in combination with neurodevelopmental and vestibular stimulation is intended to increase motor and learning abilities among children with cerebral paresis and mental retardation. The OT facilitates the child's learning though vestibular perceptual and environmental stimulation (Uyanik et al., 2003a,b; also see Chapter 34).

- *Movement schema* is a low-intensity training program combined with the administration of botulinum toxin A, which is used to improve movement patterns among children with cerebral paresis (Russo et al., 2007; also see Chapter 35).
- The management of chronic pain (see Chapter 36) and, in this connection, restoration of function (see Chapter 37), is intended to improve the client's knowledge of and ability to sustain working.

Learning Approaches for Participation in Working Life

Programs for participation in working life are based on ergonomic and practical principles as presented in Chapter 38. Numerous programs aim at teaching participation in working life (see examples in Chapters 38 to 42). Here people with mental ill-health (see Chapters 40 and 41) can get help with individual placement and support in a job (see Chapter 42). The same educational services are offered for aiding transitions from childhood to adulthood (see Chapter 42). However, some important programs are missing, such as work hardening (Ogden-Niemeyer and Jacobs, 1989) and the criterion-referenced multidimensional job-related model (Soderback and Jacobs, 2000).

Conclusion

This chapter discussed the role of the therapist as a teacher. As in all teaching, the teacher's basic aim is to create learning situations for clients with cognitive, sensory, neuromusculoskeletal, and movement-related diseases or disabilities. In the educational process, the client's current function is the basis for the teaching approach aimed at improving the client's learning and behavior of occupational performances.

References

Abreu, B.C., and Hinojosa, J. (1992). The process approach for cognitive-perceptual and postural control dysfunction for adults with brain injuries. In: Katz, N., ed. Cognitive Rehabilitation (pp. 167–194). Boston: Andover Medical Publishers.

Allen, C. (1985). Occupational Therapy for Psychiatric Diseases: Measurement and Management of Cognitive Disabilities. Boston: Little Brown.

Allen, C., Earhart, C.A., and Blue, T. (1992). Occupational Therapy Treatment Goals for the Physically and Cognitively Disabled. Rockvill, Md.: American Occupational Therapy Association.

Ayres, A.J. (1979). Sensory Integration and the Child. Los Angeles: Western Psychological Series.

Bain, B.K. (1993). Technology. In: Hopkins, H.L., and Smith, S.L., eds. Willard and Spackman's Occupational Therapy, 8th ed. (pp. 338). Philadelphia: Lippincott.

Bowman, M.H., Taub, E., Uswatte, G., et al. (2006). A treatment for a chronic stroke patient with
a plegic hand combining CI therapy with conventional rehabilitation procedures: case report.
Neurorehabilitation, 2(21), 167–176.
Boylstein, C., Rittman, M., Gubrium, J., Behrman, A., and Davis, S. (2005). Constraint-induced
movement therapy (CIMT). The social organization in constraint-induced movement therapy.
J Rehabil Res Dev, 42(3), 263–275.
Buchain, P.C., Vizzotto, A.D., Henna, N.J., and Elkis, H. (2003). Randomized controlled trial of
occupational therapy in patients with treatment-resistant schizophrenia. Rev Bras Psiquiatr,
25(1), 26–30.
Chan, S.H., Lee, S.W., and Chan, I.W. (2007). TRIP: A psycho-educational programme in Hong
Kong for people with schizophrenia. Occup Ther Int, 14(2), 86–98.
Cowls, J., and Hale, S. (2005). It's the activity that counts: What clients value in psycho-educational
groups. Can J Occup Ther, 72(3), 176–182.
Crist, P.H. (1993). Community living skills: a psycho-educational community based program. In:
Cottrell, R.P.F. ed. Psychosocial Occupational Therapy (pp. 171). Rockville, Md.: American
Occupational Therapy Association.
Gitlin, L.N., Hauck, W.W., Dennis, M.P., and Winter, L. (2005). Maintenance of effects of the
home environmental skill-building program for family caregivers and individuals with
Alzheimer's disease and related disorders. J Gerontol A Biol Sci Med Sci, 60(3), 368–374.
Govender, P., and Kalra, L. (2007). Benefits of occupational therapy in stroke rehabilitation.
Exp Rev Neurother, 7(8), 1013–1019.
Graff, M.J. (2008). Effectiveness and Efficiency of Community Occupational Therapy for Older
People with Dementia and Their Caregivers. Nijmegen, The Netherlands: Radboud Universiteit
Nijmegen.
Guiffrida, C.G. (1998). Motor relearning: an emerging frame of reference for occupational per-
formance. In: Nieistadt, M.E., and Crepeau, E.B., eds. Willard and Spackman's Occupational
Therapy (pp. 560–563). Philadelphia: Lippincott.
Hadas, N., and Katz, N. (1992). A dynamic approach for applying cognitive modifiability in
occupational therapy settings. In: Katz, N., ed. Cognitive Rehabilitation Models for Intervention
in Occupational Therapy (pp. 147). Boston: Andover Medical Publishers.
Hammond, A. (2004). What is the role of the OT? Best Pract Res Clin Rheumatol, 18(4),
491–505.
Henderson, A., Korner-Bitensky, N., and Levin, M. (2007). Virtual reality in stroke rehabilitation:
a systematic review of its effectiveness for upper limb motor recovery. Top Stroke Rehabil,
14(2), 52–61.
Institute of Education Sciences. (2008). ERIC—The Education Resources Information Center.
Thesaurus. Institute of Education Sciences of the U.S. Department of Education.
Johannesen, L.R. (2000). Encouraging Active Learning with Case Studies. Paper presented at the
Annual Spring Meeting of the National Council of Teachers of English, New York.
Katz, N. (1992). Cognitive Rehabilitation. Models for Intervention in Occupational Therapy, 1st
ed. Boston: Andover Medical Publishers.
Kwakkel, G., van Peppen, R., Wagenaar, R.C., et al. (2004). Effects of augmented exercise therapy
time after stroke: a meta-analysis. Stroke, 35(11), 2529–2539.
Lambert, R.A., Harvey, I., and Poland, F. (2007). A pragmatic, unblinded randomised controlled
trial comparing an occupational therapy-led lifestyle approach and routine GP care for panic
disorder treatment in primary care. J Affect Disord, 99(1–3), 63–71.
Lamport, N.K., Coffey, M.S., and Hersch, G.I. (1989). Activity Analysis Handbook. Thorofare,
NJ: Slack.
Levine, R.E., and Brayley, C.R. (1991). Occupation as a therapeutic medium. In: Christensen, C.,
and Baum, C., eds. Occupational Therapy. Overcoming Human Performances Deficits, Vol. 1
(pp. 597, 616–618). Thorofare, NJ: Slack.
Lieberman, M.D., Massel, H.K., Mosk, M.D., and Wong, S.E. (1993). Social skills training for
chronic mental patients. In: Cottrell, R.P.F. ed. Psychosocial Occupational Therapy. Proactive
Approaches (pp. 158–159). Rockville, Md: American Occupational Therapy Association.

Liu, K.P., Chan, C.C., Lee, T.M., and Hui-Chan, C.W. (2004). Mental imagery for promoting relearning for people after stroke: a randomized controlled trial. Arch Phys Med Rehabil, 85(9), 1403–1408.

Ludwig, F.M. (1993). Anne Cronin Mosey. In: Miller, J.M., and Walker, K.F., eds. Perspectives on Theory for the Practice of Occupational Therapy (pp. 41–63). Galtersburg, MD: Aspen.

Luria, A.R. (1980). Higher Cortical Functions in Man, 3rd ed. (B. Haigh, Trans.). New York: Basic Books.

Maitra, K.K., Telage, K.M., and Rice, M.S. (2006). Self-speech-induced facilitation of simple reaching movements in persons with stroke. Am J Occup Ther, 60(2), 146–154.

Matuska, K., Mathiowetz, V., and Finlayson, M. (2007). Use and perceived effectiveness of energy conservation strategies for managing multiple sclerosis fatigue. Am J Occup Ther. 61(1), 62–69.

Niestadt, M.E. (1998). Theories derived from learning perspectives. In: Niestadt, M.E., and Crepeau, E.B., eds. Willard and Spackman's Occupational Therapy, 9th ed. (pp. 551–553). Philadelphia: Lippincott.

Ogden-Neimeyer, L. and Jacobs, K. (1989). Work Hardening: State of the Art. Thorofare: SLACK.

Pedretti, L.W. (2001). Movement therapy: The Brunstrom approach to treatment of hemiplegia. In: Pedretti, L.W., and Early, M.B., eds. Occupational Skill for Physical Dysfunction, 5th ed. (pp. 588–605). St. Louis: Mosby.

Pope-Davis, S.A. (2001). Proprioceptive neuromuscular facilitation approach. In: Pedretti, L.W., and Early, M.B., eds. Occupational Skill for Physical Dysfunction, 5th ed. (pp. 606–623). St. Louis: Mosby.

Reed, K.L. (1998). Theories derived from occupational behavior perspective. In: Niestadt, M.E., and Crepeau, E.B., eds. Willard and Spackman's Occupational Therapy, 9th ed. (pp. 526). Philadelphia: Lippincott.

Royeen, C.B., Duncan, M., and McCormack, G. (2001). The Rood approach: a reconstruction. In: Pedretti, L.W., and Early, M.B., eds. Occupational Therapy. Practice Skills for Physical Dysfunction, 5th ed. (pp. 576–587). St. Louis: Mosby.

Russo, R.N., Crotty, M., Miller, M.D., Murchland, S., Flett, P., and Haan, E. (2007). Upper-limb botulinum toxin A injection and occupational therapy in children with hemiplegic cerebral palsy identified from a population register: a single-blind, randomized, controlled trial. Pediatrics, 119(5e), 1149–1158.

Sabari, J.S. (2001). Teaching activities in occupational therapy. In: Pedretti, L.W., and Early, M.B., eds. Occupational Therapy. Practice Skills for Physical Dysfunction. London: Mosby.

Schwartz, R.K. (1991). Educational and training strategies. In: Christensen, C., and Baum, C., eds. Occupational Therapy. Overcoming Human Deficits (pp. 666–698). Thorofare, NJ: Slack.

Simon, C.J. (1993). Use of activity analysis. In: Hopkins, H.L., and Smith, S.L., eds. Willard and Spackman's Occupational Therapy, 8th ed. (pp. 290). Philadelphia: Lippincott.

Söderback, I. (1981). Intellektuell Funktionsträning. Stockholm: Psykologiförlaget AB.

Soderback, I. (1988a). The effectiveness of training intellectual function in adult with acquired brain damage. Scand J Rehabil Med, 20, 71–76.

Soderback, I. (1988b). A housework-based assessment of intellectual functions in patients with acquired brain damage. Development and evaluation of an occupational therapy method. Scand J Rehabil Med, 20(2), 57–69.

Soderback, I. (1988c). Intellectual Function Training and Intellectual Housework Training in Patients with Acquired Brain Damage. A Study of Occupational Therapy Methods. Stockholm: Karolinska Institute.

Söderback, I. (1991). Processen i arbetsterapi. Referensram för bedömning och träning vid intellektuell funktionsnedsättning. (in Swedish). The Process of Occupational Therapy. The Frame of References of Assessment and Relearning of Intellectual Functions. Stockholm: Studentlitteratur.

Soderback, I., and Lilja, M. (1995). A study of activity in the home environment among individuals with disability following a stroke. Neurorehabilitation, 6(4), 347–357.

Soderback, I., Bengtsson, I., Ginsburg, E., and Ekholm, J. (1992). Video feedback in occupational therapy. Its effect in patients with neglect syndrome. Arch Phys Med Rehabil, 73, 1140–1146.

Soderback, I., Schult, M.-L., and Jacobs, K. (2000). A criterion-referenced multidimensional job-related model prediction capability to perform occupations among persons with chronic pain. Work, 15(1), 25–39.

Stein, F. (2002). Stress Management Questionnaire—Individual Version (Version 1 edition) [CD-ROM]. New York: Thomson Delmar Learning.

Stein, F., and Roose, B. (2000). Pocket Guide to Treatment in Occupational Therapy. San Diego: Singular.

Stein, F., Söderback, I., Cutler, S.K., and Larson, B. (2006). Occupational Therapy and Ergonomics. Applying Ergonomic Principles to Everyday Occupation in the Home and at the Work, 1st ed. London/Philadelphia: Whurr/Wiley.

Sterr, A., Szameitat, A., Shen, S., and Freivogel, S. (2006). Application of the CIT concept in the clinical environment: Hurdles, practicalities, and clinical benefits. Cogn Behav Neurol, 19(1), 48–54.

Stevenson, T., and Thalman, L. (2007). A modified constraint-induced movement therapy regimen for individuals with upper extremity hemiplegia. Can J Occup Ther, 74(2), 115–124.

Terms, K. (2001). Neurodevelopmental treatment: The Bobath approach. In: Pedretti, L.W., and Early, M.B., eds. Occupational Therapy. Practice Skills for Physical Dysfunction, 5th ed. (pp. 624–640). St. Louis: Mosby.

Uyanik, M., Bumin, G., and Kayihan, H. (2003a). Comparison of different therapy approaches in children with Down syndrome. Pediatr Int, 45(1), 68–73.

Uyanik, M., Bumin, G., and Kayihan, H. (2003b). Comparison of different therapy approaches in children with Down syndrome. Pediatr Int, 45(1), 68–73.

von Bertalanffy, L. (1968). General system theory—a critical review. In: Buckley, W., ed. Modern Systems Research for the Behavioral Scientist. Chicago: Aldine.

Walker, K.F. (1993). A. Jean Ayres. In: Miller, R.J., and Walker, K.F., eds. Perspectives on Theory for the Practice of Occupational Therapy (pp. 134–135, 142). Philadelphia: Aspen.

Warren, M. (1991). Strategies for sensory and neuromotor remediation. In: Christensen, C., and Baum, C., eds. Occupational Therapy. Overcoming Human Performance Deficits (pp. 638). Thorofare, NJ: Slack.

Wong, J.M. (2002). Management of stiff hand: an occupational therapy perspective. Hand Surg, 7(2), 261–269.

World-Health-Organization. (2008). International Classification of Functioning, Disability and Health. http://www.who.int/classification/icf/site/icftemplate.cfm?myurl = home.

Chapter 18
Problem Solving: A Teaching and Therapeutic Tool for Older Adults and Their Families

Laura N. Gitlin

> *The OT needs to have effective communication skills, respecting a family's values and understanding where they're coming from.... That's critical, even more than knowing her intervention strategies.*

> —Family caregiver

Abstract Problem solving is integral to clinical reasoning and everyday occupational therapy practices. It can also be a systematic therapeutic modality for identifying client or family caregiver concerns and teaching new approaches to self-management. This chapter presents a systematic approach to help occupational therapists identify target problem areas and potential modifiable contributing factors when working with older adults and families. The approach is applicable to a broad range of clinical problems associated with the consequences and management of chronic illness and provides therapists with an important tool for actively engage clients in self-management.

Keywords Caregiving • Cultural competence • Client-centered care • Self-management • Chronic illness • Self-efficacy.

Definitions

Problem solving is integral to the clinical reasoning process and everyday practices of occupational therapists. Problem solving, however, can also be a systematic therapeutic modality for identifying client or family caregiver concerns and teaching new approaches to self-management. Problem solving as a therapeutic tool is critical to manage complex health problems such as chronic illness or functional challenges that typically occur as people age or to identify and minimize the daily care concerns confronted by family caregivers that are burdensome and devalue quality of life. Using a systematic problem-solving approach directly involves the older adult or family member in a form of clinical reasoning making client/family equal to and a partner with a health care team.

I. Söderback (ed.), *International Handbook of Occupational Therapy Interventions*,
DOI: 10.1007/978-0-387-75424-6_18, © Springer Science + Business Media, LLC 2010

Background

The theoretical approach in problem solving is the transtheoretical model of behavioral change, which suggests that behavioral change involves small incremental steps in which individuals move from (1) a stage of precontemplation in which a problem is not recognized; (2) to contemplation, in which a problem is recognized but the course of action remains unclear or the person is ambivalent; (3) to action, in which a person is ready to try new approaches; (4) to maintenance, in which a person is ready, and has successfully made changes to enhance his or her performance; and (5) seeks strategies to maintain these gains (Prochaska and Velicer, 1997).

Purpose

Problem solving as a therapeutic tool involves the purposeful engagement of an older adult or family member in a specific process to identify and solve an identified health care challenge. The purposes of a problem-solving approach are manifold and include the following: (1) to model and instruct client as to a process for thinking about and solving everyday caregiving or health and functional problems; (2) to actively engage the client in a dynamic process to identify modifiable contributors to problems and their solutions; (3) to enhance self-efficacy and empower the client to own the health problems as well as the solutions derived from this process; and (4) to help establish a therapeutic partnership in which the occupational therapist (OT), a client, and health professionals are equal, with each bringing unique knowledge and skills to solve a complex challenge.

Method

Candidates for the Intervention

Inclusion Criteria

Problem solving as a teaching tool is a helpful therapeutic approach when working with *family caregivers of persons with dementia* who are struggling with managing *troublesome behaviors* (e.g., wandering, agitation, repetitive questioning) or functional challenges (e.g., resistance to care, ambulation difficulties); with older adults with functional difficulties (e.g., unable to bathe, climb stairs); or with individuals with chronic illness in which lifestyle modifications are necessary (Chodosh et al., 2005; Farrell et al., 2004; Gitlin et al., 2003, 2006; Lorig et al., 2001).

Exclusion Criteria

Problem solving may not be helpful with some clients who are distressed, or depressed, or for whom moving through these steps may be too confusing or overwhelming. Nevertheless, some aspects of problem solving can be helpful even in these cases. The OT would need to be careful so as to not to further overwhelm the client with too many processes, steps and strategies.

Signs of Readiness for Participation in Problem Solving

The problem-solving model suggests that older adults with health challenges in the precontemplative and contemplative stages may not fully understand the disease and the need for behavioral or environmental changes. Such changes may be viewed as stigmatizing and threatening to one's lifelong preferred self-care methods. For this stage of readiness, continued support, providing education, and suggesting small changes that can have a big impact on the presenting problem may be most appropriate.

Once a better understanding of the disease or health condition is achieved, then problem solving and brainstorming will be more useful. This is in contrast to the client at the active or maintenance phase who is proactively seeking lifestyle and environmental adjustments to reach their personal functional goals or overcome health challenges. In this case, engagement in the problem-solving–brainstorming process may be very much welcomed and embraced as a helpful tool.

Settings

The pace by which to proceed for any client remains a clinical judgment.

The Role of the Occupational Therapist

The role of the OT in facilitating problem solving and systematically engaging a client in this process is critical and consistent with emerging principles of geriatric care (Reuben, 2007). Occupational therapists have the unique combination of skills required to integrate environmental, social, and person-based factors (including cognitive and functional) in the problem-solving process from which to derive a multifactorial profile of the client and the problem and potential solutions.

Results

Clinical Application: The Problem-Solving Intervention Model

Genesis

Problem solving is central to clinical reasoning and at the heart of all health professional practices. It has been more formally and systematically developed by psychologists as an active and systematic therapeutic tool for use in psychosocial and behavioral interventions (Cuijpers et al., 2007). There are many variants of problem solving, which range from broad clinical reasoning to more structured, manualized approaches represented, for example, by problem-solving therapy (PST), which has been tested extensively in randomized trials for patients with depression (Gellis and Kenaley, 2008). However, a systematic approach to problem solving can be useful in occupational therapy encounters involving older adults or their family members, in which the focus of treatment is on functional performance difficulties or concerns stemming from the need to manage the consequences of chronic illness. The problem-solving approach presented here draws upon traditions from psychology that focus on behavior as an outcome of antecedents and consequences; its most recent variant was tested in a series of dementia caregiver interventions (Belle et al., 2006; Gitlin et al., 2003), sponsored by the National Institutes of Health (NIH) 12-year REACH (Resources for Enhancing Alzheimer's Caregiver Health) I and II initiatives.

Main Principles

A problem-solving approach is part of a larger movement toward *consumer-directed health care*. A consumer-directed approach relies on informed consumers to direct their own health care choices and participate in disease management. Emerging chronic disease care models emphasize patient-oriented care with patients and families as partners on a care team (Bodenheimer et al., 2002). Chronic disease care models entails the core content notion that patient activation or engagement in one's own care is necessary to achieve better health care outcomes (Hibbard et al., 2004). Thus, of importance are interventions that use techniques that actively engage patients and involve them in their own health management. Problem solving offers therapists a tool for actively involving and promoting the clients' engagement. It also provides a mechanism for obtaining more in-depth knowledge of a client-identified problem from which to tailor or customize strategies to fit the particularities of the person-environmental context. Tailored interventions allow for a more patient-centered focus. This focus has been shown to be more advantageous than a prescriptive, one-size-fits-all approach, which typifies current health care practices (Chee et al., 2007; Richards et al., 2007).

The problem-solving approach discussed here is based on the assumption that for any behavior or challenging problem there are identifiable antecedents or potential triggers, specific characteristics of the behavior/problem itself, and consequences or responses to the behavior/problem that potentially exacerbate the presenting problem.

Content of Problem-Solving Model: The ABC Approach

This model is referred to as the ABC approach, in which A = antecedent, B = behavior, and C = consequence. The client's functioning is examined as a consequence of each of these components and their interaction.

The *goal of problem solving* is to identify each component and fully characterize an identified problem in order to discern modifiable contributory factors. From this, *strategies* are developed and implemented to address specific modifiable factors with the goal of minimizing or eliminating the presenting problem.

Problem solving makes explicit the underlying clinical reasoning that OTs typically engage in, but in such a way as to enable clients to effectively contribute to solving their self-identified problems. Prior to actively engaging in problem solving with a client, it is important to provide a brief explanation as to its purpose, as listed in Table 18.1.

Six Basic Steps

The approach involves six basic steps outlined in Table 18.2.

Step 1 starts with an agreement on the identified problem (e.g., unable to prepare a small meal) or behavior (e.g., gets lost in neighborhood). Moving through the process, the initially identified problem is refined or modified. However, in some cases, the OT discovers underlying or different problems to be the real problem or concern. One of the strengths of this approach is that it facilitates a greater understanding of the underlying issues that are causing client distress. and helps to uncover the troublesome components of a behavior or performance deficit.

In step 2, the client is asked to tell his or her story. As the client describes the problem, the OT takes notes and probes using the questions presented in Table 18.3. It is important to be familiar with the probes so that questioning can proceed

Table 18.1 Talking points to introduce problem solving

- Let's discuss the problem area/behavior that you have identified
- As we discuss the problem area/behavior, I will take notes. This will help us identify some of the things that may be contributing to the [name the problem or behavior].
- First, can you describe the problem or what happens?

Table 18.2 Six steps in problem solving with older adults and family members

Steps	Description
1. Problem identification	Identify a specific problem area that is challenging to the client and/or family caregiver. Examples of a problem may be: Difficulty engaging in desired activities such as visiting with friends/family Climbing stairs quickly to use bathroom Managing challenging behavior associated with dementia
2. Evaluate antecedents to problem, context in which problem occurs, and consequences of problem	Understand the antecedents of a particular problem area (e.g., such as what preceded a dementia patient's catastrophic reaction), or the context in which a problem occurs (e.g., older adult takes diuretic but has difficulty climbing stairs to bathroom in a timely manner); the particular consequences (e.g., caregiver raises voice; or older adult stops taking diuretic) are important for identifying particular solutions for the target problem. Evaluation involves a semistructured questioning approach along with either role-play or direct observation of performance and assessment of the environment.
3. Brainstorming	Identify potential solutions by having client/family member help generate a list of what works and what has not worked in the past and what they might consider trying.
4. Identify potential solutions	Select those solutions from the brainstorm list that client/family member agrees to and that have therapeutic potential.
5. Implement identified strategies and modify as needed	Implement strategies, reevaluate client progress, and make adjustments as needed, always informing client/family member of why a particular strategy worked or did not work.
6. Generalize process	Name and frame process and steps so that client/family member can use them as a tool for newly emerging challenges once occupational therapy is concluded.

smoothly and occur within the flow of a conversation and the client's story telling. The questions in Table 18.3 can be asked in any order and serve to keep the client focused and engaged. The OT needs to identify the who, what, when, and where of the identified problem, and thus the probes help the OT and the client to flesh out details that may not be provided initially by the client.

Step 3 entails engaging the client in either a role play or a simulation, or making a direct observation of the performance challenge or context in which a problem behavior occurs. The purpose of this step is to obtain additional information about the context of the problem, especially environmental supports and constraints or the particular management and communication approaches or level of functionality of the client. Following a role-play or observation, the client is asked whether it represented what typically happens. From the problem-solving and observation approaches, the OT may be able to offer an immediate strategy to address the problem. In some cases, it may not be possible to observe the problem/behavior immediately following the ABC interviewing, but it is very helpful if this can occur either in the same or in a future session. The ABC approach can be used in combination with a standard observational tool, for example, to determine home safety or a standard tool to assess functional performance.

Table 18.3 Problem solving worksheet TARGET PROBLEM AREA OR
BEHAVIOR:_____

What is the behavior/problem area?	Notes

❑ Take a minute and describe what client does.

❑ Listen to the words used by clients as to how they describe the problem
area, whether they understand the disease, if they have unrealistic
expectations.

Why is this behavior/area a problem?

❑ "People react differently to problems/behaviors. What about this problem/
behavior really gets to you?"

❑ "What bothers you?"

❑ "Why does this get on your nerves?"

❑ "Can you list the reason(s)?"

❑ "What effect does this problem/behavior have on you?"

❑ "How does it make you feel?"

"How would you like this problem/behavior to change?"

❑ "When would you consider the problem solved?"

❑ "What would make it seem to you that it was better (tolerable)?"

❑ "What would make you feel better about this problem?"

"Why do you think this problem/behavior happens?"

❑ "Do you see any specific causes or triggers?"

❑ "What do you think is contributing to the behavior?"

❑ "Think about what happens right before the behavior occurs."

❑ "Can you recognize any cycles or patterns?"

❑ "What happened right before the problem occurs?"

"When does the problem/behavior happen?"

Time of day?

Days of the week?

❑ "When does the problem/behavior begin?"

❑ "Can you recognize any cycles or patterns?"

❑ "What happened right before the problem/behavior occurs?"

❑ "Does the problem/behavior happen constantly?"

❑   "How often does the problem/behavior happen?"

"Where does the problem/behavior happen?"

❑ "Is there a unique place in the house?"

❑ "Does it only happen in certain places?"

❑ "Are there places where it does not happen?"

❑ "Have you changed the surroundings? If yes, did it get worse or better
when this happened?"

"Who is around when the problem/behavior occurred?"

❑ "Do other people help care for you or your family member?"

❑ "Do you care for other people or children?"

❑ "Is the problem/behavior influenced by other family members/friends?"

❑ "How do other people react to the problem/ behavior?"

❑ "Any special sleeping arrangements?"

"What have you tried?"

❑ "What do you do when she/he does this?"

❑ "Have you tried anything that hasn't worked?"

❑ "Have you tried anything that seems to help?"

❑ "How often have you tried doing that?"

(continued)

Table 18.3 (continued)

Additional information
❑ "Has your doctor been told of this problem/behavior?"
❑ "If yes, what has your doctor recommended?"
❑ "Do you or your loved one have hearing problems?"
❑ "Do you or your loved one have vision problems?"

Adapted from the NIH REACH initiative, and retested by Jefferson's Center for Applied Research on Aging and Health through NIH and foundation grant funds. Schulz, et al. (2003)

Step 4 is referred to as "brainstorming." To initiate it, the brainstorming process is explained to the client in this way:

Now that we have discussed the different aspects of the problem/behavior and how you feel about it, let's think about possible ways of handling it. Let's spend about 10 minutes or so on thinking about possible solutions. This is called "brainstorming." The purpose of brainstorming is to consider all possible solutions without judging whether they will work or if they are doable at this point or whether you want to try it. Let's take turns thinking of possible strategies. I will record all of our ideas and then we will look at each idea we come up with to see what you think about them. Remember, for right now, we are just going to list solutions. After we have a list, we will then talk about each idea in detail to see if it would work for you.

A simple worksheet for brainstorming (adapted from the NIH REACH initiative) is shown in Table 18.4.

Here are some suggestions for conducting the brainstorming:

• It is important to emphasize that solutions that are generated be realistic. A statement such as "I wish the disease would go away or that I will be cured" is not a

Table 18.4 Brainstorming worksheet

Target behavior/ problem:_____

List possible solutions: Consider solutions that minimize complexity of the environment in which the behavior/problem occurs, tasks (setup), communication:
____1.
____2.
____3.
____4.
____5.
____6.
____7.
____8.
____9.
____10.
Note: Place * next to acceptable solutions; X next to unacceptable solutions; ? next to solutions for future consideration.
Consider organizing strategies according to categories: those that address the physical environment, task complexity, communication (relevant in caregiver-identified problems), activity engagement.

Adapted from NIH REACH II initiative. Schulz, et al. (2003)

realistic or acceptable brainstorming item. Statements such as these suggest that clients may need more help in understanding their condition, and that while there may not be a cure, there are strategies that may be helpful so that they can continue to achieve their personal goals.

- Brainstorming can be uncomfortable for some clients who may be at a loss to identify a strategy. Thus, it is helpful and important for the OT to offer the first strategy to provide a concrete example of what is meant by a potential solution. For clients who continue to have difficulty identifying potential solutions, it is helpful to ask them to describe what has worked and what has not worked in the past to address the problem. This often triggers ideas and helps the client understand that in fact they can come up with specific solutions to their problems.
- It is important to allow sufficient time for a client to generate an idea and to praise any response from the client. Some clients may need more time, whereas others will move through this exercise quickly.
- Although there is no specific number of strategies that need to be generated, anywhere from five to ten strategies are helpful to have listed. While the OT may be aware of many more potential strategies, it is important not to overwhelm a client and to proceed at a reasonable pace that allows the client to absorb the information and strategies.
- Brainstorming can be as short as 10 minutes or as long as 20 minutes, depending on the level of engagement and number of solutions a client seeks to list.
- In brainstorming, it is helpful for the OT to think in terms of overarching categories of types of strategies such as those that may address environmental barriers, communication issues, or task complexity.
- Strategies can be reorganized by the OT according to these particular modifiable factors after brainstorming as a way of further educating clients as to the different strata in their living space that are potential contributors to functional/behavioral challenges.

Most OTs can identify strategies on their own without engaging a client in a brainstorming. However, brainstorming is an important step in problem solving for several critical reasons: (1) it illustrates for clients a process they can use when new problems arise once therapy is completed; (2) the process helps to directly involve clients in their own self-management and gives them ownership of it; (3) it is empowering and validating since clients begin to see that they can generate solutions to their own problems; and (4) it provides a mechanism for securing a client's agreement to try a new approach, which in turn enhances the likelihood that the agreed upon strategy will in fact be attempted. Thus, brainstorming serves as a *therapeutic tool*.

In step 5, at the completion of the brainstorming session, the OT explains the next steps using these suggested talking points:

> We discussed different aspects of the problem area/behavior that is troublesome to you, how you are feeling, and things that you have done. Also, we now have a list of possible ways of managing the problem/behavior. Let's agree upon and take a closer look at each of the specific strategies you will try.

For each strategy generated, starting with the first, the OT reads the strategy to the client, who is asked (1) if it is a feasible one for him or her to use, and (2) if he or she would be willing to try it. The OT rules out any strategy that the client rejects outright or feels strongly that he or she would never try.

For strategies for which the client shows some hesitation, the OT can suggest returning to that strategy at another time to see if it might be helpful. For strategies that the OT believes will work, but are rejected by the client, it is important to provide a rationale for why it may be effective and suggest that the client consider it as a possible approach in the future. Each strategy is labeled on the list as (1) completely rejected by the client, by placing an X next to it; (2) a "maybe," in that the client is unsure but the OT believes it would be effective, by placing a question mark by the strategy; or (3) acceptable to the client, by placing an asterisk (*) by the strategy.

In step 6, for the strategies the client agrees to, the OT demonstrates the strategy and then observes the client performing the strategy.

Throughout, it is important to praise the client, inquire as to whether the strategy appears helpful, explain why the strategy may work, and tweak or modify the strategy to fit the client-environmental context based on the therapist's initial observation of how the client performs the strategy.

At the end of an intervention session, it is important to help clients identify when and how they will use each of the strategies.

The problem-solving questioning phase and brainstorming process should both occur sequentially within one face-to-face treatment session. This typically requires 20 to 30 minutes to complete.

If necessary, demonstrating and practicing agreed-upon strategies can occur in a separate face-to-face session, but again it is preferable if this is completed in the same session as the problem solving.

Clients should be given the brainstorming sheet so that they can refer to the list of solutions that were identified and to the agreed-upon ones that they should try prior to the next treatment session.

This process can be repeated for any number of identified problem areas. The more it is used, the easier it becomes for clients, who learns how to use the process on their own.

Clinical Considerations

There are several challenges that OTs will confront when using problem solving as an active teaching tool. First, some clients may be uncomfortable engaging in this process, and may find the process not in keeping with their expectations for a more prescriptive, top-down practice model approach. In this case, it is beneficial to fully explain (1) the purpose of the model, and (2) how it can be helpful for the client and or the caregiver. Some clients may become distracted or have difficulty concentrating or sustaining the problem-solving and brainstorming engagement process. For overwhelmed clients, there is a tendency to stray from the initial presenting problem, and it is necessary for the OT to keep the discussion on track. A primary challenge is identifying one particular problem area, as problems are often complex and multifaceted. It may be discovered that the initial identified problem really represents two or more related issues, each requiring its own problem-solving and brainstorming process. Alternately, through problem solving, it may be discovered that the problem initially identified is not actually the problem at all. This can occur with clients who may not fully grasp the nature of their conditions, or with overwhelmed clients who may not be able to disentangle the underlying problem that is causing their distress. Brainstorming too can be uncomfortable for some people who may not be able to think off the top of their head as to possible solutions. Nevertheless, clients typically find this process very validating.

Discussion

Some form of problem solving is at the core of most evidence-based interventions for family caregivers and chronic disease self-management programs. As a systematic questioning and brainstorming process, the approach helps clients clarify the characteristics of a presenting problem and potential ways it can be addressed.

The process serves as a teaching tool to uncover a client problem and the modifiable contributing factors as well as a mechanism for identifying viable solutions. Moreover, clients learn to use a tool for addressing problems that may emerge in the future. Furthermore, and perhaps most importantly, the technique itself promotes self-awareness and enhances self-efficacy (Bandura, 1986) in that clients derive control over specific behavior-event contingencies that may have previously deterred functional goal attainment. Naming and framing the process for the client following the successful completion of a problem-solving exercise is important, particularly for those in the active/maintenance phase of readiness. In this way, clients can fully own this technique and it can become part of their personal repertoire for disease self-management at the completion of a therapeutic encounter. As chronic health problems present challenges, which change over time, the therapeutic goal of problem solving is not only to solve the problem at hand but also to leave the client with a strategy for managing future challenges. While the technique outlined here has been successfully used in caregiver interventions, more research is required to evaluate the benefits of different approaches to problem solving and iterations of this technique with clients from diverse socioeconomic and cultural backgrounds and with a wider range of problem areas.

Although engagement in problem solving may not match every client's needs and abilities, therapists have the requisite professional knowledge and skill to be able to modify the process to accommodate different levels of abilities. An approach such as that proposed here, which is systematic yet flexible, is an important part of the tool kit that occupational therapists can bring to the patient/family encounter.

References

Bandura, A. (1986). Social Foundations of Thought and Action: A Social Cognitive Theory. Englewood Cliffs, NJ: Prentice-Hall.

Belle, S.H., Burgio, L., Burns, R., et al. (2006). Enhancing the quality of life of Hispanic/Latino, Black/African American, and White/Caucasian dementia caregivers: The REACH II randomized controlled trial. *Ann Intern Med*, 145, 727–738.

Bodenheimer, T., Lorig, K., Homan, H., and Grumbach, K. (2002). Patient self-management of chronic disease in primary care. *JAMA*, 288, 2469–2475.

Chee, Y., Gitlin, L.N., Dennis, M.P., and Hauck, W.W. (2007). Predictors of caregiver adherence to a skill-building intervention among dementia caregivers. *J Gerontol Med Sci*, 62(6), 673–678.

Chodosh, J., Morton, S.C., Mojica, W., et al. (2005). Meta-analysis: chronic disease self-management programs for older adults. *Ann Intern Med*, 143(6), 427–438.

Cuijpers, P., van Straten, A., and Warmerdam, L. (2007). Problem solving therapies for depression: a meta-analysis. *Eur Psychiatry*, 22, 9–15.

Farrell, K., Wicks, M.N., and Martin, J.C. (2004). Chronic disease self-management improved with enhanced self-efficacy. *Clin Nurs Res*, 13(4), 289–308.

Gellis, Z.D., and Kenaley, B. (2008). Problem-solving therapy for depression in adults: a systematic review. *Res Social Work Pract*, 18, 117–131.

Gitlin, L.N., Winter, L., Corcoran, M., Dennis, M., Schinfeld, S., and Hauck, W. (2003). Effects of the home environmental skill-building program on the caregiver-care recipient dyad: Six-month outcomes from the Philadelphia REACH Initiative. *Gerontologist*, 43(4), 532–546.

Gitlin, L.N., Winter, L., Dennis, M., Corcoran, M., Schinfeld, S., and Hauck, W. (2006). A randomized trial of a multi-component home intervention to reduce functional difficulties in older adults. *J Am Geriatr Soc*, 54, 809–816.

Hibbard, J.H., Stockard, J., Mahoney, E. R., and Tusler, M. (2004). Development of the Patient Activation Measure (PAM): Conceptualizing and measuring activation in patient and consumers. *Health Serv Res*, 39, 1005–1026.

Lorig, K.R., Sobel, D.S., Ritter, P.L., Laurent, D., and Hobbs, M. (2001). Effect of a self-management program on patients with chronic disease. *Effect Clin Pract*, 4(6), 256–262.

Prochaska, J.O., and Velicer, W.F. (1997). The transtheoretical model of health behavior change. *Am J Health Prom*, 12, 38–48.

Reuben, D.B. (2007). Better care for older people with chronic diseases: an emerging vision. *JAMA*, 298(22), 2673–2674.

Richards, K.C., Enderlin, C.A., Beck, C., McSweeney, J.C., Jones, T.C., and Roberson, P.K. (2007). Tailored biobehavioral interventions: a literature review and synthesis. *Res Theory Nurs Pract*, 21, 271–285.

Schulz, R., Burgio, L., Burns, R., et al. (2003). Resources for enhancing Alzheimer's caregiver health (REACH): Overview, site-specific outcomes, and future directions. *Gerontologist*, 43(4), 514–520.

Chapter 19
Teaching and Supporting Clients with Dementia and Their Caregivers in Daily Functioning

Maud J.L. Graff

Look, he is happy doing the gardening by himself with these adaptations. Now, I don't feel helpless anymore and I have time to do my own activities.

—A caregiver wife

Abstract Community-based occupational therapy for clients with dementia and their caregivers is a client-centered and family-centered intervention that enables clients with dementia to participate in meaningful activities of daily living (ADL) in their own environment. It enables caregivers to support these clients in ADL and reduce the caregiver's burden. Occupational therapists (OTs) achieve this outcome first by analyzing the life stories and the needs and motivations for meaningful daily activities of these clients and their caregivers in the past and present, second by enabling clients with dementia to do meaningful activities in ways that will enhance their ability to participate by using strategies to compensate for their cognitive decline, and thirdly by modifying the client's environment to better support participation. Caregivers are trained in supervision and problem solving and in using cognitive and behavioral strategies to change their coping behavior and reduce their burden of care.

Keywords Behavioral interventions • Caregiver burden • Dementia • Environmental adaptations • Home modifications.

Definition

Dementia is a chronic and degenerative disease that causes disorders of memory; behavioral problems; and loss of initiative, of independent functioning in daily activities, and of participation in social activities. These problems (1) decrease the well-being of people with dementia and their caregivers (Graff et al., 2007), (2) put pressure on family and friends' relationships (Coen, 1998; Graff et al., 2006a,b; Jepson et al., 1999) and (3) cause high health-care costs.

Community-based occupational therapy for clients with dementia and their caregivers is a *client-and-caregiver-centered intervention*. The intervention enables

I. Söderback (ed.), *International Handbook of Occupational Therapy Interventions*,
DOI: 10.1007/978-0-387-75424-6_19, © Springer Science+Business Media, LLC 2010

clients to participate in meaningful activities of daily living (ADL) in their present environment and helps caregivers to support these clients with dementia in these activities and reduce their caregiver burden. These definitions follow the World Federation of Occupational Therapists (WFOT, 2004), the Canadian Association of Occupational Therapists (CAOT, 2008), the consensus of guidelines of this community-based occupational-therapy program (Graff et al., 1998, 2000, 2003, 2006b; van Melick et al. 1998, 2000), and the Dutch Foundations of Occupational Therapy (Kuijper et al., 2006).

Development of the Intervention

This client-caregiver–centered intervention (van Melick et al., 1998, 2000) was developed in 1996 to 1998 by a workgroup of occupational-therapy experts in a consensus process (Graff et al., 1998, 2000). Its feasibility was tested (Graff et al., 1998, 2000), and the contents and process of community occupational therapy were identified through a qualitative case-study analysis (Graff et al., 2006b).

Purpose, Rationale, and Objectives

The intervention is directed to *clients* with dementia and their *caregivers*. The focuses are on conducting optimal adaptation of the limitations caused by the dementia clients' cognitive decline. The aims are improvement of problem- solving and coping behavior and maintenance of skills that enable clients to participate in meaningful everyday activities. The aims for the caregivers are to give them support and to facilitate their burden so that they in turn encourage the clients' participation in meaningful ADL. The intervention goals are based on the needs, interests, beliefs, habits, and roles of both clients and caregivers. This intervention approach is based on the model of human occupation (MOHO) (Kielhofner, 2007) and narrative methods (Hasselkus, 1990; Riopel-Smith and Kielhofner, 1998). Here, information originating from clients' and caregivers' stories, beliefs, needs, interests, habits, roles, norms, and goals are interpreted for use in the goal-setting and intervention processes.

Method

Candidates for the Intervention

The intervention is directed at all people with *mild to moderate dementia* (Mini–Mental State Examination [MMSE] score of 10 to 24) (Folstein et al., 1983), who are living in the community, and at their caregivers (partners, family members, neighbors, or friends) who support them at least one day a week, or at people living in homes for the elderly.

Epidemiology of Dementia and Caregiving

Dementia is one of the three major diseases that make the largest demands on health care (Meerding et al., 1998; Wimo et al., 1998, 2003, 2006), and is a major cause of disability and care burden in the elderly (Jönsson et al., 2006).

The world prevalence of dementia has recently been estimated at 24.3 million people. This is expected to double over the next 20 years (Ferri et al., 2005). In 2002, in the Netherlands, nearly 1% of 65-year-olds suffered from dementia. This percentage rose with increasing age to around 40% in people aged 90 and over. In 2050, it is predicted that 2.2% of 65-year-olds will suffer from dementia. Older people with dementia (age >65 years) are mostly women (80%). Of the younger people with dementia (age <65 years), the mean age is 59 years; here 50% are men and 50% are women (Dutch Health Council, 2002).

In 2003, dementia was responsible for 5.3% of the total health care costs, which was 14% of the age-specific total costs for people aged 75 to 84 and 22% for people aged 85 and older (Sobbe et al., 2006). In 2002, 39% of dementia patients needed continuous care, 38% needed home care daily, 23% needed home care occasionally, and 60% of community- dwelling dementia patients had a need for daily or continuous care.

In the Netherlands, there are 3.73 million caregivers. Most are the partners (70%) or daughters (28%) of people with dementia. About 750,000 people deliver care for more than 8 hours per week and for longer than 3 months, and 150,000 to 200,000 caregivers report a very high burden of care (Raad voor de Volksgezondheid en Zorg, 2006). Therefore, it is important to implement effective and efficient health care interventions that increase the independence and well-being of people living with dementia, decrease caregiver burden, and permit a more efficient use of scarce health care resources (Karlsson et al., 1998).

Settings

Occupational therapy aimed at clients with dementia and their caregivers is conducted at the client's home, in a community-based occupational therapy programs, or in a nursing home (Graff et al., 2006b, 2008; Kenens and Hingstman, 2003). Referrals to occupational therapy are made from outpatient services, memory clinics, hospitals, nursing homes, homes for the elderly, outpatient mental health services, and community health services, and by general practitioners.

The Role of the Occupational Therapist in Applying the Intervention

With this client-caregiver–centered intervention, the caregiver acts as the expert of his own caregiving situation. In such an extensive, interactive, and complicated intervention situations, the OT has different roles for different intervention approaches. The OT has the role of a *supervisor and teacher* when the cognitive and behavioral approach is conducted, and fulfills the role of a *coach* and a *consultant* when acting together with the caregivers and the team members.

Results

Clinical Application

Both clients and caregivers are actively involved in this process.

The Diagnostic Phase

This phase is conducted by performing interviews with the dementia client and the caregiver. Narrative techniques are used, such as the Occupational Performance History Interview (OPHI; Kielhofner et al., 1998; Riopel-Smith and Kielhofner, 1998) and the Ethnographic Interview (Hasselkus, 1990). The stories of both the client and the caregiver are analyzed in relation to needs, interests, beliefs, habits, roles, and motivation for meaningful activities. The process is completed with the clients' and the caregivers' expressed desire to choose and prioritize their most important problems in occupational performance. Each one of these interviews is interpreted together with the story of the OT.

The story of the OT is based on the observations of (1) the clients' skills in performing meaningful ADL, (2) caregivers' skills in supporting the clients' performance, and (3) the social and physical environment. This phase cover four sessions.

The Goal-Settings Phase

The goals are stated based on the results of the diagnostic phase and in cooperation with both clients and the OT during one session.

The Intervention Phase

The interventions are tailor-made to each individual client and caregiver's circumstances and adapted to their personal abilities and the actual possibility of adapting the social and physical environment. This phase contains five sessions over 5 weeks.

The following strategies, or combinations of them, are used:

- *The rehabilitation strategy.* The clients perform tasks in natural ways and thus demonstrate their skill levels.
- *The cognitive and behavioral strategy.* During these sessions, caregivers are taught how to cope with the clients' behavior and to solve problems that occur. Moreover, the caregivers are trained to support the clients' meaningful tasks. The aim is to reduce the caregivers' burden of care and to improve caregivers' participation in their own meaningful activities. The caregivers learn about the clients' disease and behavior, technical skills (task simplification and communication skills), problem solving, and home modification skills.
- *The compensation strategy* includes the clients learning how to use strategies, such as verbally rehearsing sequential steps, which compensate for their cognitive decline. For example, the OT teaches a client with dementia how to perform one of the gardening activities by using appropriate strategies such as first saying the steps that will be performed during this activity, accordingly looking around for environmental adaptations and instructions, and listening to verbal cues of the caregiver, and making use of these environmental adaptations, cues, and instructions.
- The OT conducts environmental adaptations, such as simplifications in the environment with the use of visual or hearing memory aids and written sequential task plans.

The Intervention Eases Impairments, Activity Limitations, and Participation Restrictions

The effect of occupational therapy should be based on its quality, that is, on whether or not a goal is reached. For example, if the client is able to perform only one meaningful activity several times a week, this result may improve the client's occupational performance and participation in ADL, and increase his or her and or the caregiver's quality of life, mood, and well-being (Graff et al., 2006b).

Evidence-Based Practice

Outcomes of this client-caregiver–centered intervention are diverse, client-driven, and measured in terms of participation in ADL, competence, or satisfaction derived from participation.

This client-caregiver–centered community occupational therapy program was evaluated in a pilot study that assessed its quality and practical usefulness (Graff et al., 1998, 2000). The caregiver role was identified by describing the process and contents of program (Graff et al., 2006b).

The effectiveness of community-based occupational therapy for older people with dementia and their caregivers ($n=135$) was effective in improving the participants' daily functioning (skills and need for assistance), mood and quality of life, and the caregiver's sense of competence (Graff et al., 2006a, 2007). The results were supported by Gitlin et al. (2001, 2005) and by Steultjens et al. (2004).

Moreover, community-based occupational therapy was found to be cost-effective (Slobbe, et al., 2006; Graff et al., 2008) in terms of improvement in clients' skills in daily functioning, a decrease in the need for help, and an increase in the feeling of competence in the caregivers (Graff et al., 2008).

References

Canadian Association of OTs (CAOT) Web site. (2008). The definition of the CAOT.

Coen, J. (1998). Dementia and caregiving. J Health Gain, 2, 5–6.

Dutch Health Council. (2002). Gezondheidsraad. Rapport: Dementie [Report: Dementia]. Den Haag: Gezondheidsraad, publication No. 2002/04 [in Dutch].

Ferri, C.P., Prince, M., Brayne, C., et al. (2005). Global prevalence of dementia: a Delphi consensus study. Lancet, 366, 2112–2117.

Folstein, M.F., Robins, L.N., and Helzer, J.E. (1983). The mini-mental state examination. Arch Gen Psychiatry, 40(7), 812.

Gitlin, L.N., Corcoran, M., Winter, L., Boyce, A., and Hauck, W.W. (2001). A randomised, controlled trial of a home environment intervention: Effect on efficacy and upset in care givers and on daily functioning of persons with dementia. Gerontologist, 41, 4–14.

Gitlin, L.N., Hauck, W.W., Dennis, M.P., and Winter, L. (2005). Maintenance of effects of the home environmental skill-building programme for family care givers and individuals with Alzheimer's disease and related disorders. J Gerontol A Biol Med Sci, 60, 368–374.

Graff, M.J.L. (1998). Onderzoeksrapport: Het ontwikkelen en testen van de standaard ergotherapie voor de diagnostiek en behandeling van geriatrische patiënten met niet-ernstige cognitieve stoornissen [Research report: the development and testing of a guideline for the occupational therapy diagnosis and treatment of older persons with non-severe cognitive impairments]. Nijmegen: UMC St. Radboud [in Dutch].

Graff, M.J.L., Adang, E.M.M., Vernooij-Dassen, M.J.M., et al. (2008). Community occupational therapy for older patients with dementia and their caregivers: a cost-effectiveness study. BMJ, 336, 134–138. BMJ online 2008; doi:10.1136/bmj.39408.481898.BE.

Graff, M.J.L., and van Melick, M.B.M. (2000). The development, testing and implementation of an occupational therapy guideline. The guideline for the OT diagnosis and treatment of older persons with cognitive impairments. Ned Tijdschr Ergother, 28, 169–174 [in Dutch].

Graff, M.J.L., Vernooij-Dassen, M.J.F.J., Hoefnagels, W.H.L., Dekker, J., and de Witte, L.P. (2003). Occupational therapy at home for older individuals with mild to moderate cognitive impairments and their primary caregivers: a pilot study. Occup Ther J Res, 23, 155–164.

Graff, M.J.L., Vernooij-Dassen, M.J.M., Thijssen, M., Dekker, J., Hoefnagels, W.H.L., and OldeRikkert, M.G.M. (2006a). Effects of community occupational therapy in patients with dementia: A randomised controlled trial. BMJ, 333, 1196; BMJ online 2006, doi:10.1136/bmj.39001.688843.BE.

Graff, M.J.L., Vernooij-Dassen, M.J.F.J., Zajec, J., OldeRikkert, M.G.M., Hoefnagels, W.H.L., and Dekker, J. (2006b). Occupational therapy improves the daily performance and communication of an older patient with dementia and his primary caregiver: s case study. Dementia, 5, 503–532.

Graff, M.J.L., Vernooij-Dassen, M.J.M., Thijssen, M., Dekker, J., Hoefnagels, W.H.L., and OldeRikkert, M.G.M. (2007). Effects of community occupational therapy in care givers of patients with dementia: a randomised controlled trial. J Gerontol Med Sci A, 62(9), 1002–1009.

Hasselkus, B.R. (1990). Etnografic interviewing: A tool for practice with family caregivers for the elderly. Occup Ther Pract, 2, 9–16.

Jepson, C., McCorkle, R., Adler, D., Nuamah, I., and Lusk, E. (1999). Effects of home care on caregivers' psychosocial status. Image J Nurs Sch, 31, 115–120.

Jönsson, L., Eriksdotter Jönhagen, M., Kilander, L., et al. (2006). Determinants of costs of care for patients with Alzheimer's disease. Int J Geriatr Psychiatry, 21, 449–459.

Karlsson, G., Wimo, A., Jönsson, B., and Winblad, B. (1998). Methodological issues in health economic studies of dementia. In: Wimo, A., Karlsson, G., Jonsson, B., and Winblad, B., eds. The Health Economics of Dementia. Chichester: Wiley.

Kenens, R.J., and Hingstman, L. (2003). Cijfers uit de registratie van ergotherapeuten [registration of occupational therapists] 2002. Utrecht: Nivel.

Kielhofner, G. (2007). Model of Human Occupation: Theory and Application, 4th ed. Baltimore: Williams & Wilkins.

Kielhofner, G., Malisson, T., Crawford, C., et al. (1998). A User's Manual for the Occupational Performance History Interview (version 2.1). Chicago: University of Illinois.

Kuijper, C., de Vries-Kempes, W., and Wijnties, M. (2006). Hoofdstuk 5: Betekenisvolle deelname van alledag: Wonen, werken en vrije tijd. [Meaningful participation in daily life: living, work and leisure time.] In: Kinébanian, A., and Le Granse, M, eds. Grondslagen van de ergotherapie, 2e druk [Foundations of occupational therapy.] Maarssen: Elsevier gezondheidszorg [in Dutch].

Meerding, W.J., Bonneux, L., Polder, J.J., Koopmanschap, M.A., and van der Maas, P.J. (1998). Demographic and epidemiological determinants of healthcare costs in Netherlands: cost of illness study. BMJ, 317, 111–115.

Raad voor de Volksgezondheid en Zorg (RVZ). (2006). Arbeidsmarkt en zorgvraag. Achtergrondstudies [Labour Market and Care Demand. Background Studies.] Den Haag: RVZ.

Riopel-Smith, R., and Kielhofner, G. (1998). Occupational Performance History Interview II. Chicago: University of Illinois.

Slobbe, L.C.J., Kommer, G.J., Smit, J.M., Groen, J., Meerding, W.J., and Polder, J.J. (2006). Kosten van Ziekten in Nederland 2003 [Costs of Illnesses in The Netherlands 2003]. Bilthoven: RIVM, [in Dutch].

Steultjens, E.M.J., Dekker, J., Bouter, L., Jellema, S., Bakker, E.B., and vandenEnde, C.H.M. (2004). Occupational therapy for community dwelling elderly people: A systematic review. Age Ageing 33, 453–460.

van Melick, M.B.M., and Graff, M.J.L. (2000). Ergotherapie bij geriatrische patiënten. De standaard voor de ergotherapeutische behandeling van geriatrische patiënten met niet- ernstige cognitieve stoornissen. Ned Tijdschr Ergother, 28, 176–181.

van Melick, M.B.M., Graff, M.J.L., and Mies, L. (1998). Standaard ergotherapie voor de diagnostiek en behandeling van geriatrische patiënten met niet-ernstige cognitieve stoornissen [A guideline for the OT diagnosis and treatment of older persons with cognitive impairments.] Nijmegen: UMC St. Radboud, [in Dutch].

Wimo, A., Jönsson, B., Karlsson, G., and Winblad, B. (1998). Health economics approaches to dementia. In: Wimo, A., Karlsson, G., Jönsson, B., and Winblad, B., eds. The Health Economics of Dementia. Chichester: Wiley, 1998.

Wimo, A., Jonsson, I., and Winblad, B. (2006). An estimate of the worldwide prevalence and direct costs of dementia in 2003. Dement Geriatr Cogn Disord, 21, 175–181.

Wimo, A., Winblad, B., Aguero Torres, H., and von Strauss, E. (2003). The magnitude of dementia occurrence in the world. Alzheimer Dis Assoc Disord, 17, 63–67.

World Federation of OTs (WFOT). (2008). Web site: the definition of the WFOT of 2004.

Chapter 20
Metacognitive Occupation-Based Training in Traumatic Brain Injury

Jennifer Fleming

It wasn't until the client watched the video of himself trying to cook dinner that he understood that he needed to use a checklist to keep on track.

Abstract Clients with impaired self-awareness following brain injury may benefit from an occupation-based approach to metacognitive training that uses real-life meaningful occupations in a supported therapy context. Metacognitive training aims to improve clients' intellectual awareness by demonstrating the impact of impairments on activities and participation, and thereby facilitate realistic collaborative goal setting and strategy use. Occupational performance takes place in real-life contexts to provide familiar structured experiences that allow for error recognition and error correction. Training strategies include the use of self-prediction before occupational performance; self-monitoring and self-checking during performance; and self-evaluation, verbal or video feedback, and education following performance. The occupational therapist plays a supportive role and monitors the client's emotional responses. A small but growing body of research evidence supports the use of occupation-based metacognitive training.

Keywords Brain injuries • Closed head injuries • Cognition • Human activities • Meta-cognitive strategies • Self-awareness.

Historical Development of Cognitive Teaching Approaches

Education has traditionally been incorporated as a component of cognitive rehabilitation by occupational therapists (OTs) alongside remedial and adaptive approaches to intervention (Unsworth, 1999). Teaching clients and their family members about the nature of cognitive impairments and providing feedback on cognitive performance is fundamental to assisting clients in understanding and accepting limitations in occupational performance. While most early research on the link between self-awareness and engagement in and feedback on functional performance was from

I. Söderback (ed.), *International Handbook of Occupational Therapy Interventions*, DOI: 10.1007/978-0-387-75424-6_20, © Springer Science+Business Media, LLC 2010

the field of psychology (e.g., Berquist and Jacket, 1993; Klonoff et al., 1989), this approach falls naturally within the domain of occupational therapy. Descriptions of the application of cognitive teaching approaches in the context of occupation can be found in the texts by Katz (1998, 2005).

Research evidence for a systematic occupation-based approach to the assessment and treatment of intellectual functions in people with acquired brain damage was first provided by Soderback (1988a,b). This randomized trial of 67 patients demonstrated that intellectual functions improved using intellectual training approaches that incorporated functional tasks (housework), pen-and-paper tasks, and a combination of both approaches to a greater extent than regular occupational therapy rehabilitation (Soderback, 1988a). Abreu and Toglia (1987) presented a cognitive rehabilitation model for occupational therapy, which emphasized the teaching/learning process as an important component of therapy. Since then, both authors have been pivotal in establishing the link between cognition and occupation in rehabilitation, and Katz (2005) includes chapters by each describing sophisticated models that incorporate self-awareness.

Definition

An occupation-based approach to metacognitive training (Fleming et al., 2006) uses real-life meaningful occupations in a supported therapy context to assist clients with brain injury to *develop self-awareness* and, in turn, facilitate realistic goal setting and strategy use. It is based on neuropsychological theories of the role of the frontal lobes in self-awareness. *Metacognitive strategies* and training techniques are drawn from the multicontext treatment approach proposed by Toglia (1998).

Background

Occupation-based metacognitive training emerged from work in the 1990s that emphasized the importance of timely, specific, consistent, and respectful feedback to clients about the nature of limitations in task performance (Barco et al., 1991; Mateer, 1999). Subsequently, Toglia and Kirk (2000) proposed a model of self-awareness that highlights the dynamic relationship between clients' self-knowledge and beliefs about their abilities (intellectual awareness) and the situational or "on-line" awareness generated during occupational performance (e.g., error recognition, error correction, error anticipation, and behavioral compensation). The authors recommended intervention strategies that engage the client in familiar structured experiences that allow for self-monitoring and evaluation. The premise of occupation-based metacognitive training is that the on-line experience of limitations during occupational performance facilitates the development of the client's intellectual awareness or self-knowledge.

Purpose

Occupation-based metacognitive training aims to remediate clients' metacognitive functioning by assisting them to recognize the extent of brain-injury–related impairments, and their impact on activities and participation. Gains in self-awareness can then be used as a starting point for realistic collaborative goal setting and selection of appropriate compensatory strategies, with the ultimate aim of improving occupational performance.

Method

Candidates for the Intervention

Occupation-based metacognitive training has been designed for use with adults with traumatic brain injury and other acquired brain injuries (such as stroke) that result in impairment of metacognitive functions (including self-awareness) mediated by the prefrontal cortex. It is intended to improve function including body structures of the brain (International Classification of Functioning, Disability, and Health [ICF] codes 1100 to 1103) and specific mental functions (ICF codes b140 to b189). Impairments targeted are described using various terms including *impaired self-awareness, denial of disability, lack of insight, unawareness, anosognosia,* and dysexecutive syndrome.

Epidemiology

There are no specific epidemiologic statistics as to the proportion of clients who may benefit from the intervention. However, occupation-based metacognitive training is not considered appropriate for all people with brain injury who display impaired self-awareness. In particular, clients who present with denial of disability, which is primarily the result of a psychological defense mechanism, may experience psychological distress if confronted with difficulties during occupation-based training. These clients are more likely to respond to psychological support, counseling, or psychotherapeutic approaches to facilitate adjustment (Fleming and Ownsworth, 2006). An occupation-based approach is considered more successful with clients whose impaired self-awareness is primarily due to neurologic damage such as injury to the prefrontal cortex and impaired executive function. In contrast to clients with defensive denial of disability who tend to respond to feedback in a resistant or angry manner, clients with neurologically based impaired self-awareness have a more surprised or indifferent response (Katz et al., 2002).

In a cluster analysis study of 84 participants with acquired brain injury (Ownsworth et al., 2007), only 14% were classified as having poor self-awareness, which appeared to be due to neurologic deficits in error self-regulation. Therefore, it could be assumed that this approach may be applicable to approximately 14% of people with acquired brain injury, although this requires further investigation. The investigation may also be useful for clients who have impaired self-awareness due to environmental factors such as lack of opportunity to experience injury-related disabilities either due to the recency of injury or the high levels of assistance by others (Fleming and Ownsworth, 2006).

Settings

Occupation-based metacognitive training is designed for use in real-life contexts so that activities can be meaningful and relevant to client's goals. Occupational performance in the client's natural environment allows the client to make direct comparison with preinjury performance. It is therefore most applicable to community-based rehabilitation settings where therapy occurs in the client's home, workplace, or local community. However, the intervention can be used in outpatient rehabilitation settings using simulated activities, although the effectiveness of this approach has not been evaluated.

The Role of the Occupational Therapist

The occupational therapist (OT) uses collaborative goal-setting techniques to select appropriate target occupations, and grades activities to provide sufficient challenge to the client. The OT selects and introduces metacognitive training strategies before task performance (e.g., self-prediction of numbers of errors or self-estimation of time for task completion). During the client's task performance, the OT provides prompts to encourage self-checking (e.g., stop every 2 minutes to check the recipe) and self-questioning (e.g., "Am I paying attention? Have I missed any steps?"). Following task completion, the OT encourages the client to self-evaluate, provides verbal or video feedback, educates the client about the nature of any identified problems, and facilitates selection of appropriate compensatory strategies. The OT plays a supportive role by closely monitoring the client's reaction to experiential feedback at all times, and intervening should any emotional distress or excessive frustration be displayed. The aim of the OT is to make the clients' experience a positive one of self-discovery and problem solving, which will result in gains in self-awareness being translated into productive functional gains rather than a failure experience.

Results

A Brief Guide to Clinical Application of the Intervention

The OT assists clients in choosing an activity that is relevant and meaningful to their occupational goals, and in which their current performance is limited. For clients with very low levels of self-awareness, this can be done in consultation with a family member. Examples include meal preparation, shopping, washing the car, ironing, writing a job application, taking lecture notes, or a leisure activity. It is important that the selected activity present a level of "just-right" challenge, which allows some success so as not to be overwhelmingly difficult, but at the same time provides opportunity for errors or difficulties to become apparent. Using metacognitive techniques such as self-prediction of performance before engaging in the activity, and time-monitoring, self-checking, self-evaluation, and self-questioning during and after the performance, discrepancies between the client's predicted and actual performance are highlighted (Toglia, 1998). Task performance may be videotaped to enhance the client's self-evaluation. Other techniques that are less confrontational include role reversal, in which the OT performs the task and the client detects errors (Toglia, 1998). At the end of the session, the client and OT discuss any difficulties that the client experienced, and use this improved self-knowledge as a platform to generate realistic therapy goals and choose relevant compensatory strategies. In subsequent sessions, the same process is repeated with the incorporation of compensatory strategy training.

How the Intervention Eases Impairments, Activity Limitations, and Participation Restrictions

Occupation-based metacognitive training is aimed at the remediation of impairments in metacognitive functions include error-recognition, error-correction, self-awareness, and strategy selection. It also targets activity limitations in the specific areas of occupational performance that are selected by clients as meaningful and challenging for them, by facilitating use of the appropriate strategies. This can have a flow-on effect in mitigating participation restrictions and enhancing engagement in valued occupational roles.

Evidence-Based Practice

While earlier intervention studies employing occupation-based metacognitive training have provided level IV case study evidence of its effectiveness (Fleming et al., 2006;

Katz et al., 2002; Landa-Gonzalez, 2001; Ownsworth et al., 2006), a recent randomized control has provided level II evidence supporting the intervention (Ownsworth et al., 2008). Ownsworth et al. (2008) compared an individual occupation-based intervention with group-based support and a combined group and individual intervention in a sample of 35 community-dwelling participants with acquired brain injury. Interventions were 3 hours per week for 8 weeks. Significant gains on performance self-ratings and relatives' ratings on the Canadian Occupational Performance Measure (COPM) (Law et al., 1994) were found for both the individual occupation-based intervention and the combined intervention at postintervention and 3-month follow-up assessments. Significant gains in psychological well-being were also found at follow-up for the individual occupation-based intervention.

Discussion

There is mounting research evidence that occupation-based metacognitive training is effective in improving the occupational performance of some clients with acquired brain injury. Clients are supported in the context of a safe therapeutic relationship to experience brain-injury–related activity restrictions and to develop strategies for dealing with them. Arguably, this is preferable to clients' attempting to reintegrate into the community and experiencing repeated failures without support. Nevertheless, with any attempt to facilitate the development of self-awareness, there is a *risk of emotional distress* for clients as they become aware of the extent of postinjury changes. The OTs' clinical reasoning skills are required to determine those clients for whom low self-awareness is more reflective of psychologically based denial, and to refer these clients to more intensive counseling to facilitate adjustment to their loss before participating in occupation-based training. However, further research is needed to test the suitability of occupation-based metacognitive training for particular types of clients.

References

Abreu, B.C., and Toglia, J.P. (1987). Cognitive rehabilitation: a model for occupational therapy. Am J Occup Ther, 41, 439–448.

Barco, P.P., Crosson, B., Bolesta, M.M., Werts, D., and Stout, R. (1991). Training awareness and compensation in postacute head injury rehabilitation. In: Kreutzer, J.S., and Wehman, P.H.. eds. Cognitive Rehabilitation for Persons with Traumatic Brain Injury: A Functional Approach (pp. 129–146). Baltimore, MD: Paul H. Brookes.

Berquist, T.F., and Jacket, M.P. (1993). Programme methodology: awareness and goal setting with the traumatically brain injured. Brain Injury, 7, 275–282.

Fleming, J.M., Lucas, S.E., and Lightbody, S. (2006). Using occupational to facilitate self-awareness in people who have acquired brain injury: a pilot study. Can J Occup Ther, 73, 44–54.

Fleming, J.M., and Ownsworth, T. (2006). A review of awareness interventions in brain injury rehabilitation. Neuropsychol Rehabil, 16, 474–500.

Katz, N. (1998). Cognition and Occupation Across the Lifespan. Models for Intervention in Occupational Therapy. Bethesda, MD: American Occupational Therapy Association.

Katz, N. (2005). Cognition and Occupation Across the Lifespan. Models for Intervention in Occupational Therapy, 2nd ed. Bethesda, MD: American Occupational Therapy Association.

Katz, N., Fleming, J., Keren, N., Lightbody, S., and Hartman-Maeir, A. (2002). Unawareness and/or denial of disability: implications for occupational therapy intervention. Can J Occup Ther, 69, 281–292.

Klonoff, P.S., O'Brien, K.P., Prigatano, G.P., Chiapello, D.A., and Cunningham, M. (1989). Cognitive retraining after traumatic brain injury and its role in facilitating awareness. J Head Trauma Rehabil, 4, 37–45.

Landa-Gonzalez, B. (2001). Multicontextual occupational therapy intervention: a case study of traumatic brain injury. Occup Ther Int, 8, 49–62.

Law, M., Baptiste, S., Carswell, A., and McColl, M.A. (1994). Canadian Occupational Performance Measure Manual, 2nd ed. Canada: Canadian Association of Occupational Therapist, ACE Publishers.

Mateer, C.A. (1999The rehabilitation of executive disorders. In: Stuss, D.T., Winocur, G., and Robertson, I.H., eds. Cognitive Neurorehabilitation (pp. 314–332). London: Cambridge University Press.

Ownsworth, T., Fleming J., Desbois, J., Strong, J., and Kuipers, P. (2006). A metacognitive contextual intervention to enhance error awareness and functional outcome following traumatic brain injury: a single-case experimental design. J Int Neuropsychol Soc, 12, 54–63.

Ownsworth, T., Fleming, J., Shum, D., Kuipers, P., and Strong, J. (2008). Comparison of individual, group and combined intervention formats in a randomized controlled trial for facilitating goal attainment and improving psychosocial function following acquired brain injury. J Rehabil Med, 40, 81–88.

Ownsworth, T., Fleming, J., Strong, J., Radel, M., Chan, W., and Clare, L. (2007). Awareness typologies, long-term emotional adjustment and psychosocial outcomes following acquired brain injury. Neuropsychol Rehabil, 17, 129–150.

Soderback, I. (1988a). The effectiveness of training intellectual functions in adults with acquired brain injury: an evaluation of occupational therapy methods. Scand J Rehabil Med, 20, 47–56.

Soderback, I. (1988b). A housework-based assessment of intellectual functions in patients with acquired brain damage: development and evaluation of an occupational therapy method. Scand J Rehabil Med, 20, 57–69.

Toglia, J., and Kirk, U. (2000). Understanding awareness deficits following brain injury. Neurorehabilitation, 15, 57–70.

Toglia, J.P. (1998). A dynamic interactional model to cognitive rehabilitation. In: Katz, N., ed. Cognition and Occupation in Rehabilitation. Cognitive Models for Intervention in Occupational Therapy (pp. 5–50). Bethesda MD: AOTA.

Unsworth, C. (1999). Cognitive and Perceptual Dysfunction. A Clinical Reasoning Approach. Philadelphia: F.A. Davis.

Chapter 21
Metacognitive Mental Imagery Strategies for Training of Daily Living Skills for People with Brain Damage: The Self-Regulation and Mental Imagery Program

Karen P.Y. Liu and Chetwyn C.H. Chan

The use of meta-cognitive strategies has demonstrated the positive effects to improve clients' relearning and performance of simple motor function as well as complicated daily tasks.

Abstract Meta-cognitive strategies are thought to assist people suffering from brain damage in relearning daily living tasks. The use of self-regulation and mental imagery as metacognitive strategies used in an intervention program is described. The program requires the clients' active participation. The evidence is gathered from two case reports, four randomized clinical trials, one controlled clinical trial, and one review paper.

Keywords Brain damage • Metacognition • Mental imagery • Occupational performance • Self-regulation.

Definition

Occupational performances and *task performances* include all daily activities and are interchangeably used in this chapter.

Strategies are the teaching techniques used by OTs to promote clients' active participation and problem solving during their occupational performances. *Metacognitive strategies*, such as self-regulation and mental imagery, refer to the efficient use of self-awareness to self-regulate occupational performances (Shimamura, 2000).

Self-regulation refers to the identification and correction of one's own deficits through self-reflection (Liu et al., 2002; Lucas and Fleming, 2005). Individuals applying the self-regulation strategy are able to govern their own learning by acknowledging the requirement of effort in success, apply appropriate means to utilize their efforts, and regulate their activities. Clients employing self-regulation are able to learn actively to achieve the set goals. Self-regulation is used as a cognitive strategy for (1) helping clients identify problems encountered in doing the tasks after brain damage, (2) seeking appropriate solutions based on their previous

I. Söderback (ed.), *International Handbook of Occupational Therapy Interventions*,
DOI: 10.1007/978-0-387-75424-6_21, © Springer Science + Business Media, LLC 2010

experience of the task requirement, and (3) revealing their present understanding of their dysfunction. These strategies help clients to relearn impaired functions.

Mental imagery is a process in which a performance is rehearsed mentally as if the person is actually performing it. It is believed to enhance relearning by involving the client in actively memorizing the information of how the performance is performed (Liu et al., 2004a,b).

Purpose

Clients with brain damage use metacognition, that is, cognitive strategies of self-regulation and mental imagery, for performing daily living tasks to enhance relearning, maintenance, and generalization of occupational performances.

Method

Candidates for the Intervention

Clients who have experienced problems in occupational performance due to brain damage and mainly have poor mobility functioning or a low energy level are the potential candidates for the Self-Regulation and Mental Imagery Program.

In our studies, clients suffering from a brain damage, and who meet the following inclusion criteria, are recruited to participate: (1) diagnosed as having suffered a first unilateral cerebral infarction as confirmed by a computed tomography scan, (2) over the age of 60, (3) independent in carrying out daily activities prior to the brain damage, and (4) able to communicate effectively as screened by the Cognistat (Chan et al., 2002).

Epidemiology

In Hong Kong, there are more than 20,000 clients admitted to the hospital for brain damage treatment each year. About 40 brain damage clients had entered the studies since year 2000. Thus far, approximately 200 brain damage clients have participated in the Self-Regulation and Mental Imagery Program.

Settings

The Self-Regulation and Mental Imagery Program is carried out in a rehabilitation hospital with a major brain damage unit. The intervention program is performed at the occupational therapy department.

The Role of the Occupational Therapist

The occupational therapist (OT) provides guidance to clients in developing strategies to overcome deficits in occupational performance. Throughout the intervention, the OT acts as a teaching facilitator, who engages the client into the process of the Self-Regulation and Mental Imagery Program.

Results

Clinical Application

The Rationale of the Self-Regulation and Mental Imagery Intervention Program

The rationale underlying the Self-Regulation and Mental Imagery Program is that it enables the clients to (1) evaluate his or her *ability*, and (2) *plan* how the actions of a task should be executed before it is performed in reality. This strategy is similar to *stop, think, and act*, which is commonly used by therapists working with children with special needs (Post et al., 2006).

Self-regulation involves clients' identifying the steps for a complete performance of a task, occupation, or activity. With these steps clients identify the perceived problems in the performance when compared with their ability before the brain injury occurred. The client is guided to find the solutions to these problems by looking at the issues arising with each of the steps and then brainstorming the possible solutions.

For example, a client with right hemiplegia identifies "losing balance" as the problem. This problem occurs in the "fold the laundry" task (Table 21.2), that is, when he reaches out to take a laundry item from the laundry basket. If the client is unable to identify a solution, the OT guides the client by offering various possible suggestions for the client to try out. Based on the usefulness of these various suggestions, the OT guides the client to identify the most effective solution. After trying different ways, the solution would be effective if the client puts the basket closer to his left side or holds the abdominal muscles tight when reaching for the basket. The client then practices using this solution to solve the laundry task and other tasks. Through this process, the client learns to self-regulate the task performances, which enables him to develop a deeper insight in the functioning.

Mental imagery is the platform with which clients rehearse the processes of analyzing the task, identifying problems, generating solutions, and mentally practicing the self-rectified performance on the task. Each of the steps of this process is listed in Table 21.1.

Table 21.1 Use of mental imagery in occupational performance training of clients suffering from brain damage or brain damage

Task analysis enhancement	Tell the participant the task to be trained.
	Get the participant to identify the steps in the task through mentally imagining the task.
	Present the participant with the computer-generated task steps for verification of self-identified steps.
Problem identification	Get the participant to visualize his or her own performance with the help of the steps shown in the computer program on the steps of the task.
	Get the participant to identify the problems encountered and solutions in each step by going through the mental process.
Task performance	Get the participant to imagine his or her own task performance with the rectified steps.
	Get the participant to actually perform the task and videotape the performance.
	Get the participant to evaluate the performance on the videotape so as to adjust the problems and solutions.
	Repeat the above steps until the participant learns the tasks with the proper method

The Self-Regulation and Mental Imagery Intervention Program

This program focuses on clients' active self-education for performing daily living tasks that they performed smoothly before the brain damage occurred. The client learns to perform the daily tasks (Table 21.1) by using the strategies of self-regulation and mental imagery. The OT guides the client to develop appropriate strategies to overcome the problems.

The program takes 3 weeks. The clients receive training in five 1-hour sessions each week. The client performs the specific daily tasks included in each session. These tasks include, for example, functioning of mobility, balance, and upper limb coordination. The level of difficulty of each set of tasks is organized in a demand-ascending order (Table 21.1). However, among these tasks the demands are overlapping. The training of the easiest task set (e.g., folding laundry) is practiced in the first week, while the most difficult task set (e.g., shopping and use of transportation) is practiced in the third week. This design aims to enhance generalization of skills learned from one stage to another (Liu et al., 2004a,b).

The *first* week is used for training of the clients' skills in using *self-regulations*. The client identifies the deficits in performing the various sequential steps of a task (e.g., for tearing the tea bag). Once identified, the client would need to generate the best alternatives to complete the task. Examples of the best alternatives would be stabilizing the tea bag with the weaker arm or using the better hand to manipulate the tea bag while tearing the tea bag. Tasks used in the program are presented in Table 21.1.

The second and third weeks are used for training the clients' ability to perform tasks based on mental imagery. Here, the clients mentally rehearse the solutions generated from the self-regulation, as if the task is to be executed with the process. The work process for use of mental imagery is presented in Table 21.2.

Table 21.2   The daily tasks used for training, assessment, and the evaluation criteria

	Daily tasks for training
Week 1	Put clothes on hanger
	Fold the laundry
	Prepare a cup of tea
	Wash the dishes
	Carry out a money transaction
Week 2	Prepare fruit
	Make the bed
	Take medication
	Use the telephone
	See the doctor
Week 3	Sweep the floor
	Tidy the table after a meal
	Fry vegetables with meat
	Go to a park/outdoors
	Go to the canteen

Previous studies indicate that mental imagery was composed of sequential mental processes, which include attention, memory, and visualization of images and generalization (Chow et al., 2007).

Evidence-Based Practice

The self-regulation is widely applied (1) in the field of education for behavioral management and problem solving (Post et al., 2006), (2) to enhance self-awareness of impairments (Lucas and Fleming, 2005), and (3) for conducting occupational performance tasks for a client with brain damage (Liu et al., 2002). Mental imagery is most often used in training of motor function (moving blocks, reaching for and grasping an object). An audiotape (Page, 2000; Page et al., 2001, 2005) or occupational performances (Liu et al., 2002, 2004a,b) were used to guide the imagery process. The results of a literature review showed positive effects on recovery of arm function after stroke (Braun et al., 2006; Dijkerman et al., 2004; Page, 2000; Page et al., 2001, 2005). Liu et al. (2002, 2004a,b) showed that using metacognitive strategies had positive effects on improving performance on tasks learned in the program and generalization effects to other occupations apart from those used during the training sessions. This positive effect lasted 1 month after discharge from the program.

Discussion

People with brain damage participate in rehabilitation programs. The role of OTs is to teach clients to relearn occupational performance of daily living tasks. Here, various teaching methods are used.

The most common method is demonstration and then practice. After analyzing the clients' behavioral problems, OTs generate ways of rectifying the problem and demonstrate the rectified behavior for the client, who learns through imitation. The effectiveness of this teaching method is called into question.

Instead, metacognition using the strategies of the self-regulation and mental imagery, that is, the clients' active awareness of the process of learning, is a critical ingredient in successful learning. This learning approach initiates the clients' ways of solving the problems and planning for the action. The results last over time and even generalize to new tasks.

Mental imagery is more effective if those who practice the technique have a thorough understanding of their own body capacity. This principle is applied when the strategy of the self-regulation is used to help clients to recapture their own capabilities and become familiar with their "new" body functioning.

Mentally rehearsing the performance can serve as a supplement to carrying out the task among clients who find performance of tasks too demanding because they have poor mobility functioning or a low energy level.

Conclusion

Previous studies have demonstrated the positive effects of using the meta-cognitive strategies to improve clients' understanding, relearning of performance, and motor function. This research offers further evidence concerning the role of active cortical control, which can be mediated by self-regulation and mental imagery to enhance the relearning potential of clients with brain damage.

References

Braun, S.M., Beurskens, A.J., Borm, P.J., Schack, T., and Wade, D. T. (2006). The effects of mental practice in brain damage rehabilitation: a systematic review. Arch Phys Med Rehabil, 87, 842–852.
Chan, C.C.H., Lee, T.M.C., Fong, K., Lee, C., and Wong, V. (2002). Cognistat profile for Chinese client with brain damage. Brain Injury, 16, 873–884.
Chow, K.W.S., Chan, C.C.H., Huang, Y., Liu, K.P.Y., Li, L.S.W., and Lee, T.M.C. (2007). Temporal course of vibrotactile imagery. Neuroreport, 18, 999–1003.
Dijkerman, H.C., Letswaart, M., Johnston, M., and MacWalter, R.S. (2004). Does motor imagery training improve hand function in chronic brain damage patients? A pilot study. Clin Rehabil, 18, 538–549.
Liu, K.P.Y., Chan, C.C.H., Lee, T.M.C., and Hui-Chan, C.W.Y. (2004a). Mental imagery for promoting relearning for people after brain damage: a randomized controlled trial. Arch Phys Med Rehabil, 85, 1403–1408.
Liu, K.P.Y., Chan, C.C.H., Lee, T.M.C., and Hui-Chan, C.W.Y. (2004b). Mental imagery for relearning of people after brain injury. Brain Injury, 18, 1163–1172.
Liu, K.P.Y., Chan, C.C.H., Lee, T.M.C., Li, L.S.W., and Hui-Chan, C.W.Y. (2002). Case reports on self-regulatory learning and generalization for people with brain injury. Brain Injury, 16, 817–824.

Lucas, S.E., and Fleming, J.M. (2005). Intervention for improving self-awareness following acquired brain injury. Aust Occup Ther J, 52, 160–170.

Page, S.J. (2000). Imagery improves upper extremity motor functions in chronic brain damage patients with hemiplegia: a pilot study. Occup Ther J Res, 20, 200–215.

Page, S.J., Levine, P., and Leonard, A.C. (2005). Effects of mental practice on affected limb use and function in chronic brain damage. Arch Phys Med Rehabil, 86, 399–402.

Page, S.J., Levine, P., Sisto, S. and Johnston, M.V. (2001). A randomized efficacy and feasibility study of imagery in acute brain damage. Clin Rehabil, 15, 233–240.

Post, Y., Boyer, W., and Brett, L. (2006). A historical examination of self-regulation: helping children now and in the future. Early Child Educ J, 34, 5–14.

Shimamura, A.P. (2000). Toward a cognitive neuroscience of metacognition. Consciousness Cogn, 9, 313–323.

Chapter 22
Strategies to Compensate for Apraxia Among Stroke Clients – The Cognitive Strategy Training

Caroline van Heugten and Chantal Geusgens

Apraxia influences the daily life of stroke clients. Strategy training is the preferred intervention because it is expected to include generalization; that is, training effects are established from trained to nontrained tasks and across settings.

Abstract Apraxia is a "cognitive disorder characterized by the inability to perform previously learned skills" (National Library of Medicine, 2008) that influences stroke clients' ability to perform daily life tasks (Bjorneby and Reinvang, 1985; Foundas, 1985). Treatment of apraxia should be part of a rehabilitation program because of its negative impact on daily life. *Cognitive strategy training* is the preferred form of treatment, as it focuses on improving daily life functioning by compensating for lost functions, despite the probably lasting presence of apraxia. In addition, strategy training has the advantage over skills training because of generalization of training results to other tasks and other contexts.

Keywords Apraxia • Generalization • Stroke.

Definitions

There are two types of apraxia that may cause severe disabilities in activities of daily living (ADL):

- *Ideomotor apraxia* is a condition that affects the implementation of purposeful and meaningful skills, such as the inability to carry out a complex motor activity. A client with ideomotor apraxia knows what to do, but does not know how to do it (De Renzi, 1989). The most frequent errors in ideomotor apraxia are (1) the use of body parts as objects, for example, brushing the teeth with a finger; (2) spatial orientation problems such as use of inappropriate hand postures as for example, cutting with the wrong part of a knife (Heilman and Gonzalez-Rothi, 1985; Miller, 1986; Shelton and Knopman, 1991). A client with ideomotor apraxia may not be able to perform on command, while the same activity may be executed perfectly in a natural setting (De Renzi et al., 1980).

I. Söderback (ed.), *International Handbook of Occupational Therapy Interventions*,
DOI: 10.1007/978-0-387-75424-6_22, © Springer Science+Business Media, LLC 2010

- *Ideational apraxia* is the inability to formulate mentally the processes involved when performing an action. The person does not know what to do because the idea or concept of the motor act is lacking (De Renzi, 1989). It is expressed as (1) omitting parts of an activity; (2) incorrect use of tools and things; and (3) sequence errors, that is, errors in the order in which activities are done (De Renzi and Lucchelli, 1988). Dressing apraxia may result from an inability to formulate mentally the act of placing clothes on the body (National Library of Medicine, 2008; Tate and McDonald, 1995); for example, the person first puts on his shoes and then tries to fit the socks over the shoes.

Cognitive strategy training or substitution (Donkervoort et al., 2001; van Heugten et al., 1998) uses compensatory strategies for clients with apraxia. It is based on theories of neuropsychology (such as models of human information processing) (Schiffrin and Schneider, 1997), occupational therapy practice (Kielhofner, 2004; Law, et al., 1998; Trombly and Ma, 2002), and educational psychology (Singley and Anderson, 1989). The client's independent functioning is maximized by improving ADL performance, while little change is expected in cognitive remediation that influences the severity of the apraxia itself.

Compensation is achieved by teaching clients to change their behavior to perform motor actions. Clients are taught to use *external strategies* (e.g., point-lists with one instruction for each of the movements required to carry out the motor functions for performing a specific daily-life task, such as brushing one's teeth) or *internal strategies* (e.g., verbalizing the steps of which the daily-life task consists covertly), and techniques to reach their goals in alternative ways. Strategy training is widely used and is effective in the rehabilitation of cognitive deficits such as memory, executive functioning, and apraxia (Cicerone et al., 2000; 2005). During the intervention, the client is taught to use more efficient and more independent strategies.

The newly learned strategy is expected not only to be item-specific, for example, the client is able to perform the trained task more smoothly and easily, but also to *generalize* to other, nontrained tasks. Generalization means that a strategy is not task-specific but relies on principles that are more general. Generalization is the degree to which transfer effects are found. The client is able to transfer the motor actions to different tasks and settings. Transfer relates to the way in which prior learning affects new learning or performance (Geusgens, 2007).

Cognitive strategy training is practiced in the Netherlands as the *"occupational therapy protocol for the assessment and intervention of stroke clients with apraxia"* (Stehmann-Saris et al., 1996).

Purpose

Cognitive strategy training is the occupational therapy intervention aimed at improving the clients' ability to carry out motor actions, establishing generalization effects from trained to nontrained tasks and across settings (Cicerone et al., 2000, 2005).

Method

Candidates for the Intervention

Cognitive strategy training is intended (1) for clients who present with apraxia behavior in the subacute phase of a stroke, caused by damage in the left or right hemisphere of the brain (De Renzi, 1989), and preferably with the apraxia persisting beyond the first 2 weeks and before 15 weeks post-stroke; (2) for clients diagnosed with Huntington's disease; and (3) for clients diagnosed with Alzheimer's disease. Either sex can be enrolled for the intervention. The intervention is effective in clients of average age 60 to 70 years (range 39 to 91 years). There are no reasons to exclude clients because of old age. Moreover, neither the severity of the apraxia nor the presence of cognitive comorbidity seems to cause a less favorable intervention outcome.

Epidemiology

Stroke is the second most common cause of death and a major cause of long-term disability worldwide (Doman et al., 2008). Of all survivors, 54% experience ADL disabilities. Usually apraxia follows left-hemisphere lesions and is reportedly present in 30% to 50% of all left-sided stroke clients (Zwinkels et al., 2004). Apraxia at the start of the rehabilitation period predicts a dependent ADL outcome 1 year after stroke (Sundet et al., 1988).

Setting

Cognitive strategy training is given in rehabilitation centers, nursing homes, and hospital departments. It has been offered from 8 to 15 weeks post-onset (Donkervoort et al., 2001; Van Heugten et al., 1998).

The Role of the Occupational Therapist

The role of the occupational therapist (OT) during the cognitive strategy training is to (1) determine the client's level of functioning, (2) apply the intervention individually, (3) teach the cognitive strategies, and (4) structure the various tasks used for training during the sessions.

Results

Clinical Application of the Intervention

The presence of apraxia hindering the client's execution of ADL is established by a multidisciplinary team and with the special responsibility of a neuropsychologist.

Occupational therapy assessments are used to define what tasks the client cannot execute and are important for the client to relearn. The protocol contains (1) the assessment instruments recommended for use, (2) the ADL observations (van Heugten et al., 2000), and (3) a description of the process and contents of the strategy training.

The Intervention Includes

The Individual Choice of Meaningful Activities

The individual chooses meaningful activities to perform for the training sessions. These choices are made in collaboration between the client and the family together with the OT. Any task that relates to the client's interest, lifestyle, and remaining capacities can be used. For example, the Canadian Occupational Performance Measure (COPM) (Law et al., 1998) or the Activity Card Sort (ACS) (Baum and Edwards, 2001) is suitable to use for making this choice. The COPM is an individualized outcome measure for use by OTs to detect change in a client's self-perception of occupational performance. The ACS provides an immediate impression of the client's activity patterns.

The Intervention Goals

The intervention goals are determined by investigation of the specific consequences of apraxia for the client's daily life. Clients' problems and errors in motor performance and their style of action are investigated. This is attained with ADL observations using a standardized way to assess clients' level of independent functioning. Here, the Arnadóttir OT-ADL neurobehavioral evaluation (the "A" one) (Arnadóttir, 1990) may be used. The ADL observations are performed by choosing two or more tasks and following the client's performance in a natural environment.

The client's performance of the completed task (the overall independence score) and following three sequence phases, representing the course thereof, are observed:

- *Orientation:* The OT prepares the task by explaining how the task should be performed in the actual environment.
- *Execution:* The OT observes how the client performs the actual task, with special regard to how the client starts, performs, and stops the motor functioning.
- *Control:* The OT checks the results of the actions.

The client's errors and the level of assistance needed are noted on the protocol using a scale of 0 to 3:

- 0 = no assistance needed, performance is adequate
- 1 = verbal assistance needed
- 2 = physical assistance needed to handle objects and guide hand postures
- 3 = OT takes over activity

Each of the three phases (orientation, execution, and control) is linked to a specific type of intervention, as follows:

- If the focus is on the orientation phase, the intervention will be aimed at instructions.
- If the focus is on the execution phase, intervention will be aimed at providing guidance.
- If a focus is on the control phase, the intervention will be aimed at providing feedback, or teaching the client how to use feedback.

The Specific Strategy

The specific strategy that will be used during training is the next decision the OT makes. This needs to be adjusted to the phase of task performance, and thus to the intervention type. The strategy needs to be attuned to the client's strengths and weaknesses, as follows:

- Strategies for instructions to support the preparation of the performance when the client's performances deficits occur in the *orientation* phase:

  - Give instructions more than once and use extra attention.
  - Ask questions about the performance.
  - Demonstrate the performance or its parts.
  - Give a written description of the performance.
  - Show pictures of the task performance.
  - Show objects needed for the task.
  - Hand objects to the client one by one.
  - Take over performance or its parts.

- Strategies for instructions to support the preparation for the performance when the client's performance deficits occur in the *execution* phase are guidance strategies:
  - Show pictures.
  - Guide with verbal support.
  - Guide with physical support.
  - Start with a slow tempo.
  - Start with only one object.
  - Show objects needed for the task.
  - Hand objects to the client (one by one).
  - Take over the performance or its parts.

- Strategies for instructions to support the preparation for the performance when the client's performance deficits occur in the *control* phase are feedback strategies:
  - Give verbal feedback.
  - Show the result in a mirror.
  - Make video recordings to show to the client.
  - Ask questions about the result ("Did you put on your socks?").
  - Make pictures to show to the client.

The Role of the Occupational Therapist

The OT has to monitor the client's task performance and can evaluate the effects of the intervention after each fourth training session, using the ADL observations. This evaluation will help the therapist to decide how to continue with new goals.

Evidence-Based Practice

Evidence for the effectiveness of interventions that compensate for apraxia has only been established for stroke clients with left hemisphere lesions, not for apraxia clients with Huntington's disease or Alzheimer's disease (Donkervoort et al., 2001; Edmans et al., 2000; Smania et al., 2000; Van Heugten, 2001; West et al., 2008).

The effectiveness of cognitive strategy training has been demonstrated in a non-controlled pre- and posttest study involving a 12-week intervention using the OT protocol for strategy training included left-hemisphere stroke clients with apraxia ($n = 33$) (Van Heugten et al., 1998). The findings showed that the clients had learned to compensate for their apraxia-based problems.

A randomized two-group clinical trial (cognitive-strategy training, or intervention as usual) was conducted with left-hemisphere-stroke clients with apraxia ($n = 113$). After 8 weeks, strategy training was significantly more effective in improving ADL functioning than was the usual intervention (Donkervoort et al., 2001).

In another study, the cognitive strategy training transfer (generalization) effects from trained ADL tasks to nontrained ADL tasks and from the rehabilitation setting to the clients' own home improved daily life functioning in left-hemisphere-stroke clients ($n = 29$) with apraxia. The transfer effects of ADL functioning were stable at a 5-month follow-up (Geusgens et al., 2007a).

Discussion

The OT intervention using cognitive strategy training for apraxia in stroke clients with left-hemisphere lesions demonstrably improves daily life functioning and has generalization effects. Educational psychology has considered how to promote transfer of learning. If positive transfer effects are to occur, clients should know what transfer of strategies is and how it works, and should be aware of their own functioning before they will acknowledge that a strategy is needed to improve their motor functioning, and finally to be able to judge when and where the transfer can be applied. The client needs to understand the connection between what is learned and the situation in which it is learned. This might be overcome by practicing a strategy or skill in greatly varying situations. Training that promotes transfer should be addressed during the training sessions, as transfer cannot occur automatically.

The OT should teach general knowledge because this type of knowledge is easier to transfer than specific knowledge (Geusgens et al., 2007b).

References

Arnadóttir, G.T. (1990). The Brain and Behaviour. St. Louis, MO: Mosby.

Baum, C., and Edwards, D. (2001). Activity Card Sort Test Kit. St Louis, MO: Washington University.

Bjorneby, E.R., and Reinvang, I.R. (1985). Acquiring and maintaining self-care skills after stroke. The predictive value of apraxia. *Scand J Rehabil Med*, 17, 75–80.

Cicerone, K.D., Dahlberg, C., Kalmar, K., et al. (2000). Evidence-based cognitive rehabilitation: recommendations for clinical practice. *Arch Phys Med Rehabil*, 81, 1596–1615.

Cicerone, K.D., Dahlberg, C., Kalmar, K., et al. (2005). Evidence-based cognitive rehabilitation: updated review of the literature from 1998 through 2002. *Arch Phys Med Rehabil*, 86(8), 1681–1692.

De Renzi, E. Apraxia. (1989). In: Boller, F., and Grafman, J., eds. Handbook of Neuropsychology, vol. 2. Amsterdam: Elseviers Science Publishers.

De Renzi, E., and Lucchelli, F. (1988). Ideational apraxia. *Brain*, 111, 1173–1185.

De Renzi, E., Motti, F., and Nichelli, P. (1980). Imitating gestures: a quantitative approach to ideo-motor apraxia. *Arch Neurol*, 37, 6–18.

Doman, G.A., Fisher, M., Macleod, M., and Davis, S.M. (2008). Stroke. *Lancet*, 371(9624), 1612–1623.

Donkervoort, M., Dekker, J., Stehmann-Saris, J.C., and Deelman, B.G. (2001). Efficacy of strategy training in left hemisphere stroke patients with apraxia: a randomized clinical trial. *Neuropsychol Rehabil*, 11(5), 549–566.

Edmans, J.A., Webster, J., and Lincoln, N. (2000). A comparison of two approaches in the treatment of perceptual problems after stroke. *Clin Rehabil*, 1, 230–243.

Foundas, A.L., Macauley, B.C., Rayner, A.M., Maher, L.M., Heilman, K.M., and Rothi, L.J.G. (1985). Ecological implications of limb apraxia: evidence from mealtime behaviour. *J Int Neuropsychol Soc*, 1, 62–66.

Geusgens, C.A. (2007). Transfer of Cognitive Strategy Training After Stroke: No Place Like Home? Maastricht: Neuropsych Publishers.

Geusgens, C.A., Winkens, I., Van Heugten, C.M., Jolles, J., and Heuvel, W. van den (2007b). Occurrence and measurement of transfer in cognitive rehabilitation: a critical review. *J Rehabil Med*, 39(6), 425–439.

Geusgens, C.A.V., van Heugten, C.M., Cooijmans, J.P.J., Jolles, J., and Heuvel, W.J.A. van den (2007a). Transfer effects of a cognitive strategy training for stroke patients with apraxia. *J Clin Exp Neuropsychol*, 29(8), 831–841.

Heilman, K.M., Gonzalez-Rothi, L.J. Apraxia. (1985). In: Heilman, K.M., and Valenstein, E., eds. Clinical Neuropsychology, 2nd ed. Oxford: Oxford University Press.

Kielhofner, G. (2004). Conceptual Foundations of Occupational Therapy, 3rd ed. Philadelphia: F.A. Davis.

Law, M., Baptiste, S., Carswell, A., McColl, M., Polatajko, H., and Pollock, N. (1998). Canadian Occupational Performance Measure, 3rd ed. Ottawa, ON: CAOT Publications ACE.

Miller, N. (1986). Dyspraxia and Its Management. London: Croom Helm.

National Library of Medicine. (2008). PubMed: MeSH is NLM's controlled vocabulary used for indexing articles in PubMed. http://www.ncbi.nlm.nih.gov/entrez/query.fcgi?db=PubMed.

Schiffrin, R.M., and Schneider, W. (1997). Controlled and automatic human information processing: II. Perceptual learning, automatic attending and a general theory. *Psychol Rev*, 8, 127–190.

Shelton, P.A., and Knopman, D.S. (1991). Ideomotor apraxia in Huntington's disease. *Arch Neurol*, 48, 35–41.

Singley, M.K., and Anderson, J.R. (1989). The Transfer of Cognitive Skill. Cambridge: Harvard University Press.

Smania, N., Girardi, F., Domenicali, C., Lora, E., and Aglioti, S. (2000). The rehabilitation of limb apraxia: a study in left-brain damaged patients. *Arch Phys Med Rehabil*, 81, 379–388.

Stehmann-Saris, J.C., Van Heugten, C.M., Kinebanian, A., and Dekker, J. (1996). [OT guideline for assessment and treatment of apraxia in stroke clients]. Utrecht: NIVEL, Amsterdam and Hogeschool van Amsterdam

Sundet, K., Finset, A., and Reinvang, I.R. (1988). Neuropsychological predictors in stroke rehabilitation. *J Clin Exp Neuropsychol*, 10(4), 363–379.

Tate, R.L., and McDonald, S. (1995). What is apraxia? The clinicians dilemma. *Neuropsychol Rehabil*, 5(4), 273–297.

Trombly, C.A., and Ma, H. (2002). A synthesis of the effects of occupational therapy for persons with stroke. Part I: Restoration of roles, tasks and activities. *Am J Occup Ther*, 5, 250–259.

Van Heugten, C.M. (2001). Rehabilitation and management of apraxia after stroke. *Rev Clin Gerontol*, 11, 177–184.

Van Hengten C.M., Dekker, J., Deelman, B.G., Dijk, A.J., A.J. Van Stehmann-Saries, J.C., and Kinebanian, A. (1998). Outcome of strategy training in stroke patients with apraxia: a phase II study. *Clin Rehabil,*12, 294–303.

Van Hengten C.M., Dekker, J., Deelman, B.G., Dijk, A.J., A.J. Van Stehmann-Saries, J.C., and Kinebanian, A. (2000). Measuring disabilities in stroke patients with apraxia: a validation study of an observational method. *Neuropsychol Rehabil*, 10(4), 401–414.

West, C., Bowen, A., Hesketh, A., and Vail, A. (2008). Interventions for motor apraxia following stroke (Review). *Cochrane Database Systematic Review*, 23(1),CD004132.

Zwinkels, A., Geusgens, C., Sande. P., and van Heugten, C. (2004). Assessment of apraxia: inter-rater reliability of a new apraxia test, association between apraxia and other cognitive deficits and prevalence of apraxia in a rehabilitation setting. *Clin Rehabil*, 18(7), 819–827.

Chapter 23
Delivering Energy Conservation Education by Teleconference to People with Multiple Sclerosis

Marcia Finlayson

> *The program broke things down into simple basic things that I could do to manage my fatigue—things I didn't think about before the course.*
>
> —Participant

Abstract Fatigue is one of the most common and disabling symptoms reported by people with multiple sclerosis (MS). Teaching people with MS how to manage their fatigue using energy conservation strategies is an important role for occupational therapists (OTs). Typically, these strategies are taught face to face, either in groups or on a one-to-one basis. For some people with MS, traveling to a location for this education is difficult. Therefore, teleconference delivery can be a viable option.

Keywords Multiple sclerosis • Self-management • Tele-health

Background

Fatigue is reported by 75% to 90% of people with multiple sclerosis (MS), making it one of the most common symptoms of the disease (Multiple Sclerosis Council for Clinical Practice Guidelines [MS Council], 1998). People with MS have described fatigue as frustrating, overwhelming, immobilizing, and disabling (Holberg and Finlayson, 2007; McLaughlin and Zeeberg, 1993). The MS Council (1998) defined fatigue as "a subjective lack of physical and/or mental energy that is perceived by the individual or caregiver to interfere with usual and desired activities" (p. 2).

Energy conservation education is a key part of comprehensive fatigue management in MS and is one of the primary roles of the occupational therapist (OT) on the MS care team. Energy conservation education teaches people with MS to examine their energy use and modify activities to reduce fatigue (MS Council, 1998). These modifications can occur at the level of the person, the environment, or the activity itself.

Improvements in fatigue impact, quality of life, self-efficacy for managing fatigue, and the use of energy conservation strategies have been demonstrated through face-to-face delivery of the energy conservation education program "Managing

I. Söderback (ed.), *International Handbook of Occupational Therapy Interventions*,
DOI: 10.1007/978-0-387-75424-6_23, © Springer Science+Business Media, LLC 2010

Fatigue" (Mathiowetz et al., 2005, 2007; Matuska et al., 2007; Packer et al., 1995). A group teleconference version of the program was developed in response to requests by clients with MS (Finlayson, 2005).

Purpose

The purpose of the teleconference energy conservation intervention is to maintain and promote occupational performance and engagement among people with MS by reducing fatigue severity and fatigue impact and by improving self-efficacy for managing fatigue and overall quality of life.

Method

Candidates for the Intervention

Candidates for the intervention are adults with MS (International Classification of Diseases [ICD-10] code G35). This disease is typically diagnosed in patients between the ages of 20 and 50, and is more common among women and people of Northern European descent.

Epidemiology

This intervention targets adults with MS who experience moderate to severe fatigue, as measured by a Fatigue Severity Scale score of 4 or more (Krupp et al., 1989). The short version of the Blessed Orientation Memory Concentration test (Katzman et al., 1983) is used to identify individuals who have the requisite attention and concentration to participate. Individuals who have difficulty accessing face-to-face education programs are specific targets for the intervention.

Settings

The intervention is advertised through community settings, MS clinics, and MS support groups. Interested individuals volunteer and are screened for eligibility by telephone. Because this is a teleconference intervention, individuals can participate by dialing into the sessions from the location of their choice.

The Role of the Occupational Therapist

The OT functions as an educator, coach, and facilitator by introducing and explaining energy conservation strategies, providing examples of strategy application, promoting discussion and sharing across participants, encouraging and answering questions, and supporting vicarious learning. The OT may also be involved in recruiting and screening participants and organizing program logistics.

Results

Clinical Application

The intervention is a community-based, group educational program guided by psych-oeducational group theory (Brown, 2004) and informed by existing self-management interventions for people with chronic illness (Lorig and Holman, 2003). It is a modification of the intervention published by Packer et al. (1995) to accommodate teleconference delivery (Finlayson, 2005). The intervention is a closed group that includes six sessions held once a week for 6 weeks. Ideal group size is five or six participants.

Each session is 1 hour and 10 minutes in length. Participants are provided with a telephone, a headset, and a program binder, and they dial into a toll-free conference call line at a designated time. The major topics of the six sessions are as follows:

- Rest
- Communicating with others about fatigue
- Using good body mechanics and setting up activity stations
- Activity analysis and modification
- Planning and setting priorities
- Goal setting for long-term use of strategies

Across the entire intervention, 14 energy conservation strategies are taught. (Table 23.1) (Finlayson, 2005).

Delivering an occupational therapy intervention through a group teleconference call is challenging, and requires a high level of knowledge of group dynamics and strong group facilitation skills. Participants must be provided with tips for participating in a group teleconference, and therapists must be prepared to deal with technological problems. Preintervention introductory calls from the therapist can mitigate participant anxiety, if it exists. Intervention costs include the teleconference line and associated charges, telephones, and headsets for participants, and copying and distribution of the program binders.

Table 23.1 Energy conservation strategies taught in the course (Finlayson, 2005)

Energy conservation strategies
- Adjust priorities by choosing how to spend available energy
- Change the way the body is positioned during an activity to conserve energy
- Use adaptive equipment, gadgets, or energy-saving devices to conserve energy
- Eliminate part or all of an activity to conserve energy
- Stop to take a rest in the middle of a long activity to manage energy
- Plan days to balance work and rest times to manage energy
- Ask for help from family or friends to manage energy
- Reduce standards for an activity in order to reduce the amount of energy it takes
- Change the location of equipment, furniture, or supplies at home or work to conserve energy
- Change work heights at home or at work to conserve energy
- Simplify activities so they require less energy
- Change the time of day an activity is done to manage energy
- Include rest periods in the day, or rested at least one hour/day in order to manage energy
- Delegate part or all of an activity to another person to conserve energy

How the Intervention Eases Impairments, Activity Limitations, and Participation Restrictions

Participants build knowledge of energy conservation strategies and develop confidence in their abilities to apply these strategies through peer support and vicarious learning. Participants learn, refine, and generalize the application of the strategies across a range of activities through discussion, exploration, practice, and reflection.

Evidence-Based Practice

A pilot test of the intervention was conducted in 2003–2004 with 29 people with MS. On average, they were 47 years of age and had been living with MS for 14 years (Finlayson, 2005). Pilot results demonstrated significant reductions on the Fatigue Severity Scale (Krupp et al., 1989) ($t = 2.34$, df $= 28$, $p = .03$; effect size $= 0.52$) and significant reductions on the Fatigue Impact Scale (Fisk et al., 1994) ($t = 2.09$, df $= 28$, $p = .05$; effect size $= 0.44$). Participants also reported using several strategies taught during the course, based on findings from the Energy Conservation Strategies Survey (Mallik et al., 2005). Between pre- and post intervention, the greatest percent change in strategy use was found for resting (+93%), planning the day to balance work and rest (+69%), changing work heights (+67%), and using gadgets and adapted devices (+67%). The intervention was well received, perceived as providing useful assistance for fatigue management, and was relevant to participants' everyday lives (Finlayson and Holberg, 2007; Holberg and Finlayson, 2007).

Discussion

Delivering an educational intervention without the benefit of visual feedback to gauge participant understanding is challenging. As tele-health and distance education technologies continue to advance, this challenge will eventually be remediated. The promising pilot findings have led to a randomized control trial that includes a 6-month follow-up. The study is currently underway, with funding from the National Institute of Disability and Rehabilitation Research (grant H133G070006). It will conclude in late 2010. Future research will need to compare participant outcomes and cost-effectiveness between the teleconference delivery model and a more traditional face-to-face model.

References

Brown, N.W. (2004). Psychoeducational groups: Process and practice, 2nd ed. New York: Brunner-Routledge.

Finlayson, M. (2005). Pilot study of an energy conservation education program delivered by telephone conference call to people with multiple sclerosis. NeuroRehabilitation, 20, 1–11.

Finlayson, M., and Holberg, C. (2007). Evaluation of a energy conservation course delivered by teleconference to people with multiple sclerosis. Can J Occup Ther, 74, 337–347.

Fisk, J.D., Ritvo, P.G., Ross, L., Haase, D.A., Marrie, T.J., and Schlech, W.F. (1994). Measuring the functional impact of fatigue: initial validation of the fatigue impact scale. Clin Infect Dis, 18(Suppl 1), S79–S83.

Holberg, C., and Finlayson, M. (2007). Factors influencing utilization of energy conservation strategies by people with multiple sclerosis. Am J Occup Ther, 61, 96–107.

Katzman, R., Brown, T., Fuld, P., Peck, A., Schechter, R., and Schimmel, H. (1983). Validation of a short orientation-memory-concentration test of cognitive impairment. Am J Psychiatry, 140, 734–739.

Krupp, L.B., LaRocca, N.G., Muir-Nash, J., and Steinberg, A.D. (1989). The fatigue severity scale. Application to patients with multiple sclerosis and systemic lupus erythematosus. Arch Neurol, 46, 1121–1123.

Lorig, K.R., and Holman, H. (2003). Self-management education: history, definition, outcomes, and mechanisms. Ann Behav Med, 26, 1–7.

Mallik, P.S., Finlayson, M., Mathiowetz, V., and Fogg, L. (2005). Psychometric evaluation of the Energy Conservation Strategies Survey. Clin Rehabil, 19, 538–543.

Mathiowetz, V., Finlayson, M., Matuska, K., Chen, H.Y., and Luo, P. (2005). A randomized trial of energy conservation for persons with multiple sclerosis. Multiple Sclerosis, 11, 592–601.

Mathiowetz, V.G., Matuska, K.M., Finlayson, M.L., Luo, P., and Chen, H.Y. (2007). One-year follow-up to a randomized controlled trial of an energy conservation course for persons with multiple sclerosis. Int J Rehabil Res, 30, 305–313.

Matuska, K., Mathiowetz, V., and Finlayson, M. (2007). Use and perceived effectiveness of energy conservation strategies for managing multiple sclerosis fatigue. Am J Occup Ther, 61, 62–69.

McLaughlin, J., and Zeeberg, I. (1993). Self-care and multiple sclerosis: a view from two cultures. Soc Sci Med, 37, 315–329.

Multiple Sclerosis Council for Clinical Practice Guidelines. (1998). Fatigue and Multiple Sclerosis: Evidence-Based Management Strategies for Fatigue in Multiple Sclerosis. Washington, DC: Paralyzed Veterans of America.

Packer, T.L., Brink, N., and Sauriol, A. (1995). Managing Fatigue: A Six-Week Course for Energy Conservation. Tucson, AZ: Therapy Skill Builders.

Chapter 24
Psychoeducational Groups

Sandra Hale and Jocelyn Cowls

I valued a lot of the exercises. They were all good introductions to the topic and they also got you involved.

—Participant

Abstract Clients attending psychoeducational groups report that in addition to skills learned and social benefits, the activities reinforce content, assist in establishing healthy milieus, encourage involvement in the group, and assist with the recollection of the topic discussed (Cowls and Hale, 2005).

Keywords Mental health • Psychoeducational groups • Rehabilitation

Background

The therapeutic value of group work has long been supported by a variety of disciplines, predominantly psychology, psychiatry, social work, nursing, and rehabilitation. Groups in mental health settings aid in promotion of hope, universality ("I am not alone with my problems"), and mutual support (Yalom, 1995). Psychoeducational groups often bring together people with similar illness states or health-related concerns. Effective learning can occur in group settings through individuals sharing concerns and strategies used to overcome them. This is much more powerful than didactic relaying of information (Anderson, 2001).

Definition

Psychoeducational groups are defined as groups that offer a supportive and structured environment in which to acquire new skills or focus on task accomplishment (Brown, 1998). The professionals involved can ensure that current, up-to-date information is provided.

I. Söderback (ed.), *International Handbook of Occupational Therapy Interventions*,
DOI: 10.1007/978-0-387-75424-6_24, © Springer Science+Business Media, LLC 2010

Historical Roots

Psychoeducation has its roots as a family-focused intervention. It is considered an evidence-based approach and a useful adjunct to medication wherever possible in the treatment and prevention of mental health issues (Colom et al., 2003). It is used with mental health clients interested in learning new ways of coping and problem solving. Skills learned can assist people to improve functioning in their personal and work lives. Topics addressed in psychoeducation vary and can include stress management, self-esteem, recognizing and managing symptoms of illness, strategies to stay well, and conflict-resolution.

Purpose

Psychoeducational groups can help to prevent relapses with mental health conditions by the skill teaching and information they provide. These groups can assist in maintaining wellness and can remediate recurring problems by improving knowledge of illness and coping skills and by establishing routines to restore abilities. Clients have stated that they benefit from review and repetition of information (Cowls and Hale, 2005).

Method

Candidates for the Intervention and Epidemiology

Psychoeducational groups are reportedly effective with a variety of Axis I diagnoses in the *Diagnostic and Statistical Manual of Mental Disorders* (DSM-IV), such as schizophrenia, mood disorders, anxiety disorders, eating disorders, and concurrent disorders of mental health and addiction.

The above disorders may begin in adolescence (in the case of eating disorders and anxiety disorders) and range through to adulthood. The diagnosis of schizophrenia generally varies in onset from 18 to 25 years of age. Aside from eating disorders (90% female), most illnesses mentioned affect the lives of both genders.

Psychoeducational groups have wide applicability within mental health from adolescences to older adulthood. Exclusion criteria include significant cognitive limitations that interfere with one's ability to learn and to participate in a group.

Settings

A review of the literature and clinical experience show that psychoeducational groups are used in both inpatient and outpatient settings. Although benefits have been identified in both, it can be argued that inpatients may have greater difficulty attending to, understanding, and incorporating information gained in groups into their daily life (Cowls and Hale, 2005; Sibitz et al., 2007).

Sibitz et al. (2007) found that clinical stability might be the most important prerequisite for benefiting from psychoeducational groups. They state, "This finding casts doubt on the most common recruitment setting for psychoeducational interventions, namely psychiatric hospitals, and advocates the more widespread use of psychoeducational interventions in outpatient care" (p. 914).

The Role of the Occupational Therapist in Applying the Intervention

Although a variety of health care professionals conduct psychoeducational groups, occupational therapists (OTs) bring a unique focus and method of group facilitation. When involved in a group, OTs practice as *facilitators*, empowering the client to direct and carry a large portion of group discussion. However, psychoeducational groups by definition do require structure. The OTs develop the structured content of these groups while incorporating two distinct factors: activity and link to occupational performance (participating in a task for self-care, productivity, or leisure). Recent literature suggests that OTs need to reconnect with their roots in activities. It has been stated "activity is valuable and should be promoted in order to deliver best practice for occupational therapy in mental health" (Cowls and Hale, 2005, p. 178). At present, there is a trend for many OTs to place a higher value on discussion-based groups, abandoning these roots in activity (Moll and Cook, 1997).

Results

Clinical Application

Principles for Practice

Attending a psychoeducational group should not be uniformly recommended for everyone.

An *occupationally based assessment* helps individuals to identify goals they define as central and important in their life. One such standardized assessment is the Canadian Occupational Performance Measure (COPM) (Law et al., 1998). Once occupational issues in self-care, productivity (work), or leisure have been established, goals can then be generated in partnership with the client.

The content of psychoeducational groups can be discussed to ensure that they are relevant to the clients and could assist in the recovery of identified occupations.

The assessment process is a key to developing rapport and collaborating with the client who attends a group. The results of these assessments serve as a guide for recovery and assist the client in integrating the skills from groups to their occupational goals.

If a client is reluctant to attend psychoeducational groups or uncertain of their benefits, a trial offer to try a group should be encouraged before ruling it out. Ultimately, the decision rests with the clients. Nothing will take this process further, however, than creating a collaborative, respectful working partnership. A regular review of goals and adapting them to each client's needs and abilities is central to occupational therapy practice.

Two other important principles in terms of effective group process relate to *group composition* and *readiness to attend to the content of the psychoeducational group*. People attending groups should be at comparable points in their recovery. This promotes optimal group dynamics.

Readiness to attend these groups is often dependent on where clients are in understanding, accepting, and dealing with their illness and life circumstances (Cowls and Hale, 2005).

The need for stability for participants of psychoeducational groups has been highlighted in recent qualitative studies and is understood clinically by facilitators who run them. The OTs can assist in adapting the progression from social or activity-based groups to psychoeducational groups. For example, clients may find that attendance in leisure or cooking activities gives them the opportunity to increase their comfort level for groups prior to engaging in a psychoeducational group.

Psychoeducational groups are based on the group members' having discussions or performing activities. Compared to discussion groups, clients placed higher value on groups that involve activity as either the primary function in the group or when used as a catalyst for discussion (Cowls and Hale, 2005). For example, "warm-up" activities help clients think about topics in a fun way, such as group juggling aimed at stress management, or charades for communication skills. Not only do these activities facilitate comfort and understanding of the topic, they have been noted to strengthen the memory for the content of the group. Clients often remember the activity and link this to the content of the discussion.

Evidence-Based Practice

Intervention Efficacy

The effectiveness of psychoeducational groups has been documented through research focused on outcome measures as well as client feedback (Cowls and Hale, 2005; Goldner-Vukov et al., 2007; Sibitz et al, 2007). Qualitative findings report that clients experience an increase in self-esteem, connection to others, sense of empowerment, and confidence with problem solving (Cowls and Hale, 2005; Goldner-Vukov et al. 2007).

When activity is combined with skills teaching, this process facilitates an increase in memory for the skills learned. Of special interest to OTs is that clients often experience an increase in psychosocial functioning in the spheres of self-care, productivity, and leisure (Goldner-Vukov et al. 2007).

Clients who are educated about their illness and healthy coping strategies, gain essential insight and become empowered to make healthy choices in their life. By linking clients' goals to potential benefits of psychoeducational groups, clients demonstrate increased motivation to participate in groups and implement learned skills into their daily life. For example, with the knowledge of how to manage anger assertively, clients may be more confident and perform better in the workplace knowing that they are capable of dealing with a difficult coworker. With knowledge of how to increase self-esteem, clients may take the risk of joining a community book club as a way to combine their love of reading with connecting to others and thereby increasing their leisure activities.

Evidence-Based Practice

Research provides evidence that clients often show greater improvement of measured skills when activity groups were offered (Cowls and Hale, 2005; Moll and Cook, 1997.

Typically, scientific evidence for mental health has focused on biologic therapies, namely pharmacotherapy. A growing body of evidence is emerging of the adjunctive benefit of psychosocial interventions along with pharmacotherapy. A recent study of 120 individuals diagnosed with bipolar disorder by Colom et al. (2003) demonstrated that group psychoeducation was an efficacious adjunct to lower the number of illness occurrences, detect symptoms earlier, and reduce the severity of recurrent episodic symptoms.

Qualitative studies are providing the perspective of persons who participate in these types of groups (Cowls and Hale, 2005; Goldner-Kukov et al., 2007; Sibitz et al., 2007). These findings assist in guiding practice toward what is meaningful for clients.

Discussion

Group work has been used for decades to assist people with mental health illness. Groups can be powerful change agents. Psychoeducational groups bring people together to learn life skills and new ways of solving problems (Anderson, 2001). Occupational therapists bring a unique style and vision to these groups through the use of activity and through the linking of skills to application in daily life. This is consistent with the philosophical belief that we learn by doing. Recent literature reaffirms that OTs should consider this core belief in the interventions they provide (Cowls and Hale, 2005; Eaton, 2002; Moll and Cook, 1997).

Occupational therapists aim to facilitate client's engagement in meaningful activities of occupation, in a manner that supports their health and participation in life. Bearing this in mind, the content of psychoeducational groups should fit with clients' stated goals. Skills learned needed to be meaningful and provide a link to the activity they wish to return to in the areas of self-care, productivity (work), and leisure.

A commonly recommended group size of between six to eight people represents a cost-effective treatment modality. It is recommended that OTs continue to conduct research related to the unique contributions of incorporating activity into groups and how this can facilitate returning to meaningful occupations in clients' lives.

References

Anderson, A.J. (2001). Psychoeducation. Group therapy for the dually diagnosed. Int J Psychosocial Rehabil, 5, 77–78.

Brown, N. (1998). Psychoeducational Groups. Philadelphia: Accelerated Development.

Colom, F., Vieta, E., Martínez-Arán, A., et al. (2003). A randomized trial on the efficacy of group psychoeducation in the prophylaxis of recurrences in bipolar patients whose disease is in remission. Arch Gen Psychiatry, 60, 402–407.

Cowls, J., and Hale, S. (2005). It's the activity that counts: what clients value in psychoeducational groups. Can J Occup Ther, 72(3), 176–182.

Eaton, P. (2002). Psychoeducation in acute mental health settings: Is there a role for occupational therapists. Br J Occup Ther, 65(7), 321–326.

Goldner-Vukov, M., Moore, L., and Cupina, D. (2007). Bipolar disorder: from psychoeducational to existential group therapy. Austral Psychiatry, 15(1), 30–34.

Law, M., Baptiste, S., Carswell, A., McColl, M.A., Polatajko, H., and Pollack, N. (1998). Canadian Occupational Performance Measure (COPM), 3rd ed. Ottowa, ON: CAOT Publications.

Moll, S., and Cook, J. (1997). Doing in mental health practice: therapist' beliefs about why it works. Am J Occup Ther, 51, 662–670.

Sibitz, I., Amering, M., Gossler, R., Unger, A., and Katsching, H. (2007). Patients' perspectives on what works in psychoeducational groups for schizophrenia. A qualitative study. Soc Psychiatry Psychiatr Epidemiol, 42, 909–915.

Yalom, I. (1995). The Theory and Practice of Group Psychotherapy, 4th ed. New York: Basic Books.

Chapter 25
Illness Management Training: Transforming Relapse and Instilling Prosperity in an Acute Psychiatric Ward

Sunny Ho-Wan Chan

Transforming relapse and instilling prosperity (TRIP) is a ward-based intervention program that aims to decrease treatment noncompliance and relapse rate by improving insight and health during the visits to the acute psychiatric care of clients with schizophrenia.

Abstract Participation to TRIP using the strategies learned from illness management, including knowledge enhancement, behavioral tailoring, relapse prevention development, cognitive behavioral technique, and related coping skills (Mueser et al., 2002) helps the clients adhere to treatment recommendations and minimize relapses. Moreover, TRIP is aimed at redesigning or reestablishing the clients' goal-driven healthy lifestyle. By learning how to manage the illness, the participants can be further reinforced to take part in their respective occupations.

Keywords Acute psychiatry • Healthy lifestyle • Illness management • Psycho-education • Schizophrenia.

Definition

Statements: The Theoretical Framework of the Intervention

Transforming relapse and instilling prosperity (TRIP) connotes the notions of relapse reduction and health promotion within the program (Chan et al., 2007) by using strategies. The program provides information on illness and relevant skills for coping with symptoms, and a goal-driven, healthy lifestyle is re-established or designed with the participants.

I. Söderback (ed.), *International Handbook of Occupational Therapy Interventions*,
DOI: 10.1007/978-0-387-75424-6_25, © Springer Science+Business Media, LLC 2010

Historical Development

The TRIP program has been developed to meet the needs of psychiatric inpatients. Traditionally during an acute stage of hospitalization, due to an unstable mental state, patients usually follow an activity-oriented occupational therapy program while on the ward. Such programs aim to maintain healthy activity during hospitalization by providing a normal routine selected by patients from a typical array of work, rest, and leisure activities. However, such programs cannot fully help patients reintegrate into the community on discharge. Therefore, TRIP was developed to fill this gap.

Purpose

The purpose of the intervention is to improve insight and health among clients with schizophrenia during acute psychiatric care, so that treatment noncompliance can be reduced and relapse prevented, with the ultimate aim of progressing toward personal healthy goals within clients' respective occupations.

Method

Candidates for the Intervention

Inclusion criteria for TRIP are as follows:

- Age 18–65
- Diagnosed schizophrenia or schizoaffective disorder
- Admitted to an acute psychiatric unit
- Stable mental condition after admission
- Attained primary education level or higher
- Participating voluntarily

The only exclusion criteria is a diagnosis of substance abuse, organic brain syndrome, or mental retardation.

Settings

The TRIP program is commonly carried out in a confined area or a special room in an acute psychiatric unit, equipped with a large whiteboard, notebook (with Microsoft PowerPoint), and LCD projector. Chairs are arranged in a circle.

The Role of the Occupational Therapist in Applying the Intervention

As emphasized by Eaton (2002), the occupational therapist (OT) can play a major role in delivering psychoeducational group interventions in acute mental health settings. The TRIP program is conducted mainly by an OT. Playing the roles of educator and facilitator in the group, the therapist not only teaches the clients adaptive life skills and knowledge of illness, but also facilitates the sharing of experience among clients within the group.

The therapist works with the clients to develop strategies or cues by incorporating the learning content (e.g., medication taking) into their daily routine, to connect to their respective occupation. It is also important that the therapist promote a healthy and noteworthy lifestyle within the program. This includes articulating individual personal goals and exploring how illness management (e.g., medication taking) may be useful in achieving those goals. Addressing the meaningfully personal goals among clients is crucial to motivate participation. Varieties of techniques are used to optimize learning and retention. They include interactive teaching, and emphasizing the sharing among group members. Echoing Blair and Hume (2002), the therapist in the group focuses on helping individuals to become aware of their own power by gaining life skills that give them a greater sense of personal control.

Results

A Brief Guide to Clinical Application

The TRIP program is a 2-week ward-based illness management program. It includes ten sessions, each lasting for about 50 minutes. The sessions can be further categorized into the two themes of illness orientation and health orientation.

Topics under illness orientation include the following:

- Introduction to schizophrenia
- Rehabilitation resources—residential and family services
- Rehabilitation resources—vocational and social services
- Medication management and compliance
- Relapse prevention plan development
- Symptom management
  Topics under health orientation include the following:
- Mental health
- Emotion management
- Healthy diet and lifestyle
- Stress management

The following strategies are suggested by Mueser et al. (2002, 2006) and incorporated into TRIP accordingly.

The brief goals and content of each session are as follows:

(a) Introduction to schizophrenia, which includes:

- Providing information about schizophrenia including signs and symptoms and the treatment regime
- Introducing the stress-vulnerability model
- Dispelling some myths or misconceptions about schizophrenia

(b) Rehabilitation resources—residential and family services, which include:

- Introducing the residential care services in the community
- Understanding and improving the relationship with family members

(c) Rehabilitation resources—vocational and social services:

- Introducing different kinds of vocational rehabilitation services in the community
- Introducing different kinds of social support services in the community

(d) Medication management and compliance:

- Highlighting the importance of medication compliance
- Understanding the side effects of medication
- Learning strategies to cope with the side effects
- Learning behavioral tailoring to ease medication adherence

(e) Relapse prevention plan development:

- Learning the signs and symptoms of relapse
- Recognizing environmental triggers
- Developing a contingency plan

(f) Symptom management:

- Learning preventive measure or cognitive-behavioral coping skills to deal with symptoms and related stress

(g) Mental health:

- Increasing knowledge of good mental health
- Learning methods to maintain good mental health

(h) Emotion management:

- Identifying types of unhealthy emotion
- Learning related coping methods to deal with emotion

(i) Healthy diet and lifestyle

- Building up a good habit of healthy diet
- Setting personal recovery goals
- Coestablishing a meaningfully personal goal-directed healthy lifestyle

(j) Stress management

- Increasing knowledge of sources and causes of stress
- Learning pertinent stress management methods
- Practicing related strategies

The sessions are designed in a semistructured format with didactic presentation of the topics followed by open discussion within the group. Warm-up or socialization games are introduced at the beginning of each session with homework assignments developed collaboratively with the client at the end of each session. During each session, the material is presented using an LCD projector and PowerPoint, to give the group a classroom feeling. Each participant receives educational handouts that summarize the main content of the topic, or cue cards about the strategies reviewed in every session. Visual aids used in the group can further facilitate learning and sharing among the group.

How the Intervention Eases Impairments, Activity Limitations, and Participation Restrictions

The core content of TRIP is teaching clients how to manage their illness collaboratively with treatment providers, so as ultimately to achieve their life goals. Mueser et al. (2002) reviewed ample evidence to support the effectiveness of the strategies used in the illness management program. Using those strategies, TRIP can further facilitate clients' participation in their personal occupation by underscoring goal achievement. By realizing good mental health, grasping stress management techniques, or pursuing meaningful personal goals of healthy-lifestyle building, an eventual goal of recovery with a full life beyond the illness can be achieved (Mueser et al., 2006).

Evidence from Practice

The TRIP program has positive effects on insight and health during acute psychiatric care. Kavanagh et al. (2003) emphasized the application of psychoeducation as an early intervention in the acute setting. Rebolledo and Lobato (1998) also state that the psychoeducational approach could further foster the adoption of a safer lifestyle when facing vulnerability. Health-oriented illness management can benefit patients' experiences of illness. The knowledge gained and the direct sharing of personal difficulties in various group sessions may increase patients' insight into mental health and influence their perspectives on their own well-being. Mueser et al. (2002), in a literature review, demonstrated that psychoeducation, relapse prevention, coping skills training, or a cognitive behavioral approach is effective in preventing relapse in patients with psychotic symptoms. Walling and Marsh (2000) suggested that as long as clients have learned from stress management, healthy lifestyle building, or coping skills enhancement, they can be encouraged to engage in activities to reduce the risk of relapse and improve the quality of life. In fact, both the traditional activity-based ward occupational therapy (WOT) program and TRIP can supplement each other to meet the needs of different levels of patient. During acute psychiatric care, a WOT program can be used in a very early phase for mental-state stabilization, whereas TRIP can be used in a later phase to prepare clients for discharge to the community.

Discussion

The TRIP program accepts only voluntary participants, implying that they may get better insight due to their willingness to engage in the rehabilitation program. Involuntary participants may represent a large group with "poor insight" and repeated hospitalizations. Hence further programs have to be considered to help those clients with poor insight.

The TRIP program is conducted within the hospital setting during acute psychiatric care with the aim of reducing rehospitalization; yet the effectiveness of retaining the clients in the community still awaits further systematic research. As suggested by Hornung et al. (1996) and Zygmunt et al. (2002), supportive services such as booster sessions can be an effective means of reinforcing and consolidating the knowledge taught to clients with psychiatric illness. Thus, some kinds of post-discharge program can be considered, aimed at further reducing relapse rates.

References

Blair, S.E.E., and Hume, C.A. (2002). Health, wellness and occupation. In: Creek, J., ed. Occupational Therapy and Mental Health, 3rd ed. Edinburgh, New York: Churchill Livingstone.

Chan, S.H.W., Lee, S.W.K., and Chan, I.W.M. (2007). TRIP: A psychoeducational program in Hong Kong for people with schizophrenia. Occup Ther Int, 14, 86–98.

Eaton, P. (2002). Psychoeducation in acute mental health settings: is there a role for occupational therapists. Br J Occup Ther, 65, 321–6.

Hornung, W.P., Kieserg, A., Feldmann, R., and Buchkremer, G. (1996). Psychoeducational training for schizophrenia patients background, procedure and empirical findings. Patient Educ Counsel, 29, 257–268.

Kavanagh, K., Duncan-Mcconnell, D., Greenwood, K., Trivedi, P., and Wykes, T. (2003). Educating acute inpatients about their medication: is it worth it? An exploratory study of group education for patients on a psychiatric intensive care unit. J Mental Health, 12, 71–80.

Mueser, K.T., Corrigan, P.W., Hilton, D.W., et al. (2002). Illness management and recovery: a review of the research. Psychiatr Serv, 53, 1272–1284.

Mueser, K.T., Meyer, P.S., Penn, D.L., Clancy, R., Clancy, D.M., and Salyers, M.P. (2006). The illness management and recovery program: rationale, development, and preliminary findings. Schizophr Bull, 32, 32–43.

Rebolledo, S., and Lobato, M.J. (1998). Psychoeducation for people vulnerable to schizophrenia. In: Caballo, V.E., ed. International Handbook of Cognitive and Behavioral Treatments for Psychological Disorders (pp. 571–595). New York: Pergamon.

Walling, D.P., and Marsh, D.T. (2000). Relapse prevention in serious mental illness. In: Frese, F.J., ed. The Role of Organized Psychology in Treatment of the Seriously Mentally Ill. New Directions for Mental Health Services (pp. 49–60). San Francisco: Jossey-Bass.

Zygmunt, A., Olfson, M., Boyer, C.A., and Mechanic, D. (2002). Interventions to improve medication adherence in schizophrenia. Am J Psychiatry, 159, 1653–1664.

Chapter 26
Psychosocial Intervention in Schizophrenia

Adriana D.B. Vizzotto, Patricia C. Buchain, Jorge Henna Netto,
and Hélio Elkis

*Occupational therapy intervention combined with appropriate
medication is associated with improvement in clients' condition. (Buchain et al., 2003)*

Abstract Occupational therapy as a psychosocial approach based on cognitive rehabilitation among clients with schizophrenia is discussed in this chapter. For these
clients it is demonstrated that psychopharmacologic treatment combined with
psychosocial interventions is more effective than solely psychopharmacologic
treatment. This strategy improves cognitive aspects and social functioning and consequently counteracts the deterioration caused by the illness (Huxley et al., 2000).

There is a clear evidence that clients with schizophrenia have an intensive
impairment of their executive functions (Morrice and Delahunty, 1996; Velligan
and Bow-Thomas, 1999; Wykes et al., 1999). This deficit is defined as the "negative
syndrome" of schizophrenia (Crow, 1980) and, in treatment-resistant schizophrenia,
the syndrome exhibits great intensity. Thus, occupational therapy is a complementary
treatment, which enables improvement in clients' executive functions.

Keywords Cognitive rehabilitation • Psychosocial intervention • Schizophrenia.

Background and Definitions

Disease and Symptoms

Schizophrenia is a chronic and incapacitating illness, with cognitive and interpersonal deficits (International Classification of Diseases [ICD-10], 1992). Schizophrenia
is characterized by *positive and negative symptoms*, the latter being the most critical
determinants of psychosocial functioning in schizophrenia (Pratt et al., 2005). The
positive or *productive symptoms* are characterized by delusions, hallucinations, and
disorganized thought, and the negative or *deficits symptoms* include blunting
affective and poor discourse (Crow, 1980). Schizophrenia sufferers describe problems

I. Söderback (ed.), *International Handbook of Occupational Therapy Interventions*,
DOI: 10.1007/978-0-387-75424-6_26, © Springer Science + Business Media, LLC 2010

in concentrating on simple tasks and *executive functioning deficits* (cognitive flexibility, working memory, and planning), affecting every aspect of life (Wykes et al., 1999).

Impairments

The *cognitive impairments* and thought disorder that characterize schizophrenia may interfere with the development and influence of *self-efficacy beliefs*. For example, Brekke et al. (2007) have reported that cognitive functioning moderates the relationship between subjective well-being and psychosocial functioning.

Executive functioning (Baddeley and Della Sala, 1996; Shallice et al., 1991) is closely related to good social and occupational functioning (Green et al., 2000), describing the way information is controlled and processed. These processes are essential in many different situations, such as planning the execution of tasks, making decisions, correcting errors, and responding to new information (Wykes et al., 1999). Clients with schizophrenia do poorly on neuropsychological tests reputed to tap these skills: working memory, cognitive flexibility, and planning (Wykes et al., 2002).

Complementary Therapy and Psychopharmacological Treatment

The *psychosocial intervention approach* is based on treatment without psychopharmacologic preparations and includes any activity aimed at involving the client in the social environment.

Pratt et al. (2005) suggest that the negative symptoms, and not self-efficacy, are the most critical determinants of psychosocial functioning in schizophrenia, and that psychosocial treatment should focus on the amelioration of these symptoms.

Occupational therapy is performed in mental health clinics, whereas clients with schizophrenia aim mainly at social involvement using the daily routine as an organizing axis (Benetton, 1994). These interventions using *activities* (occupations) have a pedagogic aspect, enabling clients to learn new behaviors, to face up to the possibilities and limitations of materials and processes, to develop or use specific skills, and to experience several situations transferable from the therapeutic setting to external activities (Villares, 1998).

The process of occupational therapy that focuses on the *psychosocial aspect* includes the major aims of enabling individuals to engage in meaningful occupations and to cope better with daily life (Finlay, 2004).

Occupational therapy *related to the executive functions* of schizophrenia gives participants in task activities and occupations the opportunity to plan, organize, create strategies, increase personal development, experience motivation, and learn how to solve problems (Grieve, 1993).

Psychopharmacologic Treatment Compared to Complementary Therapy

Evidence-based studies have shown that the most efficient treatment for people with schizophrenia consists of the combination of *psychopharmacologic treatment* and *psychosocial interventions*, such as psychotherapy (cognitive behaviorist therapy, cognitive remediation, social skills training, integrated psychosocial therapy), and *complementary therapy* (day hospital, family intervention, psychoeducational intervention, supported employment, and *occupational therapy*) (Buchain et al., 2003; Cook and Howe, 2003; Dickerson and Lehman, 2006; Lauriello et al., 1999; Pfammatter et al., 2006).

Psychopharmacologic treatment has made it possible to reduce psychotic symptoms and to prevent relapses, but it does not have the same convincing effect on cognitive or functional impairments (Penadés et al., 2006).

Buchain et al. (2003) concluded that for clients with schizophrenia nonresponsive to conventional neuroleptic treatment, that is, treatment-resistant schizophrenia (TRS) (Henna Neto, 1999), the combination of clozapine and occupational therapy was more effective than clozapine alone. Occupational therapy represents an additional intervention for these TRS clients. In their study, Buchain et al. demonstrated improved occupational performance and interpersonal relationships among 26 clients, as assessed on Scale for Interactive Observation in Occupational Therapy (EOITO) (Oliveira, 1995).

Purpose

The principal purpose of occupational therapy applied in the psychosocial approach is to *facilitate social involvement*. The intervention provides the client with tools for improving their *executive functions* and *social ability* and their *occupational performance*.

Method

Candidates for the Intervention

The Program of Schizophrenia, entitled PROJESQ is intended for clients of either gender who fulfill the diagnostic criteria for schizophrenia according to the ICD-10, and are between the ages of 18 and 60 years. Clients who at present show impairments in cognitive function, mainly in executive functions and disabilities in basic and instrumental activities of daily living and social functioning, are invited to participate. The PROJESQ is conducted at the Psychiatry Institute of the Clinical Hospital of the Medical School of the University of São Paulo, Brazil.

Epidemiology

In a recent revision by the World Health Organization (WHO) on the global impact of the disease, Murray and Lopez (1996) reported a prevalence of schizophrenia of 0.92% for men and to 0.9% for women. Higher prevalence rates (close to 1%) have also been reported in recent studies conducted in Latin America and Brazil (Almeida et al., 1992; Vicente et al., 1994;).

The epidemiologic studies in Brazil estimate that the incidence and prevalence are consistent with those seen in other countries. There is no consistency of the possible differences in the prevalence of schizophrenia between genders, regardless of the methodology employed in the epidemiologic surveys (Mari and Leitão, 2000).

A study of psychiatric morbidity in Brasilia, São Paulo, and Porto Alegre showed a life-prevalence of psychotic disorders of 0.3%, 0.9%, and 2.4%, respectively, in a population over 15 years of age (Almeida Filho et al., 1992).

Five hundred clients with schizophrenia are treated in the PROJESQ each year at the Psychiatry Institute of the Clinical hospital of the Medical School of the University of São Paulo (HCFMUSP) Brazil.

Settings

The occupational therapy intervention is conducted in groups and coordinated by an occupational therapist (OT). The activities are suggested by the OT, who teaches all the clients the process of execution, with well-established phases to develop initiative, organization, planning, and problem solving. The intervention is mediated by handcraft activities (paintings, mosaic, découpage, and others) and activities of daily living (ADL). The intervention takes place in the occupational therapy department.

The Role of the Occupational Therapist in Conducting the Intervention

The most important role of the OT is to improve cognitive functions, mainly executive functioning.

The triadic relationship *therapist–client–activities* creates the conditions to develop an *environment* in which clients *experience learning* and the possibility of applying their resources, in which a pathologic condition can be transformed into one of creative and structured development, thus enabling clients to deal differently with their limitations and to improve their social interaction (Villares, 1998). The

OT's role during the group intervention is to facilitate the interpersonal relationship and social interaction between the participating clients.

Results

Clinical Application

The schizophrenia program (PROJESQ) specific to the Psychiatry Institute of the HCFMUSP, Brazil, includes the following components: (1) social skill training, (2) cognitive behavior therapy, (3) occupational therapy, (4) psychoeducation with families, and (5) vocational orientation. Assessments are used to determine what an individual client's program should entail:

1. *Social skill training* includes a range of techniques founded on operant or social learning theory to enhance social performance, such as instructions, modeling, role play, reinforcement, corrective feedback, and in vivo exercise using homework assignments (Pfammatter et al., 2006).
2. *Cognitive behavior therapy* is an empathic and nonthreatening technique, in which clients elaborate their experience of schizophrenia. Specific symptoms are identified as problematic by the client and become targeted for special attention. This work may include, for example, belief modification, focusing/reattribution, and normalizing of psychotic experience (Dickerson and Lehman, 2006).
3. *Occupational therapy:* The general aim is to assist clients in maximizing their occupational performance within their localized and unique social and cultural environments. The therapy here is focused on the continual assessment of each individual's occupational performance and goal negotiation, and on the selection, grading, and adaptation of activities related to self-care, leisure, and productivity (Cook and Howe, 2003).
4. *Psychoeducational teaching with families* includes ensuring that knowledge of the disease meets the expectations of family members and clients so that they may deploy their resources in combating the disease and promoting better family interaction (Anderson et al., 1996).
5. *Vocational orientation* is useful in helping clients to develop vocational skills that can exploit their abilities in a supervised, accepting environment. To be useful for independent living, this learning must be generalized to the workplace (Gunatilake et al., 2004).

The PROJESQ program uses different methods with each of the following components. For example, OTs use the cognitive rehabilitation model.

Occupational therapy based on cognitive rehabilitation comprises (Cook and Howe, 2003):

- Continual assessment of function, skills, and environment
- Collaborative goal-setting, treatment-planning, and review
- Selection, grading, adaptation, and sequencing of activities
- Adaptation of the social and physical environments, including educational interventions and support for relatives and people at work
- Training and development of skills, education, and rehabilitation

Occupational Therapy

Clients are encouraged to perform daily tasks, to develop constructive tasks (e.g., handcraft), to have contact with each other, and to share tasks. The process is exemplified in Table 26.1.

The occupational therapy groups include verbal elements, tasks and concrete elements that are independent of the approach used, social abilities training, social interaction, and cognitive training (Finlay, 1993).

Discussion

Clinically there is agreement among mental health professionals about the effects of occupational therapy interventions among schizophrenia clients with executive dysfunction. More evidence-based studies are needed to investigate detailed cognitive areas amenable to modification with such interventions. These studies would be relevant in mental health services once they improve the prospects of rehabilitation for schizophrenia sufferers and can lead to improvement in health costs.

Table 26.1 Occupational therapy sessions exemplified

Occupational therapy session planning nr____		
Performace of activity	Daily activities	Client-chosen handcraft activity
Performance of tasks	Example is cooking	Examples is working with mosaic-stones
Analyses of the performance components	Decide the recipe	Learn the task's sequence order
	Organize the ingredients	Organize the physical space and material for task execution
	Prepare the food	
	Organize the table	Plan the individual mosaic project (object, color draw, etc)
	Organize and clean the room	Organize materials
Purposes and expected outcome	The client takes:	the client takes:
	initiative	initiative
	plans and organize the activity	plans and organize the activity
	relates to other clients	relates to other clients demonstrates mental flexibility and problem-solving
	social interaction occurs	social interaction occurs

References

Almeida, N.F., Mari, J.J., Coutinho, E.S.F., et al. (1992). Estudo Multicêntrico de Morbidade Psiquiátrica em Areas Urbanas Brasileiras. Brasília, São Paulo: Porto Alegre Rev. ABP –APAL; 14(3), 93–104. Jul-Set, 1

Anderson, C., et al. (1996). Schizophrenia and the Family. New York: Guilford

Baddeley, A., and Della Sala, S. (1996). Working memory and executive control. Philos Trans R Soc Lond, 351, 1397–1404.

Benetton, M.J. (1994). Trilhas associativas, Lemos editorial, São Paulo.

Brekke, J.S., Hoe, M., Long, J., and Green, M.F. (2007). How neurocognition and social cognition influence functional change during community-based psychosocial rehabilitation for individuals with schizophrenia. Schizophr Bull. 33(5), 1247–1256.

Buchain, P.C., Vizzotto, A.D.B., Henna Neto, J., and Elkis, H. (2003). Randomized controlled trial of occupational therapy in clients with treatment resistant schizophrenia. Rev Bras Psiquiatr, 25(1), 26–30.

Cook, S., and Howe, A. (2003). Engaging people with enduring psychotic conditions in primary mental health care and occupational therapy. Br J Occup Ther, 66(6), 236–246.

Crow, T.J. (1980). Molecular pathology of schizophrenia: more than one disease process. Br Med J, 280, 66–68.

Dickerson, F.B., and Lehman, A.F. (2006). Evidence-based psychoccupational therapy for schizophrenia. J Nerv Ment Dis, 194(1).

Finlay, L. (1993). Groupwork in Occupational Therapy. Cheltenham, UK: Stanley Thornes .

Finlay, L. (2004). The Practice Psychosocial Occupational Therapy,, 3rd ed. Cheltenham: Nelson Thornes Editorial.

Green, M.F., Kern, R.S., Braff, D.L., and Mintz, J. (2000). Neurocognitive deficits and functional outcome in schizophrenia: are we measuring the right stuff? Schizophr Bull, 26, 119–136.

Grieve, J. (1993). Neuropsychology for Occupational Therapists. Assessment of Perception and Cognition. Oxford: Blackwell Science.

Gunatilake, S., Ananth, J., Parameswaran Brow, S., and Silva, W.. (2004). Rehabilitation of schizophrenic patients. Curr Pharm Design, 10, 2277–2288.

Henna Neto, J. (1999). Esquizofrenia Refratária a Tratamento Antipsicótico: Caracterização Clínica e Fatores Preditivos. Dissertação [mestrado] São Paulo: Faculdade de Medicina da Universidade de São Paulo.

Huxley, N.A., Rendall, M., and Sederer, L. (2000). Psychosocial treatments in schizophrenia: a review of the past 20 years. J Nerv Ment Dis, 188(4), 187–201.

ICD-10 Classification of Mental and Behavioral Disorders. (1992). Clinical Descriptions and Diagnostic Guidelines. Geneva, Switzerland: World Health Organization.

Lauriello, J., Bustilo, J., and Keith, S.J. (1999). A critical review of research on psychosocial treatment of schizophrenia. Biol Psychiatry, 46, 1409–1417.

Mari, J., and Leitão, R.J. (2000). A Epidemiologia da Esquizofrenia. Rev Bras Psiquiatria, 22(supplement 1).

Morrice, R., and Delahunty, A. (1996). Frontal/executive impairments in schizophrenia. Schizophr Bull, 22, 125–137.

Murray, C.J.L., and Lopez, A.D. (1996). The Global Burden of Disease. Cambridge, MA: Harvard School of Public Health.

Oliveira, A.S. (1995). Adequação e Estudo de Validade e Fidedignidade da Escala de Observação Interativa de Pacientes Psiquiátricos Internados Aplicada às Situações de Terapia Ocupacional. Dissertação [Mestrado] Apresentado ao Departamento de Neuropsiquiatria e Psicologia Médica da Universidade de São Paulo, Faculdade de Ribeirão Preto.

Penadés, R., Catalán, R., Salamero, M., et al. (2006). Cognitive remediation therapy for out clients with chronic schizophrenia: a controlled and randomized study. Schizophr Res, 87, 323–331.

Pfammatter, M., Junghan, U.M., and Brenner, H.D. (2006). Efficacy of psychological therapy in schizophrenia conclusions from meta-analyis. Schizophr Bull, 32, S64–S80.

Pratt, S.I., Mueser, K.T., Smith, T.E., and Lu, W. (2005). Self-efficacy and psychosocial functioning in schizophrenia: a mediational analysis. Schizophr Res, 78, 187–197.

Shallice, T., Burgess, P., and Frith, C. (1991). Can the neuropsychological case-study approach be applied to schizophrenia. Psychol Med, 21, 661–673.

Velligan, D.I., and Bow-Thomas, C.C. (1999). Executive function in schizophrenia. Semin Clin Neuropsychiatry, 4, 24–33.

Vicente, B., Saldivia, S., Rioseco, P., et al. (1994). Trastornos psiquiátricos en diez comunas de Santiago: Prevalência de seis meses. Rev Psiquiatría Chile, 4, 194–202.

Villares, C.C. (1998). Terapia ocupacional na esquizofrenia. In: Shirakawa, I., Chaves, A.C., and Mari, J.J., eds. O Desafio da Esquizofrenia (pp. 183–195). São Paulo: Lemos Editorial.

Wykes, T., Brammer, M., Mellers, J., et al. (2002). Effects on the brain of a psychological treatment: cognitive remediation therapy. Functional magnetic resonance in schizophrenia. Br J Psychiatry, 181, 144–152.

Wykes, T., Reeder, C., Corner, J., Williams, C., and Everitt, B. (1999). The effects of neurocognitive remediation on executive processing in clients with schizophrenia. Schizophr Bull, 25(2), 291–307.

Chapter 27
Behavioral Approach to Rehabilitation of Patients with Substance-Use Disorders

Natalia Punanova and Tatiana Petrova

At last, I learned how to clean a potato. Before I was 40,
I never held anything heavier than a syringe in my hand.

—A former drug abuser

Abstract This chapter describes the practice of treatment and rehabilitation of persons suffering from substance-use disorders (i.e., abuse of drugs or alcohol). It uses the experience gathered in one of the departments of the Narcologic Clinic of St. Petersburg, Russia, and works as a therapeutic society (TS). Therapeutic societies are organizations, sometimes voluntary, aimed at helping drug and alcohol abusers to rid themselves of substance-use disorders.The treatment is based on the philosophical concept of the 12-step programs and the method of the cognitive behavioral therapy approach. Patients participate in three stages of treatment. During this treatment the patient is placed in an artificial environment similar to a normal society.

Keywords Cognitive behavioral therapy • Dependency syndrome • Detoxification • Group treatment • Psychoactive substances • Withdrawal.

Background

Dependency Syndrome

This syndrome is a combination of physiologic, behavioral, and cognitive phenomena in which the use of psychoactive substances (PASs) has the highest priority in the patient's system of values, while all other interests and needs are neglected. The patients spend more and more time and effort to get drugs and to recover from the usage of drugs. The main features of the dependency syndrome are (1) a very strong, often insatiable, need of getting drugs; (2) inability to control the dosage; (3) withdrawal; and (4) growing tolerance to drugs, that is, the need to increase the dosage with time to achieve the same effect that earlier could be achieved with lower dosages (Tschurkin and Martushov, 1999).

I. Söderback (ed.), *International Handbook of Occupational Therapy Interventions*,
DOI: 10.1007/978-0-387-75424-6_27, © Springer Science+Business Media, LLC 2010

Implications of Intervention

The main difficulty in dealing with such patients is their lack of *motivation*. In order to continue with drugs, they create protective mechanisms that justify their drug abuse. More often it is their relatives, rather than the patients themselves, who are interested in getting help and who ask for it. For the patient to be sincerely motivated to completely refrain from drugs, some objective conditions should be fulfilled that force the patient to make this choice. It happens when drugs or alcohol becomes a problem not only for their family but also for themselves. A typical scenario is that the family refuses to accept the person's behavior and he or she faces the choice of "the family or the drugs," and risks of being thrown out of the home. A similar situation arises if the drug user develops serious health problems or legal troubles. In order to return to normal life, the patient has to address his physical dependency, learn how to deal with his psychological dependency, and consciously refrain from drugs or alcohol even under external or internal stress factors.

Intervention

The framework of intervention among patients with dependency syndrome is in Russia based on the Order of the Ministry of Health of Russian Federation (2003). This chapter refers to the experience of one of the departments of the Narcologic Clinic of St. Petersburg.

The clinical work with patients suffering from chemical dependences is based on the concept of the 12-step programs (Wallen et al., 1987), in which (1) patients admit that they have a disease, want to recover, and agree that it is possible; (2) patients accept assistance from the team, and analyze their own behavior, including all the failures and damages inflicted on other people: and (3) patients perform self-control and correct the misbehavior. This program is conducted in an artificial environment—*a therapeutic society*—which is a model of a normally functioning society. To facilitate abstention from drugs/alcohol, the patients' environment should be free from provoking factors (substance-abusers, easily accessible drugs or alcohol);, therefore, their environment should be completely changed.

Within this concept, the *cognitive behavioral approach* is used for the intervention (Karvasarsky, 2007). This approach, as it is interpreted in the clinic, is based on the beliefs that (1) abuse of drugs or alcohol is a behavioral disorder; (2) behavioral disorder is a consequence of deficiency of education; and (3) if the patient learns the correct behavior, such as by learning a pattern (model), the symptoms of the disease will decrease or disappear. The clinic uses the system of learning called "token economy" in the following way:

- The patient is rewarded for "desired" behavior by a special token.
- The patient gets more tokens the better the behavior that he/she demonstrates.

- The tokens can be exchanged for something the patient wants, such as a trip to the theater.

The intervention program includes three stages that are carried out simultaneously: (1) disconnection and complete abstention from drugs and treatment of withdrawal and postwithdrawal syndrome with medication, (2) rehabilitation by a combination of a cognitive behavioral approach and medication, and (3) supportive and antirelapse treatment by a combination of cognitive behavioral therapy and medication.

Purpose

The main aim of the intervention for patients with dependency syndrome is learning how to return to normal life. During this process the patient first has to overcome the physical dependence on drugs or alcohol, and second to learn how to deal with the psychological dependence. Patients have to learn how to control the desire to use drugs or alcohol and to acquire new habits of normal behavior and social communication.

Method

Candidates for the Intervention

Rehabilitation from substance-use disorders is suitable for any patient and is not limited by age, type of drugs, or duration of the abuse. Contraindications are (1) developed psychopathology, and (2) behavior that is dangerous for other patients or the team members.

Admission to the Clinic

Patients are admitted to the rehabilitation program in the following ways: (1) about 40% of the patients are admitted after detoxification treatment; (2) 25% of the patients seek rehabilitation help by themselves; (3) 20% of the patients are admitted for antirelapse treatment (not necessarily after having been treated in this clinic); and (4) 15% of the patients seek help after having been informed by previous successful patients, by other medical centers, by parents visiting the meetings of Azaria, an organization for "mothers against drugs."

Each patient is accepted after a collective decision by the psychologists, social workers, and narcologists, sometimes after a trial period of 1 week.

Epidemiology

> *There are more than 300,000 registered drug abuses in Russia, but experts believe the real figure to be between five and eight times greater than this.*

(Dalziel, 2002)

In St. Petersburg there were 9,604 registered drug abusers and 35,280 alcoholics in 2006, and 10,094 drug abusers and 33,024 alcoholics in 2007. The clinic accepted about 10,000 patients in 2007, including the patients admitted several times during the same year.

Settings

The settings concern one of the departments of the clinic with a capacity of 85 patients. Thirty-five patients, mainly heroin abusers, are going through the rehabilitation stage. The other patients are treated for detoxification, withdrawal, and post-withdrawal syndrome.

The Role of the Therapists

The job title of occupational therapist does not exist in Russia. The corresponding functions with focuses on the patients' occupational performances are conducted by psychologists, social workers, and consultants on chemical dependency (i.e., people who once abused drugs or alcohol but are drug-free for several years).

The team of the present department consists of 28 members who conduct the intervention program. They represent various specialists, such as narcologists, psychologists, social workers, and consultants on substance-use disorders. They work as a *semiprofessional therapeutic society*. Medical team members conduct seminars aimed at discussing dependency, codependency, problems that occur during the first days of sobriety, and reasons for recidivism. A lot of work is also done with the patient's relatives in order to deal with possible codependency. The team members' roles are to (1) help the patient to overcome the drug dependency, and (2) to increase the patients' motivation.

The *psychologist/narcologist* prescribes medication for treatment of the withdrawal and the postwithdrawal syndrome, treats possible psychological complications such as depression, and makes decisions regarding involvement of other medical specialists. The whole process of intervention and rehabilitation is under control of this staff member.

The *social workers* are employed by the clinic, and their role is to help the patients find jobs in cooperation with employment agencies. When a job is found, they follow the client for 1 year.

The *consultants on substance-use* have a special and important role in the clinic, which is to demonstrate that the treatment can be successful. This role is extremely important for the motivation of patients in the process of overcoming the addiction and to help them gain a realistic view of the disease. The consultant's personal positive experience makes this possible because he becomes a kind of mirror for the patient. One of the functions of consultants on substance-use is psychological support for the groups.

Results

Clinical Application

Organization

Stages of Rehabilitation

The treatment is arranged in stages of rehabilitation in a hierarchical order. The extent of freedom that patients enjoy depends on the rehabilitation stage. Patients receive more freedom and responsibility the higher the stage attained. Patients can be moved between these stages depending on their progress of rehabilitation. The more that patients are trusted, the more rights and responsibilities they get. Thus, some patients from the third group (see below) are more trusted by the team and have responsible assignments.

- *Motivation stage:* The patient is not allowed to leave the facility. Even if the patient is not suffering from withdrawal, his will is still paralyzed by psychological dependency. If he returns to his environment, he will again start seeking drugs and justify it using protective psychological mechanisms. It takes time and substantial effort both by the patient and the team members to overcome these mechanisms. The patient learns how to adapt an objective view on himself and to call things by their proper names. The consultant on chemical dependency plays the main role in this stage by being both the judge and the friend who gives psychological support.
- *Limited functional mode stage:* After some time the patient earns more freedom, that is, he lives in a *limited functional mode*. He is allowed to go outside with relatives, and later on with other patients and groups. The patient obtains this stage if he complies with the ten specified criteria of expected behavior and actively cooperates with the team members. Most of the patients are allowed to spend weekends at home on the condition that they go to Narcotics Anonymous meetings (NA, 2008) when they are outside the clinic.
- When the discharge time approaches, the patient starts looking for a job and is allowed to travel to interviews. Two weeks before the discharge, the patient is allowed to spend all night at home but is expected to attend all group sessions at the clinic.

- *The follow-up stage:* The psychosocial follow-up is performed by the consultants after the discharge, within a time frame of up to 8 months. At this stage, the patients sign the "family agreement" which is similar to the therapeutic agreement (see assignments). The patient is expected to have a job and, by the end of the period, to have found an adviser/instructor in NA. The adviser is typically a person with a very long period of abstention from drugs/alcohol who regularly attends NA groups and plays a supporting role. It is recommended to attend the NA sessions daily for the first 3 months after discharge.

Groups

Patients who are at different stages participate in the program and are placed in a group.

The aim of participating in the *motivation group* is to go through detoxification and to be qualified for the rehabilitation program.

The *rehabilitation group* is a model of the society, and the therapeutic agreement is a model of the law. Therefore, to keep the agreement means to train to keep the social norms, which is of most importance for these patients. The patient learns how to predict consequences of his behavior and be responsible for them; every act leads to well-known and immediate consequences. The patients' hierarchy is reflected by badges of different colors that the patients carry; the motivation group carries white badges, and patients in the rehabilitation group carry yellow or red badges depending on the advancement of the rehabilitation process.

Assignments

A newly enrolled patient starts by signing a therapy agreement. It contains the behavioral norms for the group to which he/she belongs.

The following behaviors are prohibited:

- Use of any drugs except for tobacco and prescribed medicines
- Sexual relations, physically or verbally aggressive behavior, use of slang, displays of alcoholic or drug subculture and symbols
- Use of mobile phones
  Permitted behavior include:
- Keeping the daily routines
- Maintaining personal hygiene

It is every patient's responsibility to make sure that all patients keep these norms and do not enter any "contract relations," that is, bribery is not allowed. Keeping these rules helps to avoid conflicts in the group.

Encouragements and Punishment

The correlation between behavior and consequences is defined in a document entitled "Classification of Encouragements and Punishments." It describes in which situation a patient can earn (1) more rights and privileges, or (2) a promotion, or, on the other hand, (1) lose some or all of his privileges, or (2) be required to do extra work such as dish washing. The worst punishment is to be expelled from the group, and the money paid for rehabilitation is not returned.

Contents of the Intervention

Duties

The patients are engaged as instructors for supporting other patients who are still at a lower stage. An instructor has the responsibility for the other patients' behavior and follows them everywhere, even to the restroom. This creates a kind of surrogate family, where the newly arrived patient has the role of a younger brother or sister, the instructor has the role of an older brother/sister, and the medical team plays the parents' role. Thus, the training of everyday live and social roles is conducted. In this way, the patients earn more responsibilities for themselves and other patients, which is aimed at increasing continually during the rehabilitation program.

Duties that are part of the rehabilitation program include training of responsibility, honesty, organizational skills, and ability to resolve conflict situations.

Every patient has certain duties at all stages of the program. The duty tasks are defined by the patients themselves at the morning meeting. Usually it is different kinds of homework, such as cleaning and dish washing. For example, more advanced patients may become training instructors and also work as volunteers after their own program has ended. All these duties are elective, and the patients have to be rated by other patients on four parameters: trust, discipline, contactability, and knowledge of the program.

Habits and Daily Routine

A typical day involves several blocks of duties:

- Occupational performance of morning and afternoon housework at the ward and outside the premises
- Group therapy conducted by an instructor
- Performing small individual daily tasks, such as discussing current psychological problems.
- Participating in individual consultations.
- Free time for walks, watching TV, movies, etc.
  There are several daily features of the program:
- Morning meetings under the supervision of the consultant. The purpose is to teach the patients to act together and to define the day's focus. The participants discuss the news, encountered problems, and individual problems in the context of the "here and now," such as the use of drugs or alcohol, resolving conflicts inside the group, insults, etc. Housework for the day is also planned during these meetings. The philosophy of the group is discussed constantly.
- Meetings are conducted under direction of the patients at a higher stage.
- Afternoon discourses are conducted by the consultant. The participants discuss their performances of the housework; make comments and apologies, express

gratitude, and read the Diary of Feelings that every patient has to keep constantly. The participants fill the Mirror of Recovery ("what I did today for my recovery"), discuss the Focus of the Day, and their feelings of the moment. Every participant gets feedback and reasonable social pressure.

- A weekly meeting is held similarly to the daily meeting. A team member helps to set up the coming week's activities. The patients can apply for a leave of absence or participating in a group activity, such as going to the theater. If the group accumulated too many demerits for the week, they are made public and the corresponding measures are announced. The meeting's secretary collects applications and follows up the announced measures.

- Special discourses are conducted when necessary. Here the patients can comment on other patients' behavior. The aim is to get feedback to the patients and serve as a "valve" for socially acceptable feelings or for aggression. The instructor is usually an advanced patient and the team members are present.

- Approximately once a month the speakers' meetings are held with participation of persons with long periods of sobriety (more than 1 year) who once were patients at this clinic, or persons from one of the NA groups. They discuss their own experience of abstention from drugs/alcohol. Thus, the participants of the program can see successful cases from people from outside and thus can objectively judge their own problems and the possibilities of resolving them.

Evidence-Based Practice

The figures for the last 2 years show that 23% of the patients at the clinic who fulfilled the program have a remission period longer than 1 year. About 8% to 10% of patients return for an antirelapse treatment, and 15% have periodic relapses but with longer periods of sobriety and a better quality of life. There is no available information about 10% to 15% of the patients.

Generally speaking, the results of rehabilitation are better if the patient is connected to the clinic and participates in rehabilitation for a longer time; however, there are also some exceptions.

Acknowledgment Our thanks to Naum Purits for his translation from Russian to English, and for his everlasting kindness in arranging the publication of this manuscript.

References

Dalziel, S. (2002). Alarming rise in Russia drug abuse. BBC News World Wide. http://news.bbc. co.uk/2/hi/europe/2176504.stm.

Karvasarsky, B. Psychotherapeutic encyclopedia, 2007. Б Д. Карвасарский. Психотерапевтическая энциклопедия (in Russian). http://vocabulary.ru/dictionary/6/word/%C1%C8%D 5%C5%C2%C8%CE%D0%C8%C7%CC.

Narcotics Anonymous Word Wide (2008). 1999–2008 NA World Services, Incorporated. http://www.na.org.

Order of the Health Ministry of Russian Federation No. 500. Dated Oct. 22, 2003. Regarding treatment of people with substance abuse. Приказ Минздрава РФ 22.10.2003 N 500 об утверждении протокола ведения больных "реабилитация больных наркоманией (z50.3)" (in Russian). http://lawrussia.ru/bigtexts/law_1776/index.htm.

Tschurkin and Martushov. (1999). Short guidance regarding the use of International Classification of Diseases (ICD-10) in psychiatry and narcology. Russian translation. Moscow: Triada-X, pp. 1–232. Чуркин, А.А. и Мартюшов А. Н. Кратҡое руководство по использоованию МКБ-10 в психиатрии и нарколоии. – М.: Изд-во «Триада-X», 1–232 с (in Russian).

Wallen, M.C., Weiner, H.D., Mansi, A., and Deal, D. (1987). Utilization of 12-step theme groups in a short-term chemical dependence treatment unit. *J Psychoactive Drugs*, 19(3), 287–290.

Chapter 28
Intervention in Panic and Anxiety Disorders Through Lifestyle Modification

Rodney A. Lambert

A combination of habitual lifestyle behaviors such as diet, fluid intake, exercise, and habitual lifestyle drug use (such as caffeine, alcohol, and nicotine) may interact with altered sensitivity in body system function in some panic disorder clients. (Lambert et al., 2007)

Abstract Unhealthy habitual lifestyle behaviors add to the burden of local, national, and global health. When reviewing evidence of potential causes of panic disorder, at least six body systems are known to have altered sensitivity affected by habitual behaviors such as diet, fluid intake, exercise, and habitual lifestyle drug use (for example, caffeine, nicotine, and alcohol). This may also be true for other forms of anxiety disorder. Occupational therapists (OTs) work with everyday occupational behaviors that include habitual lifestyle factors. Negotiating a positive lifestyle change can affect anxiety symptoms through addressing systemic sensitivity. The occupational therapy lifestyle intervention discussed here centers on occupational form, performance, and synthesis related to habitual lifestyle behaviors that can therefore affect the development, experience, severity, and duration of anxiety symptoms. A recent random controlled study observed a significant short-term benefit (20 weeks). At long-term follow-up (10 months after entry into the trial), clinical results were equivalent to those achieved with full cognitive behavioral therapy (CBT). A model of the system within which the approach functions is presented.

Keywords Anxiety • Complexity science • Lifestyle • Occupation • Neuroses panic attacks • Randomized controlled trial • Therapy

Definition

Statements: The Theoretical Framework of the Intervention

For at least the past 40 years, global and national health policies in the United Kingdom have promoted the idea that modification to habitual lifestyle behaviors, including increased exercise, smoking cessation, and improved diet, benefit health (Flores and

I. Söderback (ed.), *International Handbook of Occupational Therapy Interventions*,
DOI: 10.1007/978-0-387-75424-6_28, © Springer Science+Business Media, LLC 2010

Ojea, 2002; Kennedy, 2002; WHO, 2003b). Unhealthy habitual lifestyle behaviors add to the local, national, and global burden of ill health as evidenced by the World Health Report 2003 (WHO, 2003b) and the U.K. Department of Health White Paper on smoking (Department of Health, 1998). The WHO, for example, has characterized smoking as "the world's leading preventable cause of death" (WHO, 2003b, p. 91), and has characterized the growing problems of obesity as a global epidemic (WHO, 2003a).

Occupational therapists (OTs) have developed their understanding of occupational behavior through theoretical developments such as those provided by Keilhofner's (2007) model of human occupation, Nelson's (1997) promotion of the tripartite structure of occupational form, performance, and synthesis, and in the development of occupational science (Yerxa, 1993). It has subsequently been suggested that "both lifestyle and occupation refer to broadly similar life processes, with both considering occupational form and occupational performance [and that] occupational synthesis can be achieved by a direct intervention based on lifestyle factors" (Lambert, 1998, p. 196).

In panic-disorder clients (International Classification of Diseases [ICD-10] code F41.0) (World Health Organization, 1992), at least six body systems have been shown to have an altered sensitivity (Lambert and Brown, 2007), leading to symptomatic reactions in these systems at lower levels of provocation than among people with other mental health problems and or among normal controls, and it is suggested that this may apply also to other anxiety disorders.

Applying a lifestyle intervention can provide a focus on the occupational form of lifestyle activities such as eating, drinking, and exercise, and the associated occupational performance of the habitual lifestyle behaviors, including the choices made by individuals of either health-enhancing behaviors (such as regular exercise) or health-damaging behaviors (such as smoking, drinking insufficient fluids, or the use of alcohol or caffeine as a major feature of fluid intake). This provides an opportunity for occupational synthesis through working with the client to increase awareness of, and minimize exposure to, elements to which the client has an altered sensitivity. It can also work toward improved fitness and function of specific body systems, as habitual lifestyle behaviors influence the function of bodily systems. In this way, reinterpretation of potential symptom causality can be promoted. Improved physiologic function can result, along with increased individual symptom control, thereby reducing the effect of previously misinterpreted symptoms on anxiety (such as chest pain being misinterpreted as an impending heart attack, leading to admission to the emergency department). Lifestyle review can identify a range of potentially harmful habitual lifestyle behaviors. By negotiating positive changes, these habitual lifestyle behaviors and physiologic responses within sensitive/hypersensitive body systems can be reduced, thereby reducing anxiety and panic.

Historical Development

The author first identified a potential link between habitual lifestyle behaviors and panic disorder in 1992 (Lambert, 1992), reporting this more formally in 1998

(Lambert, 1998). Between 2000 and 2003 a randomized controlled trial was conducted within the period of a National Health Service Researcher Development Fellowship (Lambert and Brown, 2007; Lambert et al., 2007).

Purpose

The *purpose* and fundamental principles for treating alteration of lifestyle for clinical use due to anxiety/panic disorders are to provide a focus on the occupational form and performance related to habitual lifestyle behaviors. This treatment approach can then examine methods of preventing, improving, and containing symptoms by occupational synthesis through active engagement with, and control over, routine habitual lifestyle behaviors. This approach aims to assist clients experiencing these symptoms to identify specific body system sensitivities, and to encourage alteration of potentially detrimental habitual lifestyle behaviors, through which they regain control over anxiety/panic symptoms, thereby improving their everyday occupational behaviors.

Method

Candidates for the Intervention and Epidemiology

The lifestyle intervention is intended for adults (16 to 65 years of age) who have been experiencing anxiety or panic attacks/disorder. Panic disorder is experienced by about 1.5% to 3% of the population (Weissman et al., 1997), and is well characterized in the *Diagnostic and Statistical Manual of Mental Disorders* (fourth edition, revised) (DSM-IV-R) (American Psychiatric Association, 2000) and in the International Classification of Diseases (10th Revision) (World Health Organization, 1992). The prevalence of all anxiety disorders in U.K. primary care services was estimated at 2.38% for men and 5.44% for women in 1998, with an upward trend (Office of National Statistics, 2000), and it has been estimated that this figure may be up to 19% (Ansseau et al., 2004).

This lifestyle intervention is intended to help clients with anxiety symptoms to recognize potential physiologic causes that may be associated with habitual behaviors. When these behaviors are identified, this intervention can then encourage clients to regain control over them.

Settings

The lifestyle intervention has been designed and tested with individual clients in primary care environments, although the principles could be applied in routine practice in other settings, and potentially also with small groups. Its effectiveness has not yet been tested in groups or other settings.

The Role of the Occupational Therapist in Applying the Intervention

The OT should become familiar with the literature (some examples are provided here, but the reference list is not comprehensive) relating to habitual lifestyle behaviors and health. Key works are those associated with diet (Benton and Nabb, 2003; Rogers, 2001), fluid intake (Gopinathan et al., 1988; Wilson and Morley, 2003), exercise (Atlantis et al., 2004; Broman-Fulks et al., 2004), and habitual lifestyle drug use, such as alcohol (Marquenie et al., 2007; Milani et al., 2004), nicotine (Goodwin et al., 2005; McLeish et al., 2008), and caffeine (Masdrakis et al., 2007; Nardi et al., 2007). These behaviors should not be considered in isolation, however, as evidence suggests high levels of interaction among these habitual lifestyle behaviors (Batra et al., 2003; Gilbert et al., 2000; Johansson and Sundquist, 1999). The OT should, in association with client diary data, identify potential habitual lifestyle behaviors that may represent a risk of increased anxiety, and then negotiate and monitor changes toward the client adopting health-promoting behaviors.

Results

A Brief Guide to Clinical Application

The intervention addresses four areas of lifestyle: diet, fluid intake, exercise, and habitual lifestyle drug use (caffeine, alcohol, and nicotine). It should provide up to ten intervention sessions over a 16-week period (three 1-hour appointments at weekly intervals, then three half-hour appointments at weekly intervals, then three half-hour appointments at biweekly intervals, and then one 1-hour appointment at a monthly interval). The intervention should be delivered in four distinct but largely concurrent stages:

- Lifestyle review using self-report mood and lifestyle diaries.
- Education to increase client awareness of the potential negative health effects of some lifestyle behaviors (such as smoking and poor diet), and the health benefits of other lifestyle behaviors (such as sufficient exercise and sufficient fluid intake).
- Specific lifestyle changes (in diet, fluid intake, exercise, or habitual lifestyle drug use) should be negotiated between therapist and client.
- Monitoring and review between therapist and client of the agreed lifestyle changes and any subsequent symptom change.

Evidence from Practice, and How the Intervention Eases Impairments, Activity Limitations, and Participation Restrictions

Results from a randomized controlled trial have been published in which the lifestyle intervention was compared with routine general practitioner (GP) care (Lambert et al., 2007). However, while this showed a significant short-term benefit, assessed at 20 weeks following 16 weeks of treatment, between-group differences were not significant at the 10-month follow-up. The conclusion was that the lifestyle intervention was at least as cost-effective as routine GP care (Lambert, 2005). It also produced improved results when compared with medication, and was equivalent in efficacy to the use of a full cognitive behavioral therapy program (Lambert et al., 2007). However, that is not the whole story, and the intervention is based on the observation that likely causes of panic and anxiety are diverse, from genetic predisposition to altered sensitivity in neurotransmitter/receptor density and function and body-system function, and include cognitive and environmental factors. As suggested by the Medical Research Council (MRC, 2000), this diversity of potential interaction between etiologic factors has been used to model the resulting complex system within which patterns of mood and behavior emerge (Lambert and Brown, 2007) (Fig. 28.1).

This model helps to identify at which point in the system an intervention can be attempted. For example, medication focuses on the physiologic functions of the

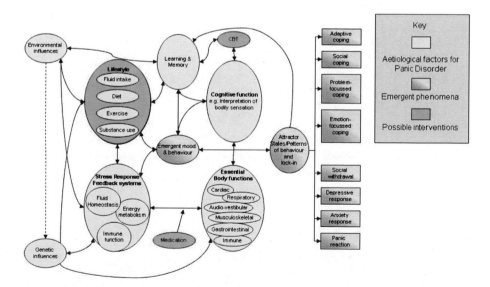

Fig. 28.1 Complex interaction and panic disorder: emergent phenomena and therapeutic implication. [Adapted from Lambert, R. (2007). Complexity, panic and primary care. In: Bogg, J., and Geyer, R., eds. Complexity Science and Society. Oxford: Radcliffe, with permission of the copyright holder.].

body, while CBT focuses on cognitive interpretation, learning, and memory. The lifestyle intervention focuses on a different and already internal part of the system, in terms of habitual lifestyle behaviors that influence emergent mood and behavior through stress-response feedback mechanisms, physiologic function, and cognitive interpretation. Another point of entry (although not shown) may be through environmental influences such as work or other occupational behaviors. Through applying the lifestyle intervention therefore, the OT can assist clients in becoming aware of individual sensitivities within their physiologic system, and to take remedial action to regain control over associated symptomatic responses. Lifestyle review can help clients gain an understanding of how their habitual lifestyle behaviors may affect symptoms of anxiety and panic. Through this, clients can learn what actions can assist them to regain control over such symptoms, and to regain control over their routine occupational behaviors. This places them in a better position to fulfill desired occupational roles and achieve an occupational balance.

Declaration of Interest

The main trial results from the wider study were presented at the 33rd North American Primary Care Research Group meeting held in Quebec City on October 15 to 18, 2005.

This research was supported by a National Health Service (NHS) Research and Development (R&D) National Primary Care Researcher Development Award Fellowship (grant RDA99/062) and by a NHS R&D Eastern Region Health Services and Public Health Research Scheme Grant (HSR/0500/1).

Acknowledgment I am indebted to the grant-awarding bodies whose financial support made the research possible. The long-term support of the patients, the GP practices, and occupational therapists who participated in the research, enabled completion of the research.

Clinical trial registration details: Controlled-trials.com—ISRCTN51562655
http://www.controlled-trials.com/isrctn/search.asp.

References

American Psychiatric Association. (2000). Diagnostic and Statistical Manual of Mental Disorders (DSM-IV-TR). Washington, DC: American Psychiatric Association.
Ansseau, M., Dierick, M., Buntinkx, F., et al. (2004). High prevalence of mental disorders in primary care. J Affect Dis, 78, 49–55.
Atlantis, E., Chow, C.M., Kirby, A., and Fiatarone Singh, M. (2004). An effective exercise-based intervention for improving mental health and quality of life measures: a randomized controlled trial. Prev Med, 39, 424–434.
Batra, V., Patkar, A.A., Berrettini, W.H., Weinstein, S.P., and Leone, F.T. (2003). The genetic determinants of smoking. Chest, 123, 1730.

Benton, D., and Nabb, S. (2003). Carbohydrate, memory, and mood. Nutr Rev, 61, S61–S67.

Broman-Fulks, J.J., Berman, M.E., Rabian, B.A., and Webster, M.J. (2004). Effects of aerobic exercise on anxiety sensitivity. Behav Res Ther, 42, 125–136.

Department of Health. (1998). Smoking Kills: A White Paper on Tobacco. London: The Stationery Office.

Flores, R., and Ojea, A. (2002). The WCRF Expert Panel Report as a model for advice and policy analysis for other (non-cancer) chronic disease, with specific note on WHO Technical Report 797 on diet, nutrition and prevention of chronic disease: Summary of Working Group 4. Asian Pac J Clin Nutr, 11, 777.

Gilbert, D.G., Dibb, W.D., Plath, L.C., and Hiyane, S.G. (2000). Effects of nicotine and caffeine, separately and in combination, on EEG topography, mood, heart rate, cortisol, and vigilance. Psychophysiology, 37, 583–595.

Goodwin, R.D., Lewinsohn, P.M., and Seeley, J.R. (2005). Cigarette smoking and panic attacks among young adults in the community: the role of parental smoking and anxiety disorders. Biol Psychiatry, 58, 686–693.

Gopinathan, P.M., Pichan, G., and Sharma, V.M. (1988). Role of dehydration in heat stress-induced variations in mental performance. Arch Environ Health, 43, 15–17.

Johansson, S.E., and Sundquist, J. (1999). Change in lifestyle factors and their influence on health status and all-cause mortality. Int J Epidemiol, 28, 1073–1080.

Kennedy, E. (2002). Healthy lifestyles, healthy people—the Mega Country Health Promotion Network. Asian Pac J Clin Nutr, 11 (Suppl 8), S738–S739.

Kielhofner, G. (2007). Model of Human Occupation: Theory and Application. 4th ed. New York/ Amsterdam Wolters Klüver/Lippincott Williams & Wilkins.

Lambert, R. (1992). An evaluation of the use of lifestyle change as a therapeutic tool with clients presenting with mental health problems with specific reference to caffeine use and fluid balance. MA in Health Research (unpublished), University of Lancaster.

Lambert, R. (1998). Occupation and lifestyle: implications for mental health practice. Br J Occup Ther, 61, 193–197.

Lambert, R. (2005). A pragmatic, unblinded randomised controlled trial and economic evaluation of an occupational therapy led Treating Alternation of Lifestyle and routine care of panic disorder presenting in primary care. Unpublished PhD dissertation, School of Allied Health Professions, University of East Anglia, Norwich.

Lambert, R., and Brown, C. (2007). Health and complexity. In: Bogg, J., and Geyer, R., eds. Complexity Science and Society. Oxford: Radcliffe.

Lambert, R.A., Harvey, I., and Poland, F. (2007). A pragmatic, unblinded randomised controlled trial comparing an occupational therapy-led treating alternation of lifestyle and routine GP care for panic disorder treatment in primary care. J Affect Disord, 99, 63–71.

Marquenie, L.A., Schade, A., van Balkom, A.J., et al. (2007). Origin of the comorbidity of anxiety disorders and alcohol dependence: findings of a general population study. Eur Addict Res, 13, 39–49.

Masdrakis, V.G., Papakostas, Y.G., Vaidakis, N., Papageorgiou, C., and Pehlivanidis, A. (2007). Caffeine challenge in clients with panic disorder: baseline differences between those who panic and those who do not. Depression Anxiety, 25, E72–E79.

McLeish, A.C., Zvolensky, M.J., Yartz, A.R., and Leyro, T.M. (2008). Anxiety sensitivity as a moderator of the association between smoking status and anxiety symptoms and bodily vigilance: replication and extension in a young adult sample. Addict Behav, 33(2), 315–327 (Epub 2007 Sep 29).

Medical Research Council. (2000). A Framework for Development and Evaluation of RCTs for Complex Interventions to Improve Health. London: MRC.

Milani, R.M., Parrott, A.C., Turner, J.J., and Fox, H.C. (2004). Gender differences in self-reported anxiety, depression, and somatization among ecstasy/MDMA polydrug users, alcohol/tobacco users, and nondrug users. Addict Behav, 29, 965–971.

Nardi, A.E., Lopes, F.L., Valenca, A.M., et al. (2007). Caffeine challenge test in panic disorder and depression with panic attacks. Comprehens Psychiatry, 48, 257–263.

Nelson, D.L. (1997). Why the profession of occupational therapy will flourish in the 21st century. The 1996 Eleanor Clarke Slagle Lecture. Am J Occup Ther, 51, 11–24.

Office of National Statistics. (2000). Key Health Statistics from General Practice 1998. London: Office of National Statistics.

Rogers, P.J. (2001). A healthy body, a healthy mind: long-term impact of diet on mood and cognitive function. Proc Nutr Soc, 60, 135–143.

Weissman, M.M., Bland, R.C., Canino, G.J., et al. (1997). The cross-national epidemiology of panic disorder. Arch Gen Psychiatry, 54, 305–309.

Wilson, M.-M.G., and Morley, J.E. (2003). Impaired cognitive function and mental performance in mild dehydration. Eur J Clin Nutr, 57(Suppl 2), S24–S29.

World Health Organization. (1992). The ICD-10 Classification of Mental and Behavioural Disorders: Clinical Description and Diagnostic Guidelines. Geneva: WHO.

World Health Organization. (2003a). Report of a Joint WHO/FAO Expert Consultation World Health Organization & Food and Agriculture Organization of the United Nations. Geneva: WHO.

World Health Organization. (2003b). The World Health Report 2003: Shaping the Future. Geneva: WHO.

Yerxa, E.J. (1993). Occupational science: a new source of power for participants in occupational therapy. Occup Sci Aust, 1, 3–10.

Chapter 29
Trunk Restraint: Physical Intervention for Improvement of Upper-Limb Motor Impairment and Function

Mindy F. Levin

The physical intervention discussed here is task-related training combined with trunk restraint to limit motor compensation during reaching-and-grasping training.

Abstract Children and adults with hemiparesis use excessive trunk movement to compensate for limitations in arm movement during reaching activities. Reaching and grasping with physical limitation of trunk movements (trunk restraint) leads to improvements in the quality of arm motor patterns (shoulder and elbow) and of upper-limb function. The intervention consists of task-oriented upper-limb therapy performed while movements of the trunk are limited by strapping the trunk to the back of a chair. The trunk restraint limits forward and lateral trunk displacement and rotation but allows scapular movement.

Keywords Cerebral palsy • Exercise movement techniques • Rehabilitation • Recovery

Background

The Theoretical Framework of the Intervention

Task-related training (Carr and Shepherd, 2000) delivered at the same time as trunk restraint (Michaelsen et al., 2004, 2006) combines physical restraint of trunk movement (flexion and rotation) with repetitive meaningful unimanual and bimanual reaching and grasping tasks using objects of different sizes, weights, and shapes (task-related training).

I. Söderback (ed.), *International Handbook of Occupational Therapy Interventions*,
DOI: 10.1007/978-0-387-75424-6_29, © Springer Science+Business Media, LLC 2010

Definitions and Historical Development

Functional gains may be accompanied by increased compensatory movements of the trunk (anterior/lateral displacement and rotation), to compensate for arm motor impairments (Levin et al., 2002). Practice of a movement without restriction of trunk motor compensations or feedback of motor performance may lead to increased motor compensation (Cirstea and Levin, 2000). When motor compensation occurs during movement production, the central nervous system receives nonoptimal sensory information from the trunk and limb (Adkins et al., 2006). This would interfere with the recovery of premorbid movement patterns, as has been suggested for the control of posture (Nashner et al., 1983) and precision grasping (Eliasson et al., 1992, 1995; Gordon and Duff, 1999). Restraint of trunk movement during performance of upper-limb activities combined with task-specific upper-limb training (Carr and Shepherd, 2000) improves functional outcomes after stroke more than unrestrained upper-limb training (Michaelsen et al., 2004, 2006). By restraining the excessive movements of the trunk during reaching and grasping training, more relevant somatosensory input from the arm joints can be provided and used to modulate the reaching pattern. This can be achieved by increasing the intensity of the afferent input (Hadders-Algra et al., 1999) or by increasing the frequency of exposure to task-appropriate somatosensory information.

Purpose

The purpose of the application of trunk restraint during the practice of upper limb tasks is to improve arm motor function by providing more appropriate, afferent information to the central nervous system from the affected arm to facilitate the reappearance of more efficient premorbid movement patterns.

Method

Candidates for the Intervention

Trunk restraint therapy is intended to remediate upper-limb motor control dysfunctions including body structures (International Classification of Functioning Disability and Health (ICF) (2007).

The technique is indicated for adults or children with moderate-to-severe hemiparesis who use excessive compensatory trunk movement when attempting to reach and grasp objects (Michaelsen et al., 2006; Thielman et al., 2004). Diagnoses include cerebral palsy, hemiplegia, quadriplegia, and stroke.

Settings

The technique may be used in rehabilitation health care settings or in home-exercise programs.

The Role of the Occupational Therapist in Applying the Intervention

The occupational therapist (OT) develops a training program consisting of uni-manual and bimanual upper-limb and hand activities in the workspace of the arm. The workspace is defined by the length of the arm and is divided into four basic quadrants: ipsilateral, contralateral, near field (proximal half of arm's length), and far field (distal half of arm's length). The length of the arm is defined as the distance between the medial border of the axilla and the fingertips of the outstretched hand for pointing activities, or the distance between the medial border of the axilla and the wrist crease for activities involving grasping. However, since trunk compensation is most likely to be greater when objects to be manipulated are placed further from the body, most of the activities should be done in the far workspace. The range of the activities should be varied and should include different combinations of wrist, elbow, and shoulder-joint movements. The number of repetitions should be high and the activities should be challenging to drive plastic changes in the nervous system (Kwakkel, 2006; Shepherd, 2001).

Results

Clinical Application

Fundamental Principles for Clinical Use

When motor compensations occur during movement production, the central nervous system receives nonoptimal sensory information from the trunk and limb (Adkins et al., 2006). This would interfere with the recovery of premorbid movement patterns, as suggested for the control of posture (Nashner et al., 1983) and for precision grasping (Eliasson et al., 1992, 1995; Gordon and Duff, 1999).

A Brief Guide to Clinical Practice

The technique is most effective in clients with moderate-to-severe hemiparesis who use more trunk compensation than do those who have mild hemiparesis (Michaelsen et al., 2006; Thielman et al., 2004). Trunk anterior displacement and rotation are restricted by a harness (de Oliveira et al., 2007) or two 3- to 4-inch-wide straps diagonally across the trunk from the right shoulder to the left hip and from the left shoulder to the right hip (Michaelsen et al., 2004, 2006). Straps can be secured around the body to a high-backed chair with buckles or Velcro closures. For adults, the straps should be applied so that no more than 2 cm of trunk anterior displacement in the sagittal plane and no more than 5 degrees of trunk rotation are permitted while shoulder girdle movement is relatively unrestricted. If trunk restraint is used in children with cerebral palsy, up to 5 cm of trunk movement should be permitted depending on the age of the child (Schneiberg et al., 2002).

How the Intervention Eases Impairments, Activity Limitations, and Participation Restrictions

Permitting the use of motor compensations could lead to a pattern of learned nonuse (Allred et al., 2005; Taub et al., 1993), limiting the capacity for subsequent gains in motor function of the paretic arm. Interventions that include the restriction of trunk motor compensations by physical trunk restraint may encourage the nervous system to find new motor solutions to task accomplishment and to overcome learned nonuse. These motor solutions may be more effective in improving upper-limb function through the emergence of new motor patterns. Improvement in upper-limb function will decrease activity limitations and social participation restrictions.

Evidence-Based Practice

Trunk restraint therapy is beneficial for motor recovery in adults (16 to 80 years of age) with chronic acquired brain damage (stroke) leading to disrupted motor control of the trunk and arms (Michaelsen et al., 2006). The principles should be equally applicable to adults with other types of acquired brain damage such as traumatic brain injury, and to children with developmental motor disorders such as cerebral palsy.

Trunk restraint combined with task-related training improved arm motor function in adults with stroke in one randomized control study (Michaelsen et al., 2006) and one pre- and postdesign study (de Oliveira et al., 2007). Michaelsen et al. (2006) compared arm motor impairment and function in clients with stroke practicing task-related training with trunk restraint ($n = 15$) or task-related training without trunk restraint ($n = 15$). Clients in the trunk-restraint group made greater improvements in motor function than those in the control group. Improvements were accompanied by increased active joint range and were greater in clients with greater initial severity of hemiparesis. In these clients, task-related training with trunk restraint led to less trunk movement and increased elbow extension during reaching, while clients in the control group increased compensatory trunk movement. In addition, changes in arm functions were correlated with changes in arm and trunk kinematics in the trunk-restraint group.

Discussion

Further research needs to prove the effectiveness of trunk restraint during task-related training of the upper limb in children with cerebral palsy. The effectiveness of combining the approach with other approaches or as an element in shaping arm movement during constraint-induced therapy has not yet been evaluated.

Recommended Reading

For a description of the content and clinical application of the intervention: Michaelsen et al., 2006.
For fundamental concepts on which the intervention is based: Cirstea and Levin, 2000; Levin, 2000; Levin et al., 2002; Michaelsen et al., 2001, 2004; Michaelsen and Levin, 2004; van der Lee et al., 1999.
The originator(s) of the intervention: Mindy F. Levin, PhD, PT, Associate Professor and Director, Physical Therapy Program, School of Physical and Occupational Therapy, McGill University.

References

Adkins, D.L., Boychuk, J., Remple, M.S., and Kleim, J.A. (2006). Motor training induces experience-specific patterns of plasticity across motor cortex and spinal cord. J Appl Physiol, 101, 1776–1782.
Allred, R.P., Maldonado, M.A., Hsu, J.E., and Jones, T.A. (2005). Training the 'less-affected' forelimb after unilateral cortical infarcts interferes with functional recovery of the impaired forelimb in rats. Restor Neurol Neurosci, 23, 297–302.
Carr, J.H., and Shepherd, R.B. (2000). A motor learning model for rehabilitation. In: Carr, J.H., and Shepherd, R.B., eds. Movement Science. Foundations for Physical Therapy in Rehabilitation, 2nd ed. Gaithersburg, MD: Aspen.
Cirstea, M.C., and Levin, M.F. (2000). Compensatory strategies for reaching in stroke. Brain, 123, 940–953.
de Oliveira, R., Cacho, E.W., and Borges, G. (2007). Improvements in the upper limb of hemiparetic clients after reaching movements training. Int J Rehabil Res, 30, 67–70.
Eliasson, A.C., Gordon, A.M., and Forssberg, H. (1992). Impaired anticipatory control of isometric forces during grasping by children with cerebral palsy. Dev Med Child Neurol, 33, 216–225.
Eliasson, A.C., Gordon, A.M., and Forssberg, H. (1995). Tactile control of isometric finger forces during grasping in children with cerebral palsy. Dev Med Child Neurol, 37, 72–84.
Gordon, A.M., and Duff, S.V. (1999). Fingertip forces during object manipulation in children with hemiplegic cerebral palsy. I. Anticipatory scaling. Dev Med Child Neurol, 41, 166–175.
Hadders-Algra, M., van der Fits, I.B.M., Stremmelaar, E.F., and Touwen, B.C.L. (1999). Development of postural adjustments during reaching in infants with cerebral palsy. Dev Med Child Neurol, 41, 766–776.
Kwakkel, G. (2006). Impact of intensity of practice after stroke: Issues for consideration. Disabil Rehabil, 28, 823–830.
Levin, M.F. (2000). A model of sensorimotor deficits in clients with central nervous system lesions. Hum Mov Sci, 19, 107–132.
Levin, M.F., Michaelsen, S., Cirstea, C., and Roby-Brami, A. (2002). Use of the trunk for reaching targets placed within and beyond the reach in adult hemiparesis. Exp Brain Res, 143, 171–180.
Michaelsen, S.M., Dannenbaum, R., and Levin, M.F. (2006). Task-specific training with trunk restraint on arm recovery in stroke. Randomized control trial. Stroke, 37, 186–192.

Michaelsen, S.M., Jacobs, S., Roby-Brami, A., and Levin, M.F. (2004). Compensation for distal impairments of grasping in adults with hemiparesis. Exp Brain Res, 157, 162–173.

Michaelsen, S.M., and Levin, M.F. (2004). Short-term effects of practice with trunk restraint on reaching movements in clients with chronic stroke: a controlled trial. Stroke, 35, 1914–1919.

Michaelsen, S.M., Luta, A., Roby-Brami, A., and Levin, M.F. (2001). Effect of trunk restraint on the recovery of reaching movements in hemiparetic clients. Stroke, 32, 1875–1883.

Nashner, L.M., Shumway-Cook, A., and Marin, O. (1983). Stance postural control in select groups of children with cerebral palsy: deficits in sensory organization and muscular organization. Exp Brain Res, 49, 393–409.

Schneiberg, S., Sviestrup, H., McFadyen, B., McKinley, P., and Levin, M.F. (2002). Development of coordination for reaching in children. Exp Brain Res, 146(2), 142–154.

Shepherd, R.B. (2001). Exercise and training to optimize functional motor performance in stroke: driving neural reorganization? Neural Plasticity, 8, 121–129.

Taub, E., Miller, N.E., Novack, T.A., et al. (1993). Technique to improve chronic motor deficits after stroke. Arch Phys Med Rehabil, 74, 347–354.

Thielman, G.T., Dean, C.M., and Gentile, A.M. (2004). Rehabilitation of reaching after stroke: task-related training versus progressive resistive exercise. Arch Phys Med Rehabil, 85, 1613–1618.

van der Lee, J.H., Wagenaar, R.C., Lankhorst, G.J., Vogelaar, T.W., Deville, W.L., and Bouter, L.M. (1999). Forced use of the upper extremity in chronic stroke clients: Results from a single-blind randomized clinical trial. Stroke, 30, 2369–2375.

World Health Organization (2007). International classification of functioning, disability and health. ICF introduction (home page). http://www.who.int/classification/icf/site/icftemplate.cfm?myurl = home.

Chapter 30
Constraint-Induced Movement Therapy for Restoration of Upper-Limb Function: Introduction

Mary H. Bowman, Victor W. Mark, and Edward Taub

Before starting Constraint-Induced Movement Therapy, it was hard to remember to use my weaker hand for everyday things, but now I just use it without having to think about it.

—Client

Abstract Constraint-Induced Movement Therapy (CIMT) is a research-originated, behavioral approach to neurorehabilitation of limb function after neurologic damage. The intervention utilizes a combination of motor training elements and psychological concepts to facilitate increased use of the affected limb as well as improved movement quality and control. Importantly, CIMT is designed to achieve real-world improvements by behavioral methods which facilitate the incorporation of regained abilities into the persons' spontaneous behavior. Constraint-Induced Movement Therapy is composed of three primary elements: (1) repetitive, unilateral training procedures (e.g., shaping, task practice); (2) a set of behavioral techniques, termed the "transfer package," that promote transfer of therapeutic gains to the life situation; and (3) constraint of the less-affected hand by one of several techniques. Evidence shows that CIMT improves functional use and occupational performance of the more affected upper extremity by reversing learned nonuse and facilitating use-dependent brain plasticity.

Keywords Motor skills • Neuronal plasticity • Rehabilitation • Stroke

Definition and Background

Constraint-Induced Movement Therapy (CIMT) (Taub et al., 1993) improves the functional use of the more affected arm after neurological injury by overcoming learned nonuse and facilitating use-dependent cortical reorganization. It is an intervention based on a behavioral neurorehabilitation model employed with individuals following central nervous system damage (e.g., stroke, traumatic brain injury [TBI]). Basic neuroscience studies with monkeys (Taub, 1977, 1980) preceded studies with humans for (CIMT), and laid the foundation both for discovering the existence of

I. Söderback (ed.), *International Handbook of Occupational Therapy Interventions*,
DOI: 10.1007/978-0-387-75424-6_30, © Springer Science+Business Media, LLC 2010

learned non-use as a mechanism contributing importantly to the deficit in monkeys with single deafferented forelimbs, and for providing methods to overcome it (Taub et al., 2006a). This phenomenon is found in humans as well after neurologic insult, so that the individual has reduced use of the limb despite motor capability for occupational performance (Taub et al., 1993, 1999). The efficacy of (CIMT) is considered based on two independent but linked mechanisms (Taub et al., 2006a): (1) practice-based counterconditioning of learned nonuse, and (2) use-dependent plastic brain reorganization.

Purpose

Constraint-Induced Movement Therapy has been shown to enhance a client's occupational performance through improved motor ability and remediation of symptoms of learned nonuse. Used both in rehabilitation and habilitation of the more affected arm, (CIMT) has been shown to significantly change not only the more affected arm use and motor ability but also brain function and structure, as demonstrated by neuroimaging (Gauthier et al., 2008; Liepert et al., 2000).

Method

Candidates for the Intervention

Because the clinical practice of (CIMT) is derived from a research foundation that continues to expand, the principles and procedures of (CIMT) will likely continue to be revised. The amount of impairment of candidates has been classified in (CIMT) research by using active range of motion (AROM) of the upper extremity (UE) as a primary criterion (Bowman et al., 2006; Taub et al., 1993, 1999). Early (CIMT) research had recruited participants with only mild-to-moderate stroke deficits (Taub et al., 1993, 1999, 2006b). The research then progressed to treating clients with moderate or moderately severe upper extremity impairment (Taub et al., 1999). More recently, work has been carried out with stroke clients with plegic or nearly plegic hands (Bowman et al., 2006).

The original (CIMT) protocol has also been modified and extended to individuals with traumatic brain injury (TBI) (Shaw et al., 2005), multiple sclerosis (Mark et al., 2008), focal hand dystonia (Candia et al., 1999), lower extremity paresis following stroke or spinal cord injury (Taub et al., 1999), aphasia (CI language therapy) (Pulvermüller et al., 2001; Taub, 2002), or cerebral palsy (pediatric CIMT) (Taub et al., 2004, 2007).

In addition to the upper extremity AROM criterion, selection of research participants has taken into consideration postural balance, cognitive integrity, presence of pain that might interfere with administration of the therapy, and illness chronicity, to ensure homogenous populations. However, in clinical practice, greater flexibility may be appropriate to treat clients with learned nonuse (Mark and Taub, 2004).

Stroke chronicity of >1 year was used for most research studies, but preliminary evidence suggests that clients in the acute to subacute phases may also benefit (Boake et al., 2007; Dromerick et al., 2000; Wolf et al., 2006).

The use of the AROM criteria assists the therapist with selecting the appropriate CIMT protocol. Clients with mild or moderate upper extremity paresis are usually treated for 3,5 hours per day for 10 consecutive weekdays, while clients with more severe upper extremities paresis are usually treated 3,5 hours per day for 15 consecutive weekdays (Mark and Taub, 2004).

Epidemiology

The prevalence of stroke-associated disability in the general population has been reported to range from 173 to 200 per 100,000 (SASPI Project Team, 2004), while the estimated proportion of stroke survivors who are dependent in their activities of daily life (ADL) ranges from 30% to 50% (Carroll, 1962; Gresham et al., 1975).

Seventy percent of chronic stroke survivors are estimated to have motor deficit (Anderson et al., 2004). Studies have not yet determined what proportion of adult stroke clients with an acute hemiparesis in a subacute or a chronic stage will meet inclusion criteria for CIMT.

In a recent prospective study, 41 out of 87 people suffering from a stroke had moderate to severe hemiparesis (Prabhakaran et al. 2008). The great majority of these 41 clients (83%) recovered to at least 70% of the maximum motor gain possible by 3 months after stroke onset. These findings suggest that most acutely hemiparetic stroke clients eventually regain substantial movement ability that would appear adequate for training tasks. However, further research is needed to determine what proportion of stroke patients who are in a subacute or a chronic stage and having persistent learned nonuse of the paretic upper extremity, and therefore would be recommended to undergo CIMT.

Individuals with diagnoses other than stroke who meet the AROM criteria may also be appropriate for CIMT.

Settings

Research to date indicates that CIMT is well suited for implementation among outpatient and in home health settings. Studies have suggested that CIMT in an acute inpatient rehabilitation setting may be efficacious (Boake et al., 2007; Dromerick et al., 2000).

The Role of the Occupational Therapist

Constraint-Induced Movement Therapy may be conducted by an occupational therapist or a physiotherapist. The role of the therapist in CIMT is to ensure the integrity of the standard intervention while focusing on the unique needs and goals of each client. The occupational therapist (OT) may be required to adopt a variety of roles, including evaluator, tester, trainer, coach, problem solver, and encourager. Therapists must employ therapeutic skills in observation, listening, problem solving, behavioral management, task analysis, strategy development, safety awareness, and risk assessment, especially with regard to appropriate mitt use. Splinting, adaptive equipment selection, adaptive strategy development, and other conventional interventions are also employed to the CIMT.

In the clinical application of CIMT, it is important to duplicate the procedures that were used in the research protocols, including ensuring that prospective clients have similar movement deficits. Enrolling clients who do not meet the minimal movement requirements for the specific protocol may lead to poor results as well as frustration on the part of both the therapist and the clients.

It should be noted that many procedures in CIMT are not typically employed in conventional rehabilitation. In our experience, therapists have often voiced their unfamiliarity with the types of procedures utilized in CIMT, particularly with the techniques of the transfer package. It is important that therapists who plan to implement CIMT should first be adequately trained.

At the University of Alabama at Birmingham, CIMT training consists of a semiannual 5-day continuing education course that includes 2 days of a hands-on lab practicum accompanied by feedback on performance of procedures to ensure proper administration of the CIMT treatment.

Results

Clinical Application

Constraint-Induced Movement Therapy consists of three main components, which are demonstrated in Fig. 30.1:

- Repetitive, functionally relevant, task-oriented training of the more impaired limb.
- Employment of a set of behavioral techniques known as the *transfer package* that are designed to facilitate carryover of gains made in the research laboratory or clinic to the generalized life situation.
- Procedures to constrain use of the more affected extremity, including physical restraint of the less affected arm (Taub et al., 1993; Uswatte et al., 2006a).

Shaping (Taub et al., 1993; 1994), one of the primary training technique employed, is a systematic behavioral procedure whereby progress is achieved in small steps by successive approximations throughout multiple timed trials that use frequent detailed

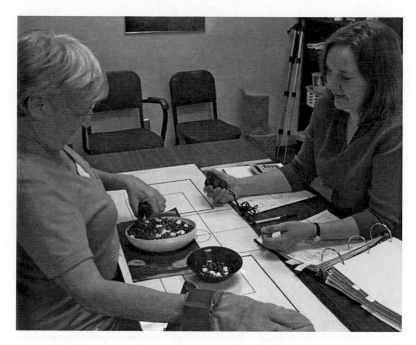

Fig. 30.1 An example of administering shaping with a client who had suffered from a stroke. The mitt on the less-affected hand greatly reduces the ability to use that extremity.

feedback and encouragement. With adults, the shaping process is usually broken up into blocks of ten trials each, and the repetitions of the task are timed or the number of repetitions completed in a set timed period, (e.g., 30 sec.). The data from each trial are recorded and reported immediately to the client. Progression of the shaping task requires consistent improvement in previous performance.

The transfer package (Taub et al., 2006a) utilizes selected behavioral techniques: home diary, behavioral contract, home skill assignment, daily administration of the Motor Activity Log (MAL) (Uswatte et al., 2006b), problem solving, and maintenance of a daily schedule. In the transfer package, protocol adherence is bolstered by maximizing client accountability, engaging the client in problem solving, and prompting the client to use the more affected limb during occupational performance. The transfer package makes compliance with the CIMT protocol the responsibility of the client; therefore, the functional achievements are his own.

A *signature feature* of CIMT protocols is the use of a padded safety mitt on the less affected hand as a physical restraint. The mitt is worn for a target of 90% of waking hours during the therapy period and is removed during personal hygiene and where safety might be comprised through its use. Mitt use is only one way of constraining the client's behavior to increase use of the more affected upper extremity and appears not to be the most important feature (Uswatte et al., 2006a).

Two outcome measures with established reliability and validity have been consistently used with CIMT research:

- The MAL (Taub et al., 1993; Uswatte et al., 2006b), a structured, scripted interview that measures the amount and quality of spontaneous arm use during activities of daily living (ADL) in the real world.
- The Wolf Motor Function Test (WMFT) (Morris et al., 2001; Wolf et al., 2001, 2005), which is a standard laboratory test of motor ability. The WMFT is not required when providing CIMT in clinical practice (Mark and Taub, 2004).

How the Intervention Addresses Impairments, Activity Limitations, and Participation Restrictions

After CIMT, motor impairments of the more affected upper extremity show positive changes, in a large majority of cases and the client is better able to engage the limb in occupational performance. In addition to the motor and functional use gains, evidence has shown that clients report quality of life improvements that are sustained for at least 2 years after undergoing CIMT (Wolf et al., 2008).

Evidence-Based Practice

Constraint-Induced Movement Therapy is an evidence-based approach that is grounded in a strong empirical foundation that has been evolving over the last two decades. Randomized controlled trials (RCTs) have been published with positive results (Shaw et al., 2005; Taub et al., 1993, 1999, 2004, 2006b, 2007). The Extremity Constraint-Induced Therapy Evaluation (EXCITE) trial (Wolf et al., 2006), a large, multisite RCT of CIMT for the upper extremity after stroke, was the first of its kind for rehabilitation of the upper extremity in the United States. Additional evidence continues to emerge from around the world, with over 200 papers published that have examined CIMT all yielding to our knowledge successful findings.

Discussion

The CIMT model brings with it engaging concepts and challenging principles that offer new perspectives and opportunities for rehabilitation. As this model has been disseminated, criticisms of CIMT have been voiced, including concerns with safety, questions about the distinctiveness of the intervention, concerns for the acceptability of CIMT to clients, and reimbursement issues. Mark and Taub (2004) discuss these issues in detail.

Constraint-Induced Movement Therapy is cost-effective in that it has proven outcomes. With proper implementation, one can anticipate a specific amount of average functional recovery. CIMT enables a breakthrough for participants toward real-world functional recovery and not only symptom management after stroke. Automated forms of CIMT have also been successfully studied to reduce the cost of administration of shaping by a therapist, which may allow the therapist to work with more than one client at a time (Taub et al., 2005)

Future studies should more closely examine the factors responsible for the therapeutic effect of CIMT, as well as attempt continued extension of CIMT to new populations of clients who display learned nonuse. Studies that combine traditional therapeutic modalities and approaches with CIMT to maximize gains for lower functioning clients are also needed.

References

Anderson, C.S., Carter, K.N., Brownlee, W.J., et al. (2004). Very long-term outcome after stroke in Auckland, New Zealand. Stroke, 35, 1920–1924.

Boake, C., Noser, E.A., Ro, T., et al. (2007). Constraint-Induced Movement Therapy during early stroke rehabilitation. Neurorehabil Neural Repair, 21, 14–24.

Bowman, M.H., Taub, E., Uswatte, G., et al. (2006). A treatment for a chronic stroke patient with a plegic hand combining CI therapy with conventional rehabilitation procedures: case report. NeuroRehabilitation, 21, 167–176.

Candia, V., Elbert, T., Altenmüller, E., et al. (1999). Constraint-Induced Movement Therapy for focal hand dystonia in musicians. Lancet, 353, 42.

Carroll, D. (1962). The disability in hemiplegia caused by cerebrovascular disease: serial studies of 98 cases. J Chron Dis, 15, 179–188.

Dromerick, A.W., Edwards, D.F., and Hahn, M. (2000). Does the application of Constraint-Induced Movement Therapy during acute rehabilitation reduce arm impairment after ischemic stroke. Stroke, 82, 2984–2988.

Gauthier, L.V., Taub, E., Perkins, C., et al. (2008). Remodeling the brain: plastic structural brain changes produced by different motor therapies after stroke. Stroke, 39, 1520–1525.

Gresham, G.E., Fitzpatrick, T.E., Wolf, P.A., et al. (1975). Residual disability in survivors of stroke—the Framingham Study. N Engl J Med, 293, 954–956.

Liepert, J., Bauder, H., Miltner, W.H.R., et al. (2000). Treatment-induced cortical reorganization after stroke in humans. Stroke, 31, 1210–1216.

Mark, V.W., and Taub, E. (2004). Constraint-Induced Movement Therapy for chronic stroke hemiparesis and other disabilities. Restor Neurol Neurosci, 22, 317–336.

Mark, V.W., Taub, E., Bashir, K., et al. (2008). Constraint-Induced Movement Therapy benefits hemiparetic multiple sclerosis. Mult Scler, 14, 992–994.

Morris, D., Uswatte, G., Crago, J., et al. (2001). The reliability of the Wolf Motor Function Test for assessing upper extremity motor function following stroke. Arch Phys Med Rehabil, 82, 750–775.

Prabhakaran, S., Zarahn, E., Riley, C., et al. (2008). Inter-individual variability in the capacity for motor recovery after ischemic stroke. Neurorehabil Neural Repair, 22, 64–71.

Pulvermüller, F., Neininger, B., Elbert, T., et al. (2001). Constraint-induced therapy of chronic aphasia after stroke. Stroke, 32, 1621–1626.

SASPI Project Team. (2004). Prevalence of stroke survivors in rural South Africa: results from the Southern Africa Stroke Prevention Initiative (SASPI) Agincourt Field Site. Stroke, 35, 627–632.

Shaw, S.E., Morris, D., Uswatte, G., et al. (2005). Constraint-induced movement therapy for recovery of upper-limb function following traumatic brain injury. J Rehabil Res Dev, 42, 769–778.

Taub, E. (1977). Movement in nonhuman primates deprived of somatosensory feedback. Exerc Sports Sci Rev, 4, 335–374.

Taub, E. (1980). Somatosensory deafferentation with monkeys: implications for rehabilitation medicine. In: Ince, L.P., ed., Behavioral Psychology in Rehabilitation Medicine. Clinical Applications. New York: Williams & Wilkins.

Taub, E. (2002). CI therapy: a new rehabilitation technique for aphasia and motor disability after neurological injury. Klin Forsch, 8, 48–49.

Taub, E., Cragp, J.E., Burgio, L.D., Groomes, T.E., Miller, N.E. (1994). An operant approach to rehabilitation medicine: overcoming learned non-use by shaping. J Exp Anal Behv. 61(2):281–293.

Taub, E., Burgio, L., Miller, N.E., et al. (1994). An operant approach to overcoming learned non use after CNS damage in monkeys and man: The role of shaping. J Exper Anal Behav 61:281–293.

Taub, E., Griffin, A., Nick, J., et al. (2007). Pediatric CI therapy for stroke-induced hemiparesis in young children. Dev Neurorehabil, 10, 3–18.

Taub, E., Lum, P., Hardin, P., et al. (2005). AutoCITE: Automated delivery of CI therapy with reduced effort by therapists. Stroke, 36, 1301–1304.

Taub, E., Miller, N.E., Novack, T.A., et al. (1993). Technique to improve chronic motor deficit after stroke. Arch Phys Med Rehabil, 74, 347–354.

Taub, E., Ramey, S.L., DeLuca, S.C., et al. (2004). Efficacy of Constraint-Induced (CI) Movement therapy for children with cerebral palsy with asymmetric motor impairment. Pediatrics, 113, 305–312.

Taub, E., Uswatte, G., King, D.K., et al. (2006b). A placebo controlled trial of Constraint-Induced Movement Therapy for upper extremity after stroke. Stroke, 37, 1045–1049.

Taub, E., Uswatte, G., Mark, V.W., et al. (2006a). The learned nonuse phenomenon: implications for rehabilitation. Eura Medicophys, 42, 241–255.

Taub, E., Uswatte, G., and Pidikiti, R. (1999). Constraint-Induced Movement Therapy: a new family of techniques with broad application to physical rehabilitation—a clinical review. J Rehabil Res Dev, 36, 237–251.

Uswatte, G., Taub, E., Morris, D., et al. (2006a). Contribution of the shaping and constraint components of Constraint-Induced Movement Therapy to treatment outcome. NeuroRehabilitation, 21, 147–156.

Uswatte, G., Taub, E., Morris, D., et al. (2006b). The Motor Activity Log-28: A method for assessing daily use of the hemiparetic arm after stroke. Neurology, 67, 1189–1194.

Wolf, S.L., Catlin, P., Ellis, M., et al. (2001). Assessing Wolf Motor Function Test as outcome measure for research in patients after stroke. Stroke, 32, 1635–1639.

Wolf, S.L., Thompson, P.A., Morris, D.M., et al. (2005). The EXCITE trial: attributes of the Wolf Motor Function Test in patients with subacute stroke. Neurorehabil Neural Repair, 19, 194–205.

Wolf, S.L., Winstein, C.J., Miller, J.P., et al. (2006). Effect of Constraint-Induced Movement Therapy on upper extremity function 3 to 9 months after stroke: the EXCITE randomized clinical trial. JAMA, 296, 2095–2104.

Wolf, S.L., Winstein, C.J., Miller, J.P., et al. (2008). Retention of upper limb function in stroke survivors who have Constraint-Induced Movement Therapy: the EXCITE randomized trial. Lancet Neurol, 7, 33–40.

Chapter 31
Constraint-Induced Movement Therapy for Restoration of Upper-Limb Function: Hemiparesis Application

Annette Sterr, Katherine Herron, and Jennifer Sanders

*CIT has helped me mentally as well as physically.
In the 2-week period, I kept finding I could do things
every day. I feel it's given me more confidence.*

—Client

Abstract Constraint-induced movement therapy (CIT) is a highly specialized
form of rehabilitation for those with upper-limb paresis. The intervention uses a
combination of motor training elements and psychological concepts to facilitate
increased use of the affected limb as well as improved movement quality and
control. Importantly, CIT is designed to achieve real-world improvements through
behavioral measures that facilitate the incorporation of regained abilities into the
person's spontaneous behavior.

Keywords Constraint-induced movement therapy • Learning • Neuronal plasticity
• Shaping • Rehabilitation • Upper extremity paresis.

Definition and Background

Constraint-induced movement therapy (CIT) works on the premise that the brain
can reorganize itself after sustaining damage to the motor area, and that these
processes are facilitated through the two treatment principles: (1) extensive
upper-limb training, and (2) constraining the unaffected limb. The intervention
encourages brain reorganization to increase its motor capacities (Kim et al., 2004)
and the cortical space devoted to the affected upper limb (Liepert et al., 2000).

The upper-limb-training component of CIT involves the massed practice of
everyday tasks or parts thereof under the guidance of and with the feedback from a
CIT therapist. Here, the therapist implements the principles of shaping, a psychological
concept derived from the behaviorist tradition, which involves: (a) quantifying and
very frequent immediate feedback concerning improvements in the speed and quality
of movement (QOM), (b) selecting tasks that were tailored to address the motor

I. Söderback (ed.), *International Handbook of Occupational Therapy Interventions*,
DOI: 10.1007/978-0-387-75424-6_31, © Springer Science+Business Media, LLC 2010

deficits of the individual client, (c) modeling, prompting, and cuing of task performance, and (d) systematically increasing the difficulty level of the task performed in small steps when five trials of improved performance occurred. (Taub et al., 2006, p. 1046)

In addition to the training of the affected arm, the unaffected limb is constrained so as to encourage the use of the affected arm outside the treatment setting and to reverse "learned nonuse." The latter is a learned behavior established during the diaschisis phase in early recovery, and it occurs when the affected limb is associated with failure to achieve goals; therefore, unaffected arm use, associated with successful functioning, is reinforced. Constraining the unaffected arm enforces the use of the affected arm and breaks the chain of reward contingencies, which establish and sustain the learned nonuse.

Constraint-induced movement therapy aims to increase the use, quality, and control of movement in the affected limb. The functional improvements obtained through the intervention enhance clients' confidence in using the affected limb in everyday situations, thus contributing to an enhancement of well-being and quality of life.

Method

Candidates for the Intervention

Candidates are clients with upper-limb paresis who have sustained brain damage because of stroke, traumatic brain injury, cerebral palsy, or tumor. Although CIT-based clinical trials to date use strict inclusion criteria, CIT has been successfully applied to clients with various causes and prognoses of hemiparesis, and at various stages postincident. Brain trauma is often associated with other persisting symptoms, ranging from physical ailments to psychological and cognitive disturbances, which may be possible areas for concern when considering a client for CIT. This is particularly true concerning the use of the unaffected-arm constraint, which forces patients to face the incapacities of their affected arm and the consequences thereof. Adequate psychological supervision alongside CIT provision is therefore mandatory, in particular when residual abilities are very poor and the incapacitation through the unaffected arm constraint is severe.

Most importantly, clients must have *some* residual movement in the arm and hand of the affected limb. Minimal movement is usually 10 degrees for digits and 10 degrees for the wrist. However, this criterion is not mandatory. Gross arm movement must also have some functioning to enable carrying out activities of daily living. High spasm can be challenging for the shaping training, and present difficulties with everyday living activities while wearing the constraint. Persons with full paralysis of the affected limb will not benefit from the CIT protocols currently available.

Constraint-induced movement therapy is a versatile intervention from which children, adults, and older adults can all benefit.

Settings

At present, CIT is available privately at the Taub Therapy Clinic in Birmingham, Alabama, and interested persons can apply to participate in various clinical trials worldwide. Implementation of CIT as a widely available form of rehabilitation is the current aim. In some countries, such as Germany, this is well underway. Other than this, CIT is applied in a research context in some European and American research centers (including the University of Surrey, England). Furthermore, practitioners presently use some components of CIT, but rarely in the formalized and systematic way that underlie all successful clinical trials of CIT.

The Role of the Therapist Applying the Intervention

The therapist-client interaction (Fig. 31.1) in CIT therapy is very intense, not only because of the length of daily treatment but also because of the therapist's functions, which are as follows:

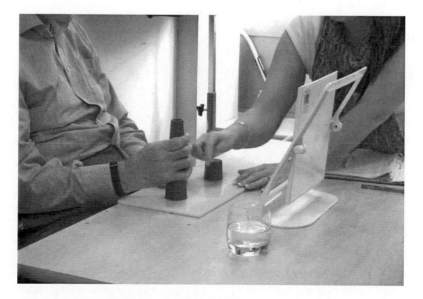

Fig. 31.1 A constraint-induced movement therapy (CIT) session. The therapist helps guide the client's movement toward the desired goal.

- Setting realistic goals and agreeing to these in a treatment contract.
- Specifying the task program for the behavior shaping in accordance with the goals, and reviewing the task in accordance with progress.
- Providing psychological support in problem-solving sessions. Monitoring the client's progress within and between sessions.

Setting Realistic Goals

Realistic goals for CIT tasks and functional aims at home are based on what the therapist and client feel is achievable. The goals are agreed upon and formulated in a treatment contract. The client input in goal-setting is an important motivational factor, and may actually encourage CIT recipients to work toward more complex goals in the longer term.

Behavior Shaping

The application of *positive reinforcement* allows the therapist to shape affected limb use toward the desired behavior. Positive reinforcement may be in the form of verbal praise, visual feedback, or quantifying actual improvement. The latter is particularly important and is reflected in the design of CIT tasks, which entails a high level of formalization and the provision of measurable performance indices.

Psychological Support

Constraint-induced movement therapy directly addresses disability, which is usually paired with psychological consequences. Therefore, good client relation skills are essential to promote a psychologically supportive environment. Encouraging clients to reflect on their experience during sessions is a good opportunity to reinforce progress and judge clients' psychological and physical state. This enables the therapist to help ease any frustration and decide whether a rest is required. Ample motivation and positive feedback are an essential part of CIT to further reinforce affected arm use with a favorable outcome.

Monitoring Progress

Constraint-induced movement therapy session content and patient achievement are documented for each task. This is usually reported as the number of repetitions per trial, the number of rests, and time to complete the task. A diary of activities is used to support and track affected arm use at home, and can further be used to highlight areas of difficulty that are subsequently addressed during problem solving.

Results

Clinical Application

During the training sessions, clients practice motor tasks with the affected upper limb with the supervision and encouragement of the therapist. Traditionally, training is administered for 6 hours a day over ten consecutive weekdays. The shaping technique is used to elicit the desired movement from the affected limb by gradually increasing task difficulty. Tasks can be directed at elements of upper-limb movement (e.g., using a spoon involves the elbow, wrist, and grip) or at specific movements (e.g., concentrating on moving individual fingers), and are practiced in a repetitive fashion using tangible feedback on task performance. The unaffected arm constraint, typically a forearm splint (Fig. 31.2), is worn for 90% of waking hours in order to force the use of the affected limb throughout this time.

Thus, clients are encouraged to employ their affected arm in functional tasks at home. These tasks are initially outlined in a treatment contract and reviewed daily. Difficulties or successes in the home environment are addressed in problem-solving sessions, which proceed every training day.

How the Intervention Eases Impairments, Activity Limitations, and Participation Restrictions

Following CIT, participants experienced a significant increase in real-world arm use, measured by the Motor Activity Log (Unswatte et al., 2006).

Recent research has extended the traditional motor outcome measures to include quality of life. Participants in a modified CIT program reported greater holistic recovery from the effects of their stroke on the Stroke Impact Scale, compared to

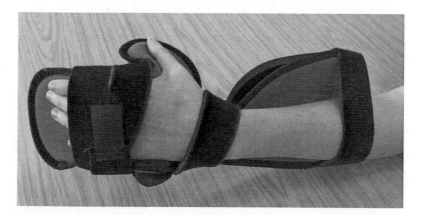

Fig. 31.2 The constraint inhibits full use of the arm and fingers, thus forcing the use of the affected arm.

those who received a traditional form of rehabilitation (Wu et al., 2007). Dettmers et al. (2005) found improvements in psychosocial domains such as social participation and communication from pretreatment to 6-month follow-up.

Evidence-Based Practice

Scientific Support

The empirical evidence for the efficacy of CIT is strong. CIT increases motor ability and real-world arm use compared to control treatment, and these changes persist for up to 2 years (Taub et al., 2006). The effectiveness of CIT was further demonstrated in a multicentered clinical trial (Wolf et al., 2006). Comparable findings have been obtained in a traumatic brain injury (TBI) population (Shaw et al., 2005). Modified protocols are also effective. Shorter daily therapy time produced lesser but significant improvements in objective and subjective motor function (Sterr et al., 2002). A shaping-only protocol involving 90 minutes of daily training over 3 consecutive weeks also increased motor function and arm use compared to a control group (Sterr and Freivogel, 2003).

Other Considerations

The Reality of Constraint-Induced Movement Therapy

A particular issue surrounding CIT is use of a constraint, which may pose safety risks for some clients. One way to overcome this is for clients to sign a treatment contract by which they agree not to wear the constraint in situations that compromise their safety, such as with the use of walking aids. In addition, it has been shown that improvements in upper-limb use can be obtained even if constraint is not used (Sterr and Freivogel, 2003). However, longer follow-ups are needed to assess the long-term outcome of shaping-only protocols.

Another area of concern is the high demand of the intervention, which may increase sleepiness and mental exhaustion. Clients therefore need to take extra caution when returning home, ensuring appropriate rest after CIT, and getting a good night's sleep for subsequent sessions.

Discussion

Wider Application of Constraint-Induced Movement Therapy

The adaptive nature of CIT allows the traditional protocol to be applied to patients with varying needs, time constraints, and health care resources. CIT has also been successfully applied to other motor movement problems including lower-limb paresis and balance (Vearrier et al., 2005). The foundations of CIT theory have strong potential in nonmotor conditions such as aphasia (Meinzer et al., 2007) and chronic pain syndrome (Pruimboom and van Dam, 2007).

Future Research

In realistic circumstances, the original protocol of 6 hours of CIT per day is likely to exhaust resources and not be applicable in all patients. The systematic testing of more practical CIT variants is therefore essential for CIT to become a standard health care procedure. Novel forms of treatment delivery, such as online CIT, have shown promising results and warrant further exploration (Page and Levine, 2007).

Conclusion

"So now I have finally overcome the major drawbacks in my life so that they have driven me forwards, and that's all because I undertook CIT." CIT, a truly life-changing intervention, has been termed the most successful treatment for those suffering from upper-limb hemiparesis. More and more rehabilitation consultants are taking an interest in CIT, making it available for the clients who need it. CIT is an interdisciplinary intervention that marries social sciences and psychology with physiotherapy and occupational therapy. Fusing disciplinary boundaries in education and practice will be the key to the successful translation of this intervention into clinical practice.

References

Dettmers, C., Teske, U., Hamzei, F., Uswatte, G., Taub, E., and Weiller, C. (2005). Distributed form of constraint-induced movement therapy improves functional outcome and quality of life after stroke. Arch Phys Med Rehabil, 86(2), 204–209.
Kim, Y.H., Park, J.W., Ko, M.H., Jang, S.H., and Lee, P.K. (2004). Plastic changes of motor network after constraint-induced movement therapy. Yonsei Med J, 45(2), 241–246.
Liepert, J., Bauder, H., Wolfgang, H.R., Miltner, W.H., Taub, E., and Weiller, C. (2000). Treatment-induced cortical reorganization after stroke in humans. Stroke, 31(6), 1210–1216.
Meinzer, M., Elbert, T., Djundja, D., Taub, E., and Rockstroh, B. (2007). Extending the constraint-induced movement therapy (CIMT) approach to cognitive functions: constraint-induced aphasia therapy (CIAT) of chronic aphasia. NeuroRehabilitation, 22(4), 311–318.
Page, S.J., and Levine, P. (2007). Modified constraint-induced therapy extension: using remote technologies to improve function. Arch Phys Med Rehabil, 88(7), 922–927.
Pruimboom, L., and van Dam, A.C. (2007). Chronic pain: a non-use disease. Med Hypotheses, 68(3), 506–511.

Shaw, S.E., Morris, D.M., Uswatte, G., McKay, S., Meythaler, J.M., and Taub, E. (2005). Constraint-induced movement therapy for recovery of upper-limb function following traumatic brain injury. J Rehabil Res Dev, 42(6), 769–778.

Sterr, A., Elbert, T., Berthold, I., Kolbel, S., Rockstroh, B., and Taub, E. (2002). Longer versus shorter daily constraint-induced movement therapy of chronic hemiparesis: an exploratory study. Arch Phys Med Rehabil, 83(10), 1374–1377.

Sterr, A., and Freivogel, S. (2003). Motor-improvement following intensive training in low-functioning chronic hemiparesis. Neurology, 61(6), 842–844.

Taub, E., Uswatte, G., King, D.K., Morris, D., Crago, J.E., and Chatterjee, A. (2006). A placebo-controlled trial of constraint-induced movement therapy for upper extremity after stroke. Stroke, 37(4), 1045–1049.

Unswatte, G., Taub, E., Morris, D., et al. (2006). The Motor Activity Log-28. A method for assessing daily use of the hemiparetic arm after stroke. Neurology, 67, 1189–1194.

Vearrier, L.A., Langan, J., Shumway-Cook, A., and Woollacott, M. (2005). An intensive massed practice approach to retraining balance post-stroke. Gait Posture, 22(2), 154–163.

Wolf, S.L., Winstein, C.J., Miller, J.P., et al. (2006). Effect of constraint-induced movement therapy on upper extremity function 3 to 9 months after stroke: the EXCITE randomized clinical trial. JAMA, 296(17), 2095–2104.

Wu, C., Chen, C., Tsai, W., Lin, K., and Chou, S. (2007). A randomized controlled trial of modified constraint-induced movement therapy for elderly stroke survivors: changes in motor impairment, daily functioning, and quality of life. Arch Phys Med Rehabil, 88, 273–278.

Chapter 32
Strategies for Curing with Self-Speech in People Living with Parkinson's Disease

Kinsuk Maitra

I can turn and not shuffle when I say three times "Turn-Turn-Turn"; this is wonderful.

—Client

Abstract Strategies for cuing with self-speech (known as the RehabSelfCue-Speech program) is a systematically organized intervention. It addresses how clients living with Parkinson's disease learn to use self-cuing to initiate movement-related actions (Maitra, 2007; Maitra and Dasgupta, 2005). The client reads action-words, which are semantically related to occupational performance of daily living tasks (e.g., get up from a chair, reach tools or food, or grasp a pen and a paper). The RehabSelfCue-Speech program is based on Pulvermüller et al.'s (2005) language-perception-action theory and empirical data on movement disorder related to Parkinson's disease (Maitra, 2007; Maitra et al., 2006).

Keywords Activities of daily living • Attention • Cuing • Dyskinesia • Self-speech

Definition

Parkinson's disease is a common neurodegenerative disease characterized by tremor, rigidity, slowness of movement (bradykinesia), and postural instability (Murphy and Tickle-Degnen, 2000). Progressive difficulty in movement initiation and bradykinesia affect sequential arm movements necessary for optimally performing many common occupations involving upper extremity, including cooking, eating, dressing, or grooming (for a review, see Murphy and Tickle-Degnen, 2000). Parkinson's disease is caused by a degenerative lesion in the substantia nigra, a basal ganglia component in the brain. The dopamine-producing ability of the substantia nigra progressively declines, resulting in typical symptoms of Parkinson's disease (Steece-Collier et al., 2002). The predominant pharmacologic intervention is levodopa (or dopamine replenishment) therapy, and most of the parkinsonian symptoms are highly responsive to this therapy. However, following long-term use,

I. Söderback (ed.), *International Handbook of Occupational Therapy Interventions*,
DOI: 10.1007/978-0-387-75424-6_32, © Springer Science+Business Media, LLC 2010

both effectiveness (quality of life) and longevity (the duration of the effect) of levodopa diminish, and the risk of developing drug-induced dyskinesia increases (Marsden and Parkes, 1977). Furthermore, although there is an immediate and significant improvement of quality of life following pharmacologic intervention, difficulties in performing activities of daily living, including gait and balance problems, still persist (Nieuwboer et al., 2007). For example, spatial characteristics (e.g., stride length) but not temporal characteristics (e.g., stride cadence) of gait improve with drug therapy (Nieuwboer et al., 2007). Therefore, there is a consistent need for physical and occupational therapy in Parkinson's disease patients to address issues of activities of daily living (ADL) and instrumental activities of daily living (IADL). With the increased understanding of pathophysiology of the disease, a range of efforts is being pursued to develop effective rehabilitative programs that work in conjunction with dopaminergic therapy.

External Cuing

Clients with Parkinson's disease have specific difficulty in internally generating motor actions in a timely manner (Praamstra et al., 1998). To address the temporal difficulty in initiating movement, over the past several years, one important aspect of Parkinson's disease rehabilitation research involves experimenting with the use of an *external cue* to initiate gait movement and gait training. These experiments suggest that *external cuing* may significantly and immediately improve gait initiation and gait performance in people with Parkinson's disease (for more discussion on cuing, see Background, below). As Lim et al. (2005) pointed out, a precise definition of *cue* needs to contrast with that of simple stimuli. This is because *cues* provide "information about how an action should be carried out and hence [is] more specific than a simple stimulus" (Lim et al., 2005). For the purpose of the present protocol, *cuing* is defined as "temporal or spatial stimuli associated with the initiation and ongoing facilitation of motor activity" or movement (Lim et al., 2005; Nieuwboer et al., 2007).

Cognitive Impairment and Parkinson's Disease

It is also now widely recognized that clients with Parkinson's disease exhibit *cognitive impairment* as a central feature of the disease even in its early stage (Mindham and Hughes, 2000). A number of cognitive difficulties that include attention, working memory, learning, visual perception, and visuospatial and executive skills have been described in Parkinson's disease (Mindham and Hughes, 2000). These cognitive impairments also contribute to the difficulties in ADL and IADL performance. For example, executive skills, specifically sequencing ability, was found to be a significant predictor of IADLs, and simple motor functioning was found to be a significant predictor of physical ADLs (Cahn et al., 1998).

Background

Parkinson's disease is a chronic and progressive neurologic disorder resulting in significant motor and cognitive disability. Parkinson's disease is associated with progressive loss of independence and increasing financial burden. Although mortality and morbidity of Parkinson's disease are delayed with modern pharmacologic intervention, a high rate of decline in motor ability and an increase in disability make the disease a public health concern (Nieuwboer et al., 2007). Nonpharmacologic interventions such as occupational, physical, and speech therapy are therefore sought to promote independence and functionality (Johnson and Almeida, 2007).

As mentioned earlier, external cues have been found useful in helping clients with Parkinson's disease to initiate movements. Many of these studies involved gait performance. External cues used for clients with Parkinson's disease for gait improvement were generally of three types: visual, auditory, or somatosensory. Examples include the following: (1) mild *tactile sensory shock* as a somatosensory cue (Burleigh-Jacobs et al., 1997), (2) rhythmic auditory cues using a metronome (Enzensberger and Fischer, 1996), and (3) *visual step cues of* high-contrast transverse lines on the floor (Majsak et al., 1998).

The intervention of the RehabSelfCue-Speech program as presented below is based on these concepts of cuing movement initiation by self-cuing via semantically related words (see Evidence for Practice, below, for further information).

Purpose

Clients with Parkinson's disease have difficulty in performing many ADLs, despite medication, due to cognitive impairments and impairments in movement initiation and performance. The purpose of the RehabSelfCue-Speech intervention is to utilize the client's semantic memory to facilitate everyday motor performance necessary for completing ADLs and IADLs.

Method

Candidates for the Intervention

The RehabSelfCue-Speech program is aimed at people who are in the mild to moderate stages of Parkinson's disease or if stage III on the Hoehn and Yahr scale. The Hoehn and Yahr scale (Hoehn and Yahr, 1967) is commonly used to classify the stages of disability with Parkinson's disease. The scale rates the severity of Parkinson's disease from 0 to 5 as follows:

- Stage 0: no disability or symptoms
- Stage 1: symptoms are present only on one side of the body

- Stage 2: symptoms are present on both sides of the body, but there is no impairment in balance
- Stage 3: the disease is at the mild to moderate stage, with balance impairment, but the patient is still independent
- Stage 4: the patient is severely disabled but is still able to walk or stand without assistance
- Stage 5: the patient is wheelchair bound

Epidemiology

Parkinson's disease occurs worldwide in all ethnic groups and socioeconomic classes. The incidence and occurrence of Parkinson's disease increases with age and is about 1% in people over the age of 65 years around the world (Singhal et al., 2003). Parkinson's disease and other neurodegenerative diseases (e.g., Alzheimer's disease) combined could surpass cancer as the second most common cause of mortality by 2040 (Singhal et al., 2003). Despite extensive and focused research, causes of Parkinson's disease remain unresolved, although genetic and environmental factors such as exposure to pesticides have been strongly suspected (Steece-Collier et al., 2002).

Settings

The RehabSelfCue-Speech intervention is a technique of promoting functional independence utilizing one's own semantic memory to facilitate one's motor performance. The technique does not require any equipment or specific environment. Thus, the client can practice the technique in any setting—at home, in the clinic, or in the community—to initiate and maintain a motor performance.

The initial RehabSelfCue-Speech technique is used in clinical settings to facilitate upper extremity and lower extremity dressing, and simple meal preparation.

The Role of the Occupational Therapist

The role of occupational therapist (OT) is to organize the context in which the client practices the RehabSelfCue-Speech intervention technique. Following client-centered practice principles, the OT collaborates with the client to choose the tasks that the client is interested in performing. For example, if the client chooses to perform tasks of simple meal preparation, the OT helps the client to select action words the client needs to read aloud during the activity to facilitate the performance.

Results

A Brief Guide to Clinical Application

RehabSelfCue-Speech techniques can be applied to facilitate ADL, work, or leisure activities. OTs use motor learning principles to organize individual training sessions to the three times a week for 30 minutes to 1 hour each time. Clients read aloud different action words three times and will then perform the action with three repetitions.

The practice of RehabSelfCue-Speech for a client with Parkinson's disease is organized along the following guidelines:

To get up from a chair, the action word is *SWAY* and then *RISE*. The OT shows a card with the word *SWAY* on it. The client reads the word aloud three times, and then does a swaying motion while sitting on a chair. This action is repeated three times. After three sways the OT shows the client another card with the words *SWAY* and *THEN RISE*. The client reads the words aloud three times and tries to rise from the chair following the sway. The client does three attempts to perform this action (Fig. 32.1). This strategy of priming the action with words can be applied to any daily tasks, such as dressing, self-care, or preparing a light meal

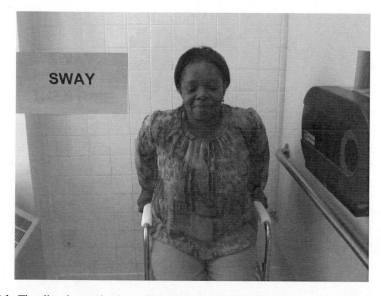

Fig. 32.1 The client is swaying by reading aloud the word *SWAY* three times in preparation to rise from the toilet seat.

How the Intervention Eases Impairments, Activity Limitations, and Participation Restrictions

RehabSelfCue-Speech is intended primarily for clients with Parkinson's disease to compensate for dysfunctions including body structures of brain (International Classification of Functioning, Disability, and Health [ICF] codes 1100 to 1103) and specific mental functions (ICF 34 b140 to b189) (World Health Organization, 2007).

Evidence-Based Practice

Recent reviews of experimental studies suggest that external cues are effective for short-term improvement of gait performance, especially in walking speed, step length, and step frequency (Lim et al., 2005; Rubinstein et al, 2002). Dam et al. (1996) compared sensory-enhanced gait therapy with conventional therapy in gait training in clients with Parkinson's disease. Sensory-enhanced therapy included both external visual cues, such as footprints on which patients walked, and auditory cues, such as high and low tones synchronized with foot lift and foot drop. Although both conventional and sensory-enhanced therapy produced significant improvement in gait characteristics, the improvements were maintained longer in sensory-enhanced therapy (12 months) than in conventional therapy (4 months).

Positive effects of exercise and external cuing on motor performance, ADLs, and cardiovascular fitness in clients with Parkinson's disease has also been reported (Gage and Storey, 2004). Most of the studies involving external cuing are a single-session experimental study, and long-term training effects of cues for ADLs and gait in familiar contexts, such as the home, are not substantiated. One study systematically investigated a 3-week home cuing program for gait training followed by 3 weeks without training among 153 clients with Parkinson's disease. Small but significant improvement in posture and gait scores was found (Nieuwboer et al., 2007). The study raised the possibility that cuing training may have long-term therapeutic benefit in the management of ADLs at home.

Cues are contextually or spatially relevant stimuli that, through experience, are associated with expected behavior. External and contextually relevant cues have been theorized to guide internally the cognitive functions necessary for ADL and IADL performances (Gage and Storey, 2004; Praamstra et al., 1998). Neurologic and motor control research has shown that the brain goes through cognitive programming or ideation before making any action or movement. Within the past few years, priming of this cognitive programming is possible through *external cuing* via semantically related language (Gentilucci, 2000; Gentilucci and Dalla Volta, 2008; Maitra and Telage 2004; Maitra et al., 2003; Manita and Dasgupta, 2005; Manita, 2007).

For example, participants performed reaching and grasping tasks with a wooden block while they silently read the words *near, far, small*, and *large* written on the block. Results of this study showed that the participants reached faster when they reach for a block with the word *far* written on it compared to reaching for a block with word *near* written on it. Similarly, the grasping aperture was larger when the participant grasped a block with the word *large* on it than when the word *small* was written on it. The conclusion was that the participants automatically associated the meaning of the word with the planning of the action (Gentilucci et al., 2000).

Studying clients with Parkinson's disease and stroke (Maitra et al., 2006), the results showed that prereading of the word is semantically related to the expected motor performance, which was performed faster, and thus positively influences the performance. Speed and smoothness of the reaching or grasping task ($n = 24$) were significantly facilitated when the words *REACH* or *GRASP* were preread (Grossi et al., 2007). The word-based contextual cues have to be in congruency with the movement performances if the expected effect is to provide the contextual cues to prime the cognitive processes related to performance. For example, a reaching performance is not influenced by an unrelated action word such as *RETURN* or nonsense word such as *GA* (Miller et al., 2005).

Pulvermüller et al. (2005) explained the mechanism by which action words can cue and facilitate a motor performance. He proposed that words are represented in the brain by a neuronal network (or cell assemblies). The network is formed by neurons that represent a word's meaning (sensory perception) as well as the neurons that represent the word's content (motor action). Thus, for example, visually seeing the word *REACH* (perception), or saying the word *REACH* would stimulate the neural network governing the reach action, which is proved by the use of functional magnetic resonance imaging (fMRI) data of the brain. Here, the subjects read the words *lick, pick,* and *kick*. The fMRI showed activation in the sensory association areas of the mouth (for *lick*), hand (for *pick*), and leg (for *kick*) for interpretation of the meaning of the word. The fMRI also showed simultaneous activation of the motor areas of the mouth, hand, and leg responsible for licking, picking, and kicking actions (Pulvermüller et al., 2005). These studies provide a strong rationale for the present protocol.

Conclusion

The evidence for the RehabSelfCue-Speech program is supported by studies with people suffering from stroke (Maitra et al., 2006) or Parkinson's disease (Maitra, 2007), and several empirical studies with older adults provided sufficient rationale to use the protocol in practice (Grossi et al., 2007; Maitra et al., 2003; Maitra and Telage, 2004).

References

Burleigh-Jacobs A., Horak, F.B., Nuttm J.G., and Obeso, J.A. (1997). Step initiation in Parkinson's disease: influence of levodopa and external sensory triggers. Mov Dis, 12, 206–215.

Cahn, D.A., Sullivan, E.V., Shear, P.K., Pfefferbaum, A., Heit, G., and Gerald, S. (1998). Differential contributions of cognitive and motor component processes to physical and instrumental activities of daily living in Parkinson's disease. Arch Clin Neuropsychol, 13, 575–583.

Dam, M., Tonin, P., Casson, S., et al. (1996). Effects of conventional and sensory-enhanced physiotherapy on disability of Parkinson's disease clients. Adv Neurol, 69, 551–555.

324   K. Maitra

Enzensberger, W., and Fischer, P.A. (1996). Metronome in Parkinson's disease [Letter]. Lancet, 347, 1337.

Gage, H., and Storey, L. (2004). Rehabilitation for Parkinson's disease: a systematic review of available evidence. Clin Rehabil, 18, 463–482.

Gentilucci, M., Benuzzi, F., Bertolani, L., Daprati, E., and Gangitano, M. (2000). Language and motor control. Exp Brain Res, 133, 468–490.

Gentilucci, M., and Dalla Volta, R. (2008). Spoken language and arm gestures are controlled by the same motor control system. Q J Exp Psychol (Colchester), 61(6), 944–957.

Grossi, J., Maitra, K.K., and Rice, M. S. (2007). Semantic priming of a daily motor performance. Am J Occup Ther, 61, 311–320

Hoehn, M., and Yahr, M. (1967). Parkinsonism: onset, progression and mortality. Neurology, 17, 427–442.

Johnson, A.M., and Almeida, Q.J. (2007). The impact of exercise rehabilitation and physical activity on the management of Parkinson's disease. Geriatr Aging, 10, 318–321.

Lim, I., van Wegen, E., de Goede, C., et al. (2005). Effects of external rhythmical cueing on gait in clients with Parkinson's disease: a systematic review. Clin Rehabil, 19, 695–713.

Maitra, K.K. (2007). Enhancement of reaching performance via self-speech in persons with Parkinson's disease. Clin Rehabil, 21, 418–424.

Maitra, K.K, Curry, D., Gamble, C., et al. (2003) Evidence using speech sound to enhance a daily occupational performance in older adults. Occup Ther J Res, 23(1), 35–44.

Matira, K.K., and Dasgupta, A.K. (2005). Incoordination of a sequential motor in Parkinson's disease. Occup Ther Int, 12(4), 218–233.

Maitra, K.K., and Telage, K.T. (2004). Influence of action word on the control of reaching-grasping movements. J Sports Exerc Psychol 2004 NASPSPA Proc, 26 (Suppl S129).

Maitra, K.K., Telage, K.M., and Rice, M. (2006). Self-speech induced facilitation of occupational performance in persons with stroke. Am J Occup Ther, 60(2), 146–154.

Majsak, M.J., Kaminski, T., Gentile, A.M., and Flanagan, J.R. (1998). The reaching movements of clients with Parkinson's disease under self-determined maximal speed and visually cued conditions. Brain, 121(Pt 4), 755–766.

Marsden, C.D., and Parkes, J.D. (1977). Success and problems of long-term levodopa therapy in Parkinson's disease. Lancet, 1, 345–349.

Miller, L.M., Maitra, K.K., and Rice, M.S. (2005). Effect of speech and arm movement in an occupational performance in older adults. Presented at the American Occupational Therapy Association Annual Meeting, Long Beach, CA.

Mindham, R.H.S., and Hughes, T.A. (2000). Cognitive Impairment in Parkinson's disease. Int Rev Psychiatry, 12, 281–289.

Murphy, S., and Tickle-Degnen, L. (2000). The effectiveness of occupational therapy-related treatments for persons with Parkinson's disease: a meta-analytic review. Am J Occup Ther, 55, 385–392.

Nieuwboer, A., Kwakkel, G., Rochester, L., et al. (2007). Cueing training in the home improves gait-related mobility in Parkinson's disease: the RESCUE trial. J Neurol Neurosurg Psychiatry, 78, 134–140.

Praamstra, P., Stegeman, D.F., Cools, A.R., and Horstink, M.W. (1998). Reliance on external cues for movement initiation in Parkinson's disease. Brain, 121, 167–177.

Pulvermüller, F., Hauk, O., Nikulin, V.V., and Ilmoniemi, R.J. (2005). Functional links between motor and language systems. Eur J Neurosci, 21, 793–797.

Rubinstein, T.C., Giladi, N., and Hausdorff, J.M. (2002). The power of cueing to circumvent dopamine deficits: a review of physical therapy treatment of gait disturbances in Parkinson's disease. Mov Disord, 17, 1148–1160.

Singhal, B., Lalkaka, J., and Sankhla, C. (2003). Epidemiology and treatment of Parkinson's disease in India. Parkinsonism Rel Disord, 9, S105–S109.

Steece-Collier, K., Maries, E., and Kordower, J.H. (2002). Etiology of Parkinson's disease, genetics and environment revisited. Proc Natl Acad Sci USA, 99, 13972–13974.

World Health Organization. (2007). International Classification of functioning, disability and health: version 10. http://www.who.int/classifications/apps/icd/icd10online/.

Chapter 33
Joint Protection: Enabling Change in Musculoskeletal Conditions

Alison Hammond

The problem is changing habits of a lifetime. Joint protection principles are easy to learn; the difficulty is changing habits sufficiently to make a difference.

Abstract Joint protection includes applying ergonomic principles in daily life, altering working methods, using assistive devices, and modifying environments. It is taught to people with musculoskeletal conditions, such as rheumatoid arthritis (RA), osteoarthritis, and soft tissue rheumatisms. Common principles are to distribute load over several joints, to reduce effort using assistive devices, to pace activities, to use orthoses, and to exercise regularly. Cognitive-behavioral, self-efficacy, and motor-learning approaches are employed. Trials demonstrate that using these approaches is significantly more effective than advice and demonstration alone in changing joint-protection behavior, improving function, and reducing pain in both early and established RA. When joint protection is combined with hand exercises, there is evidence that it improves grip strength in hand osteoarthritis, but there is still conflicting evidence for its effectiveness in soft-tissue rheumatisms.

Keywords Arthritis diseases • Assistive devices • Energy conservation • Ergonomics • Joint protection • Musculoskeletal conditions.

Definition and Background

Joint protection is a core component of occupational therapy interventions for musculoskeletal conditions. Joint protection is an active coping (or self-management) strategy to improve clients' perceived control of their condition, psychological and health status, daily activities, role performance, and social participation (Hammond, 2004).

Joint protection intervention includes educating in (1) altering working methods, (2) use of proper joint and body mechanics through applying ergonomic principles, (3) use of assistive devices, and (4) modifying occupational performance and environments. It is often integrated with energy conservation, working splints and mobility, and strengthening hand exercises.

I. Söderback (ed.), *International Handbook of Occupational Therapy Interventions*, DOI: 10.1007/978-0-387-75424-6_33, © Springer Science+Business Media, LLC 2010

Joint protection was first developed in the 1960s, based on increased understanding of pathophysiologic changes in rheumatoid arthritis (RA), and on biomechanics. Principles were extended to other inflammatory arthropathies, osteoarthritis (OA), and soft tissue rheumatisms (Brattstrom, 1987; Chamberlain et al., 1984; Cordery, 1965; Melvin, 1989; Sheon, 1985). At that time, clients were encouraged to regularly practice joint protection in the expectation that they would apply this to their personal situation (Chamberlain et al., 1984; Cordery, 1965). The focus was on improving body structures and function, and maintaining the ability to perform daily activities.

Research in the past 15 years has used structured self-management education and skills training to promote attitudinal, cognitive, and behavioral changes for improving protection of the joints. These cognitive-behavioral approaches further affect personal factors (e.g., increased self-efficacy, perceived control of the condition, problem-solving abilities, and reduced frustration). Additionally, they aim to enable clients to change habits and routines in their daily activities, work, and leisure.

Purpose

Joint protection is an active self-management strategy aiming to *maintain or improve* (1) occupational performance in daily life, (2) role performance and participation in social life, (3) perceptions of control, and (4) psychological and health status (Hammond, 2004).

The aims of joint protection are as follows:

1. *For people with RA, reduce* (a) load and effort during daily activity performance, thus reducing strain on joint structures weakened by the disease process; (b) pain; (c) irritation of the synovial membrane; (d) local inflammation; and (e) fatigue.
2. *For people with osteoarthritis*, (a) reduce loading on articular cartilage and subchondral bone, (b) strengthen muscle support, and (c) improve shock-absorbing capabilities of joints (Cordery and Rocchi, 1998).
3. *For people with soft tissue disorders* (e.g., de Quervain's disease, carpal tunnel syndrome) to reduce (a) pain, (b) inflammation, and (c) strain on soft tissues.

Method

Candidates for the Intervention

Joint protection is provided to clients with the following:

- *Inflammatory polyarthropathies*, such as RA, and seronegative and psoriatic arthritis. These diseases affect three times more women than men, most commonly in the 40- to 60-year age range, but they may start at any age. RA affects on average 1% of people globally (Kvien, 2004).
- *Osteoarthritis* (OA) affects the hand, hip, knee, or several joints of the body simultaneously (i.e., generalized OA). Nearly twice as many (1.8:1) women as

men live with OA, and 10% of people over the age of 60 years are symptomatically affected (Dennison and Cooper, 2003).
- *Upper-limb soft tissue disorders:* (1) *de Quervain's disease* is more common in women than in men, with peak onset between 30 and 50 years of age. (2) *Carpal tunnel syndrome* occurs in 5.8% of women and 0.6% of men, with peak onset between 45 and 54 years of age (Fam, 2003).

Epidemiology

The numbers of people potentially benefiting from joint protection can be estimated from percentages of those with activity limitations. Among people living with RA, about 60% have activity limitations, particularly related to hand function (Young et al., 2000). A community survey by Jordan et al. (2000) found that 43% of people over 65 years of age with arthritis (mainly OA) experienced difficulty with household activities. The number of people living with *soft tissue disorders* who could benefit from joint protection interventions is unknown. These figures suggest many people with musculoskeletal conditions could benefit from joint protection advice.

Settings

Joint protection is most often provided in rheumatology and occupational therapy departments, to both in- and outpatients, as well as in community settings.

The Role of the Occupational Therapist

In providing joint protection, occupational therapists (OTs) have both *facilitatory and teaching roles.* The OT has knowledge of (1) pathophysiology of musculoskeletal conditions, (2) ergonomic and biomechanical principles for protecting joints, and (3) cognitive-behavioral methods. This knowledge constitutes the theoretical base for joint-protection interventions, which are clinically applied using educational and facilitatory strategies.

Result

Clinical Application

The commonest principles taught to clients are the following:
- *Joint protection*: Respect pain; distribute load over several joints; use the strongest, largest joint to perform an activity; avoid working in positions of potential

deformity; reduce effort by using assistive devices and avoiding lifting and carrying; and avoid prolonged periods of working in the same position.

- *Energy conservation*: Pacing by balancing rest and work, and alternating heavy and light activities; use work simplification; use correct working positions and postures.
- *Orthoses*: Use working orthoses appropriately to reduce pain and improve grip function.
- *Exercise:* Exercise regularly to maintain range of motion and muscle strength.

The educational and facilitatory strategies used include motivational, cognitive-behavioral, self-efficacy, and motor learning approaches. These enable clients to overcome barriers to changing behavior and to maximize performance of joint protection so that therapeutic aims are achieved.

These strategies include the following:

- *Discuss* health beliefs and attitudes to the disease.
- *Identify* clients' expectations, worries, or concerns, and their valued activities and life goals.
- *Teach cognitive-behavioral strategies*, such as self-monitoring, goal setting, and how to develop action plans for practicing techniques at home. Regular review of such home programs with clients is essential.
- *Teach* using effective educational techniques to enhance recall of joint protection principles and methods, such as simplification, use of advance organizers, and explicit categorization.
- *Teach* joint-protection techniques using effective skills training methods (e.g., practicing simple and then more complex activities using joint protection, feedback, and mental rehearsal).
- *Enable modeling*, that is, teaching in small groups, encouraging members to observe each other. Seeing others perform successfully increases self-efficacy and problem-solving ability (Hammond, 2003).

Joint protection can be taught using (1) self-help booklets; (2) individual education, or (3) group education.

How the Intervention Eases Impairments, Activity Limitations, and Participation Restrictions

Joint protection reduces pain and the likelihood of deformities, and maintains activity and participation (Hammond and Freeman, 2001, 2004)

Evidence-Based Practice

A *survey* of United Kingdom practice found that joint protection education typically lasts for 1.5 hours over two treatment sessions and does not use behavioral approaches. The usual content is (1) education about RA, (2) how joints are affected,

(3) joint-protection principles, (4) demonstrations with short (e.g., 15- to 30-minute) practice of hand joint protection methods commonly used in cooking and housework activities (e.g., making a cup of tea), and (5) discussion of solutions to specific problems, supported by a self-help booklet (Hammond, 1997). This is still the typical practice.

Trials Investigating Joint Protection Education

A randomized controlled trial ($n = 55$; 6-month follow-up) of 1 hour of individual education, similar to the typical content described above, but not compared to an intervention, improved clients' knowledge of joint protection methods (Barry et al., 1994). Similarly, a pretest, posttest trial of a group program ($n = 21$; 3-month follow-up) providing this typical intervention for 2.5 hours as part of an 8-hour arthritis education program also found improved knowledge of joint protection, but no significant changes in joint-protection behavior occurred. Barriers to changing behavior were identified through interview as (1) being unable to recall methods sufficiently during daily activity performance; (2) considering these as not applicable, as "my hands are not that bad yet" or using techniques on bad days only; (3) difficulty getting used to the different actions; and (4) difficulty changing the habits of a lifetime (Hammond and Lincoln, 1999).

Many early trials had small sample sizes but indicated that, in established RA, structured group programs emphasizing active learning, problem solving, behavioral approaches, frequent practice, and home programs gave significant improvements: balance of rest and activity (nonrandomized trial; $n = 25$; Furst et al., 1987); use of assistive devices (pretest, posttest trial, $n = 53$;, (Nordenskiold, 1994); and functional ability (pretest, posttest trial, $n = 21$; Nordenskiold et al., 1998).

More recent trials have been larger and methodologically sounder. A randomized trial with people with early RA (average 18-month disease duration, age 50 years, $n = 127$) compared a behavioral joint protection program with a standard arthritis education program (including 2.5 hours of typical joint-protection education). At 12 months, those in the behavioral group had significantly improved use of joint protection, less hand and general pain, improved functional ability (e.g., less early morning stiffness), and fewer flare-ups in comparison to the standard education group (Hammond and Freeman, 2001). At 4-year follow-up, the behavioral group continued to have significantly greater use of joint protection, less early morning stiffness, better activities of daily living (ADL) scores, and fewer hand deformities than the standard education group, who had continued to deteriorate (Hammond and Freeman, 2004).

The joint protection program was also tested in people with very early RA (average 4.5-month disease duration; age 51 years; $n = 54$) with little pain or functional difficulty. At 6-month follow-up, no significant differences between groups or over time occurred (Freeman and Hammond, 2002).

Trials Investigating the Effects of Joint Protection Combined with Exercise

A randomized controlled trial with clients with moderate-severe RA (average 15-year disease duration, age 53 years; $n = 85$) receiving a behavioral joint-protection and exercise program also identified significant improvements at 8-month follow-up in pain and functional and physical ability in comparison to those receiving usual care (Masiero et al., 2007). Both groups were receiving anti-tumor necrosis factor-a (TNF-a) drugs (e.g., Infliximab, Etanercept), indicating that benefits from joint protection occur even with such biologic drugs.

A randomized controlled trial in clients with hand OA (average age 60 years, $n = 40$) identified significant improvements at 3 months in grip strength and self-perceived hand function, although not in pain control or functional ability, in comparison to a control group receiving education about OA (Stamm et al., 2002). There is conflicting evidence for the effectiveness of ergonomic interventions in soft tissue rheumatisms (Verhagen et al., 2006).

Discussion

These studies highlight three issues: (1) How the joint protection education is provided makes a significant difference to whether patients gain benefits. The use of educational, cognitive, and behavioral approaches is significantly more effective. (2) Providing information does not seemingly help clients with the tools to make changes when the need arises, as the standard intervention group provided with typical joint protection advice continued to deteriorate without making changes longer-term in response. (3) People need to perceive the relevance of using joint protection; it may be too early to use it if clients have few or no problems.

Conclusion

Joint protection intervention is effective if it is taught effectively. To date, research has focused on developing effective group joint-protection programs for RA clients. However, individual education is more often provided, and thus individual behavioral programs need to be developed and evaluated in RA. Hand OA research has to date combined joint protection and exercise. It is thus unclear whether joint protection is effective if provided without hand exercises. Long-term benefits in hand OA are unknown. Joint protection in lower-limb RA and OA has been little evaluated. In soft tissue rheumatism, randomized trials are needed using clearly defined conditions and interventions. The cost-effectiveness of joint protection has not been evaluated.

References

Barry, M.A., Purser, J., Hazleman, R., et al. (1994). Effect of energy conservation and joint protection education in rheumatoid arthritis. *Br J Rheumatol*, 33, 1171–1174.
Brattstrom, M. (1987). Joint Protection and Rehabilitation in Chronic Rheumatic Diseases, 3rd ed. London: Wolfe Medical.
Chamberlain, M.A., Ellis, M., and Hughes, D. (1984). Joint protection. *Clin Rheum Dis*, 10(3), 727–743.

Cordery, J.C. (1965). Joint protection; a responsibility of the occupational therapist. *Am J Occup Ther*, 19, 285–294.

Cordery, J., and Rocchi, M. (1998). Joint protection and fatigue management. In: Melvin, J., and Jensen, G., eds. Rheumatologic Rehabilitation, Vol. 1: Assessment and Management. Bethesda, MD: American Occupational Therapy Association.

Dennison, E., and Cooper, C. (2003). Osteoarthritis: epidemiology and classification. In: Hochberg, M.C.et al, eds. Rheumatology, 3rd ed. (pp. 1781–1791). Edinburgh: Mosby.

Fam, A.G. (2003). Regional and widespread pain: the wrist and hand. In: Hochberg, M.C.et al, eds. Rheumatology, 3rd ed. (pp. 641–650). Edinburgh: Mosby.

Freeman, K., and Hammond, A. (2002). Use of cognitive-behavioural arthritis education programmes in newly diagnosed rheumatoid arthritis. *Clin Rehabil*, 16, 828–836.

Furst, G.P., Gerber, L.H., Smith, C.C., et al. (1987). A program for improving energy conservation behaviours in adults with rheumatoid arthritis. *Am J Occup Ther*, 41(2), 102–111.

Hammond, A. (1997). Joint protection education: what are we doing? *Br J Occup Ther*, 60(9), 401–406.

Hammond, A. (2003). Patient education in arthritis: helping people change. *Musculoskel Care*, 1(2), 84–97.

Hammond, A. (2004). What is the role of the occupational therapist? In: Sambrook, P., and March, L., eds. How to Manage Chronic Musculoskeletal Conditions. Best Pract Res Clin Rheumatol, 18(4), 491–505.

Hammond, A., and Freeman, K. (2001). One year outcomes of a randomised controlled trial of an educational-behavioural joint protection programme for people with rheumatoid arthritis. *Rheumatology*, 40, 1044–1051.

Hammond, A., and Freeman, K. (2004). The long term outcomes from a randomised controlled trial of an educational-behavioural joint protection programme for people with rheumatoid arthritis. *Clin Rehabil*, 18, 520–528.

Hammond, A., and Lincoln, N. (1999). Effect of a joint protection programme for people with rheumatoid arthritis. *Clin Rehabil*, 13, 392–400.

Jordan, J.M., Bernard, S.L., Callahan, L.F., et al. (2000). Self-reported arthritis related disruptions in sleep and daily life and the use of medical, complementary and self-care strategies for arthritis: The National Survey of Self-Care and Ageing. *Arch Fam Med*, 9, 143–149.

Kvien, T.K. (2004). Epidemiology and burden of illness in rheumatoid arthritis. *PharmacoEconomics*, 22(2) Suppl. 1, 1170–1176.

Masiero, S., Boniolo, A., Wassermann, L., et al. (2007). Effects of an educational-behavioural joint protection program on people with moderate to severe rheumatoid arthritis: a randomized controlled trial. *Clin Rheumatol*, 26, 2043–2050.

Melvin, J.L. (1989) Rheumatic disease in the adult and child. In: Occupational Therapy and Rehabilitation, 3rd ed. Philadelphia: F.A. Davis.

Nordenskiold, U. (1994). Evaluation of assistive devices after a course of joint protection. *Int J Technol Assess Health Care*, 10(2), 293–304.

Nordenskiold, U., Grimby, G., and Dahlin-Ivanoff, S. (1998). Questionnaire to evaluate effects of assistive devices and altered working methods in women with rheumatoid arthritis. *Clin Rheumatol*, 17, 6–16.

Sheon, R.P. (1985). A joint protection guide for non-articular rheumatic disorders. *Postgrad Med*, 77, 329–337.

Stamm, T., Machold, K.P., and Smolen, J.S. (2002). Joint protection and home hand exercises improve hand function in patients with hand osteoarthritis: a randomized controlled trial. *Arthritis Care Res*, 47, 44–49.

Verhagen, A.P., Karels, C., Bierma-Zeinstra, S.M.A., et al. (2006) Ergonomic and physiotherapeutic interventions for treating work-related complaints of the arm, neck or shoulder in adults. Cochrane Database of Syst Rev 3: CD003471. DOI: 10.1002/14651858.CD003471.pub3.

Young, A., Dixey, J., Cox, N., et al. (2000) How does functional disability in early rheumatoid arthritis (RA) affect patients and their lives? Results of a 5 year follow-up in 732 patients from the Early RA Study (ERAS). *Rheumatology*, 39, 603–611.

Chapter 34
Neurodevelopmental Therapy: Sensory Integration and Vestibular Stimulation Intervention in Mentally Retarded Children

Mine Uyanik, Hulya Kayihan, Gonca Bumin, and Gul Sener

Mentally retarded children's development is influenced by their participation in programs containing a sensory integrative intervention, such as the vestibular stimulation and neurodevelopmental treatment.

Abstract Mental retardation is a disability characterized by significant limitations both in intellectual functioning and in adaptive behavior as expressed in conceptual, social, and practical adaptive skills. Sensory integration is the brain's organization of sensory input.

The degree of sensory integration and postural control dysfunctions in mentally retarded children has great variations. The function of learning depends on the child's ability to make use of environmental sensory information and to integrate this information to perform purposeful behaviors.

The use of neurodevelopmental treatment emphasizes the children's active participation in goal-oriented activities. The sensory integration frame of reference is critical to treating deficits in the nervous system before other issues can be addressed.

Keywords Mental retardation • Neurodevelopmental treatment • Sensory integration • Vestibular stimulation

Definitions and Background

Children's Normal Motor Development

Normal development of movement and function is essential for the child's development of motor control and learning abilities. Motor learning develops in stages during the child's general development. Movement and posture are learned in sensory states for the child in a suitable environment.

Physical activity is necessary for motor development. Therefore, the child should move actively to gain basic motor skills such as turning, sitting, crawling, and walking.

I. Söderback (ed.), *International Handbook of Occupational Therapy Interventions*,
DOI: 10.1007/978-0-387-75424-6_34, © Springer Science+Business Media, LLC 2010

The *development of postural control* occurs in stages comparable to the child's ability to integrate sensory information.

Between the *ages of 1 and 3 years*, the sense of sight is the dominant source, nessesary for achieving and maintaining the orientation of the upright position. At these ages, the proprioceptive system generates simple and incomplete information. Therefore, training of the somatosensorial system is needed if the child is able to utilize proprioceptive information effectively.

Between the *ages of 4 and 6 years*, somatosensorial and vestibular input's are the dominating sources for effective motor control.

Between the *ages of 7 and 10 years*, response according to those of adults is observed. The fundamental source of postural stability in children and adults is somatosensorial. General movements and reflexes enable voluntary and adaptive motor control. However, postural control develops first and provides the basis for movement whereas well-balances and coordinated movements occur (Martin, 1989).

Mental Retardation

Brain damage during the intrauterine period of life results in severe neurologic dysfunctions, such as mental retardation and cerebral palsy. Individuals have mild, moderate, severe, or profound retardation, based on intellectual impairments (American Psychiatric Association, 1994; World Health Organization, 2008).

Mental retardation is a disability characterized by significant limitations in intellectual functioning and adaptive behavior as expressed in conceptual, social, and practical adaptive skills, which originates before the age of 18 (American Association on Intellectual and Developmental Disabilities [AAIDD], 2008). Adaptive behavior signifies the quality of daily performance in dealing with environmental needs. Ten adaptive areas are considered critical to the diagnosis of mental retardation: communication, self-care, home living, social skills, community use, self-direction, health and safety, functional academics, leisure, and work (Lambert et al., 1993).

The motor control in these children commonly shows (1) joint and muscular *hypotonicity*; (2) a decrease in deep tendon and maintenance of primitive *reflexes*; (3) delays in *motor development*, such as slow reaction time, nonequilibrium reactions, and laterality; and (4) deficits in *visual motor control*, such as deficits in eye-hand coordination.

Sensory Integration Theory

The neurodevelopmental treatment uses automatic and voluntary components of postural control and skill acquisition as treatment mediator (Shumway-Cook and Woollacott 1985; Uyanik et al., 2003).

Sensory integration is *"the organization of sensory input for use"* (Ayres, 1979), which signifies a neurologic process. This enables spatial-temporal integration and use of the sensory information that children get from their body and environment. This is the prerequisite for children to be able to plan and design organized motor behaviors. According to the sensory integration theory, mild and moderate problems in learning are related to a defective motor coordination and a weak sensory process (Ayres, 1972; Scheerer, 1997). Moreover, sensory integration is significantly related to the development of hearing and language skills in addition to motor coordination (Ayres, 1979).

Sensory integration theory is based on the view that *neural plasticity* and sensory integration occur as long as the brain functions integrate with the hierarchically related systems. Adaptive motor response is the most significant parameter of sensory integration. "An adaptive response is a purposeful, goal directed response to a sensory experience" (Ayres, 1979).

A child's growth and development is dependent of the development of the tactile, vestibular, and proprioceptive systems (Williamson and Anzalone, 2001):

- The *tactile system* provides information about the environment through the sense of touch. The tactile system constitutes the protective system (informs when touching is harmful) and the discriminative system (informs of the difference between harmful and beneficial touch).
- The *proprioceptive system* receives sensory stimulus from the muscles and joints. Push and pull activities provide maximum stimulus to this system. The proprioceptive system is also important for the development of fine and gross motor muscles. An insufficient proprioceptive system negatively affects motor planning ability.
- The *receptors of the vestibular system* are situated in the inner ear and are related to hearing. The receptors in this system respond both to movement and to gravity. The vestibular system affects balance, eye movements, posture, muscle tone, and attention.

The Role of the Vestibular System in Motor Development

The vestibular system is important in the achievement of normal motor development (Shumway-Cook, 1992). Vestibulo-ocular inputs are significant in eye-hand coordination, which is important for enabling looking at one point in space. Vestibulospinal inputs are significant in maintaining postural stability with visual and somatosensory inputs. Vestibular dysfunction is observed in many developmental disorders, such as deficit in motor coordination and learning disabilities (Ayres, 1972; Shumway-Cook, 1992).

Purpose

Intervention programs including sensory integration and vestibular stimulation are aimed at increasing mentally retarded children's development of perceptual-motor abilities, normal movement patterns, postural reactions, functional balance, gross motor coordination, reflex integration, intellectual functions, language-hearing abilities, and social and emotional functions.

Method

Candidates for the Intervention

Neurodevelopmental programs based on sensory integration or vestibular stimulation are aimed at *children* who are diagnosed with (1) mental retardation, such as Down syndrome; (2) cerebral palsy; (3) delayed development; (4) schizophrenia; (5) immature central nervous system (CNS) disorders, as in some premature infants; (6) a specific learning difficulty; (7) difficulties in speech and receptive language; and (8) behavior problems. These programs are also appropriate for *adults* who have suffered brain damage causing a hemiplegia.

Epidemiology

The prevalence and incidence of mental retardation vary with how it is defined. It is estimated that approximately 89% of children with mental retardation have mild mental retardation, 7% have moderate mental retardation, and 4% have severe to profound mental retardation. In addition, it was reported that the prevalence of mental retardation appears to increase with age up to about the age of 20, with significantly more males than females identified (Biasini et al., 2003).

Settings

Environments that allow personal and active play aimed at stimulating the child's adaptive responses are appropriate for neurodevelopmental interventions. Examples are the snoezelen or controlled multi-sensory stimulation rooms, (Wikipedia, 2008), i.e, specially organized therapeutic rooms situated at occupational therapy units, schools, hospitals, special education settings, inpatient/outpatient, day centers, or at home (Fig. 34.1).

The Role of the Occupational Therapist

The occupational therapist (OT) is responsible for enabling and arranging the environmental stimuli that are used to allow the child to demonstrate appropriate behaviors, and to develop self-care, play, and school skills. During the acquiring process of motor skills, the OT uses oral, supportive, or visual stimuli, as well as positioning of the child and passive movement schema. The child focuses on the goal rather than on the specific motor components of the task. This intervention approach is sequentially performed by qualified professionals (Bumin and Kayihan, 2001; DeGangi et al., 1993; Uyanik et al., 2003).

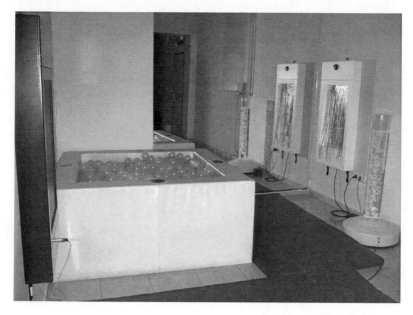

Fig. 34.1 An example of a snoezelen therapeutic room used for active play.

Clinical Application

The fundamental principle in the intervention using sensory integration is that planned and controlled sensory stimuli with adaptive responses enable improvements in brain function.

Sensory Integration Intervention

The Process

- *Sensory integration* includes *assessments* of the processes of (1) sensory motor integration, (2) adaptation of the individual, (3) effect of the maturation and behavior, and (4) defining the individual's developmental profile. The results of the assessments are analyzed, synthesized, and interrelated to the individual's sensory-perceptual motor behaviors.
- The *goal* of the first stage is to enable the learning of the skills.
- An *individually specialized intervention program* should follow the sensory integration activity training (Ayres, 1979; Bumin and Kayihan, 2001; Lerner, 1985; Scheerer, 1997; Uyanik et al., 2003).

Planning of the intervention should be done according to the following factors:

- The level of function of the child
- The developmental status of sensory integration process of the child
- The primary goals of the intervention
- The intervention methods used
- The frequency of the child's participation in the intervention
- The home programs that are used

The intervention should *follow the order of children's normal development*. Highly controlled behaviors such as running, hopping, bilateral integration, and sequence, writing, and reading, are included with expected improvement in the assimilation and adaptation process of the visual, tactile, proprioceptive, and vestibular stimuli.

The intervention should *depend on intersensory integration process*. The organization of sensory stimuli, which are internalized by the adaptation of the body, and the sensory integration process are the main steps of the intervention.

Home training of child should be provided by the parents and family, including emotional and social development. Here, the child's success depends on the therapist's communication and coordination with the family and with other disciplines while planning the intervention program.

The Content

The appropriate adaptation of the child's *environment* is very important. The following activities are recommended to stimulate the various body sensory systems:

- *Development of gross motor skills* is stimulated by activities such as running, hopping, jumping, and walking in unusual patterns.
- *Body awareness* (enables correct and coordinated movement patterns) is stimulated by activities directed at the vestibular, tactile, and proprioceptive systems.
- The *proprioceptive system* provides information about the movements of the body, and it is stimulated by activities such as climbing, pushing, pulling, carrying heavy objects, and working against resistance and pressure.
- The *tactile system* is stimulated by massage, rolling up in a blanket, having heavy or soft items rolled on top of the child, and deep pressure.
- *Motor planning* (the brain's ability to conceive, organize, and carry out a sequence of unfamiliar actions necessary for learning new skills) is stimulated by following instructions written on cards, ball games, obstacle courses, walking like different animals, and cutting out various shapes on paper.
- *Ocular control* is stimulated by throwing and catching a ball, and by drawing.
- *Bilateral motor coordination* (important for the purposeful use of the hands) is stimulated by task performances that cross the midline of the body.

- *Visual-spatial perception* is stimulated by activities directed toward vestibular and ocular controls, such as recognizing the position of objects in space.
- *Fine motor skills* are stimulated by arrangement of appropriate postural stability; good co-contraction of head, neck, and arm muscles; and good ocular control and performances of activities (Ayres, 1979; Bumin and Kayihan, Lerner, 1985; Scheerer, 1997; 2001; Uyanik et al., 2003).

Vestibular Stimulation Intervention

Content

The structure and position of the vestibular stimulus is important for reaching efficiency. The stimuli may be of an excitatory nature, such as rapid movement, or of an inhibitory nature, such as slow, rhythmic, and passive movement. Rotational movement and linear acceleration-deceleration, turning, and swinging back and forth stimulate all types of receptors. In addition, positioning upside down, lying prone and supine, and sitting activate different parts of the vestibular canals at different degrees. The horizontal position and especially the prone position are more stimulating than the upright position. Shifting between different head positions is necessary for the stimulation of the vestibular receptors (Ayres, 1979; Kelly, 1989).

Types of Intervention

- Linear activities are used to normalize *extensor muscle tone* by increasing stimulation input of the otolith organ. The recommended activities are the following:
  - Bouncing and jumping (while sitting, kneeling, or standing)
  - Linear swinging (using a platform and swing, glider, hammock, and barrel; swinging in the kneeling, standing, sitting, creeping, prone, and supine positions)
  - Other linear activities (jumping or falling onto pillows or mattress in the sitting, prone, and supine positions)

The center of gravity is changed to create disorganization for a short time, and thus phasic head movements appear, which help develop *equilibrium reactions* by increasing semicircular canal responses. The recommended activities are the following:

- Moving the support surface, so that the center of gravity is changed from active to passive.
- Pushing-pulling activities, so that displacement of the center of gravity is created. These are activities that enable active equilibrium on steep surfaces such as stairs, ramps, and other surfaces by using equipment such as balance boards, therapy balls, and a barrel.

- Linear vestibular stimulation is applied at tolerable speeds and durations and in unthreatening positions to *lessen the fear of movement or positional change* by increasing the weak passage of otolith input (Fisher and Bundy, 1989).

Vestibular stimulation should be carefully used and the child should be assessed before, during, and after the intervention session to avoid overstimulation, which in the most serious cases causes dysfunction of vital organs, seizures, and or cyanosis (Fisher and Bundy, 1989).

Neurodevelopmental Treatment Approach

The neurodevelopmental treatment (NDT) is aimed at facilitating and normalizing (1) the hyper- or hypotonic muscle reflexes (postural tonus), with focus on a complex facilitation-inhibition process; (2) reaction and movement patterns; and (3) managing the specific reactions to the treatment equilibrium. NDT uses inhibition as a major factor for the control of movement and posture (Bobath and Bobath, 1967).

The child's functional skills are observed and analyzed, and the intervention is customized with functional activity education. Automatic and voluntary activities, normal postural tonus, normal reciprocal interaction of the muscles, and automatic movement patterns are intervention priorities because all upper motor neuron lesions are disturbances to this mechanism (Mayston 1992).

Combined Intervention Approaches

In children with mental retardation and with attention and emotional problems, cognitive and perceptive skills and motor development are stimulated by a combination of sensory stimulation interventions, such as sensory integration, perceptual-motor activities, neurodevelopmental activities, vestibular stimulation, and play therapy (Ayres, 1972, 1979; Bobath and Bobath, 1967; Bumin and Kayihan, 2001; Uyanik et al., 2003).

The purpose of this intervention is to develop children's appropriate activity experiences that provide stimulus to normal movement patterns and motivate children to participate in the intervention program. The children's interactive participation in the environment is important for the acquisition of skills.

The child actively participates in the intervention process. The skills and roles are practiced, and the child becomes able to discover and integrate sensory information received from the environment by forming meaningful relations with people and objects (Lindquist et al., 1982). This child-centered intervention starts with the observation and facilitation of the child's play in the snoezelen therapeutic rooms or other multimodal sensory rooms. A safe environment is arranged using toys and materials (Bumin and Kayihan, 2001; DeGangi et al., 1993; Uyanik et al., 2003).

The general principles of combined intervention programs are as follows:

- A child's mental development level is considered. Activities that are easy to learn and the comprise the easiest possible movement components are chosen.
- A child's normal reflex motor development is followed for planning the intervention and choosing the appropriate activities. The activities are adapted to the supine-prone, quadruped, sitting, and standing positions.
- The intervention should be performed with the child working alone to avoid confusing effects that may be caused by other people or the room arrangement.
- Equipment is used gradually so that the amount of stimulation is adjusted to the tolerance level of the child.
- In the improvement of sensory-perception-motor responses, the development of proprioceptive feedback is beneficial. Motor responses of the child are increased by using methods such as positioning and movement activities, applying resistance, and by utilizing touch and equilibrium stimuli.
- The program is carried out step by step, from easy to difficult, and should only be changed when the child's skill in the previous step has been accomplished (Bumin and Kayihan, 2001; Uyanik et al., 2003).

Evidence-Based Practice

The sensory integration approach is effective in reducing self-stimulating behaviors, which interfere with the ability to participate in more functional activities (Smith et al., 2005). A meta-analysis of the NDT showed improvement in 62.2% of the disabled children compared with the children who do received the intervention (Ottenbacher et al., 1986). However, evaluation of the sensory integration approach aimed with children who have sensory processing disorders is still an ongoing process whereas its effectiveness needs further investigations (Miller, et al., 2007; Patel, 2005).

Discussion

Mentally retarded children present complex problems including sensory, perceptual, motor, and vestibular dysfunctions. Therefore, the use of sensory integration, vestibular stimulation, and NDT interventions in sequential, parallel, or combined programs conducted by an experienced OT is proved to be effective for improvements that correspond to children's needs for occupational performances.

References

American Association on Intellectual and Developmental Disabilities. (2008). Definition of Mental Retardation. http://www.aamr.org/Policies/faq_mental_retardation.
American Psychiatric Association. (1994). Diagnostic and Statistical Manual of Mental Disorders, 4th Ed. Washington, DC: American Psychiatric Press.

Ayres, A.J. (1972). Sensory Integration and Learning Disorders. Los Angeles: Western Psychological Services.

Ayres, A.J. (1979). Sensory Integration and the Child. Los Angeles: Western Psychological Services.

Biasini, F.J., Grupe, L., Huffman, L., et al. (2003). Mental retardation: a symptom and syndrome. In: Netherton, S., Holmes, D., and Walker, C.E., eds. Comprehensive Textbook of Child and Adolescent Disorders. New York: Oxford University Press.

Bobath, K., and Bobath, B. (1967). The neurodevelopmental intervention of cerebral palsy. Dev Med Child Neurol, 9, 373–390.

Bumin, G., and Kayihan, H. (2001). Effectiveness of two different sensory-integration programmes for children with spastic diplegic cerebral palsy. Disabil Rehabil, 23(9), 394–399.

DeGangi, G.A., Wietlisbach, S., Goodin, M., et al. (1993) A comparison of structured sensorimotor therapy and child-centered activity in the intervention of preschool children with sensorimotor problems. Am J Occup Ther, 47(9), 777–786.

Fisher, A.G., and Bundy, A.C. (1989). Vestibular stimulation in the intervention of postural and related deficits. In: Payton, O.D., ed. Manual of Physical Therapy. (pp. 239–258) New York, Edinburgh: Churchill Livingstone.

Kelly, G. (1989). Vestibular stimulation as a form of therapy. Physiotherapy, 75(3), 136–140.

Lambert, N., Nihira, K., and Leland, H. (1993). AAMR Adaptive Behavior Scale-School, Second Edition, Examiner's Manual. Austin, TX: American Association of Mental Retardation: Pro-ed.

Lerner, J.W. (1985). Motor and perceptual development. In: Learning Disabilities Theories, Diagnosis and Teaching Strategies. (pp. 264–307) Boston: Haughton Mifflin.

Lindquist, J.E., Mack, W., and Parham, L.D. (1982). A synthesis of occupational behavior and sensory integration concepts in theory and practice, Part 2. Clinical applications. Am J Occup Ther, 36, 433–437.

Martin, T. (1989). Normal development of movement and function: neonate, infant, and toddler. In: Scully, R.M., and Barnes, M.R., eds. Physical Therapy. (pp. 63–82) Philadelphia: Lippincott.

Mayston, M.J. (1992). The Bobath concept—evolution and application. In: Forssberg, H., and Hirschfeld, H., eds. Movement Disorders in Children, Vol 36 (pp. 1–6) Basel: Karger, S. Inc.

Miller, L.J., Schoen, S.A., James, K., Schaaf, R.C. (2007). Lessons learned: a pilot study on occupational therapy effectiveness for children with sensory modulation disorder. Am J Occup Ther, 61(2), 161–169.

Ottenbacher, K.J., Biocca, Z., DeCremer, G., et al. (1986). Quantitative analysis of the effectiveness of pediatric therapy. Emphasis on the neurodevelopment treatment approach. Physical Therapy, 66 (7), 1095–1101.

Patel, D.R. (2005). Therapeutic interventions in cerebral palsy. Indian J Pediatr, 72(11), 979–983.

Scheerer, C.R. (1997). Sensory Motor Groups. Activities for School and Home. San Antonio, TX: Therapy Skill Builders.

Shumway-Cook, A. (1992). Role of the vestibular system in motor development: theoretical and clinical issues. In: Forssberg H., and Hirschfeld, H., and (eds) Movement Disorders in Children, Vol 36 (pp. 209–216) Basel: Karger, S. Inc.

Shumway-Cook, A., and Woollacott, M.H. (1985). Dynamics of postural control in the child with Down's syndrome. Physical Therapy, 65(9), 1315–1322

Smith, S.A., Press, B., Koenig, K.P., et al. (2005). Effects of sensory integration intervention on self-stimulating and self injurious behaviors. Am J Occup Ther, 59(4), 418–425.

Uyanik, M., Bumin, G., and Kayihan, H. (2003). A comparison of different therapy approaches in children with Down's syndrome. Pediatr Int, 45(1), 68–73.

Williamson, G.G., and Anzalone, M.E. (2001). Sensory systems and sensory integration. In: Sensory Integration and Self Regulation in Infants and Toddlers: Helping Very Young Children Interact With Their Environment. (pp. 1–15) Washington, DC: Zero to Three Publications.

Wikipedia. The Free Encyclopedia. (2008). Snoezelen. http://en.wikipedia.org/wiki/Snoezelen, Retrieved 7/3/2009

World Health Organization. (2008). http://www.who.int/classifications/apps/icd/icd10online.

Chapter 35
Upper-Limb Movement Training in Children Following Injection of Botulinum Neurotoxin A

Brian Hoare and Remo N. Russo

After injection and intensive therapy, the client was really happy to be able to catch and throw a ball with his school friends.

Abstract Botulinum Neurotoxin A (BoNT-A) is a useful medication for the reduction of spasticity and dystonia in the upper limb of children with cerebral palsy (CP). The method of toxin delivery, dose, and muscle selection criteria are established. Children who are being treated require appropriate assessment at the impairment and activity levels of functioning. Once injected, children require specific therapy delivered by an occupational therapist (OT) according to the specified goals of the intervention set out, prior to injection, by the child, family, and health care workers. Botulinum neurotoxin injection offers the child with cerebral palsy a window of opportunity in which to develop further skills in upper limb functioning. Further research using rigorous scientific design evaluating specific therapy regimes and other interventions is required to enable more specific protocols to be established.

Keywords Botulinum Neurotoxin • Child • Cerebral palsy • Upper limb

Definition and Background

Cerebral palsy is a static lesion of the immature brain (Taft, 1995) leading to disorders of tone, posture, and movement (Bax et al., 2005). Affected children can experience varying degrees of positive (e.g., increased tone) and negative (e.g., sensory impairment) features of the disorder, and each can have impact on functioning (Graham, 2000). The predominant disorders of tone in cerebral palsy are *spasticity* (Graham, 2000) and *dystonia* (Autti-Ramo et al., 2001). The topography of involvement can affect the upper limb in children with all forms of cerebral palsy, and impact on function.

Both spasticity and dystonia can be influenced by botulinum Neurotoxin A (BoNT-A) injection (Brin, 1997).

I. Söderback (ed.), *International Handbook of Occupational Therapy Interventions*,
DOI: 10.1007/978-0-387-75424-6_35, © Springer Science+Business Media, LLC 2010

BoNT-A is a protein product of *Clostridium botulinum*, an anaerobic bacterium (Jankovic and Brin, 1997). Its action is to block the release of acetylcholine from the motor nerve terminal to the muscle cell, causing a chemical denervation (Brin, 1997). The pharmacologic effect of BoNT-A lasts up to 12 weeks (Graham, 2000); however, functional benefits lasting much longer can be experienced (Lowe et al., 2006; Russo et al., 2007).

BoNT-A is injected directly into the affected muscles, which are targeted according to clinical evaluation and desired functional goals (Russman et al., 1997). In the upper limb these muscles usually include the elbow flexors, wrist flexors, pronators, thumb adductor and opponens, and finger flexors (Lowe et al., 2006; Russman et al., 1997). Dosing regimes and dilution volumes for BoNT-A are established (Russman et al., 1997). The child usually has some form of analgesia for the procedure (Lowe et al., 2006; Russman et al., 1997; Russo et al., 2007), and the muscles to be injected are usually identified by surface anatomy, palpation, and some form of localization (such as with a stimulator, electromyography, or ultrasound) to ensure correct needle placement (O'Brien, 1997).

Purpose

BoNT-A injected directly into the affected muscle results in relaxation of the muscle, providing a window of opportunity to allow for therapy intervention. The overall aim of the occupational therapy intervention in children with cerebral paresis is to improve occupational performance, and whatever changes are achieved in capacity are best achieved in the context of improving skills (Kielhofner, 1995).

Method

Candidates for the Intervention

For children with cerebral palsy with *more severe upper limb impairment* (i.e., Manual Ability Classification System [MACS] level IV to V) (Eliasson et al., 2006), BoNT-A is injected to reduce muscle spasticity and muscle tone, increase range of motion, improve agonist-antagonist balance, delay the need for or complement orthopedic procedures, improve tolerance to splinting, maintain hygiene and skin integrity, improve cosmesis, manage pain, and prevent long-term deformity.

For children with *less severe upper limb impairment* (i.e., MACS level I to III) (Eliasson et al., 2006), hand skill development, improved occupational performance, and functional goal attainment are often the goals for treatment.

Epidemiology

Cerebral palsy occurs with an incidence of approximately 2 to 2.5 per 1000 live births (Reddihough and Collins, 2003). Upon careful and thorough clinical assessment, it is estimated that up to 50% of the population of children with cerebral palsy will benefit from upper limb injection of Botulinum Neurotoxin A.

The Role of the Occupational Therapist in Applying the Intervention

The role of the occupational therapist (OT) is integral in the identification of appropriate children for Botulinum Neurotoxin A injection, the selection of muscles for injection, pre- and postinjection assessment, goal setting, and the provision of adjunct interventions following injection.

Results

Clinical Application

Assessment of the Upper Limb Before Injection of BoNT-A

Assessment of impairment level should occur in larger muscle groups in the upper limb in children who receive BoNT-A injection. These measures assist in (1) identifying muscles with significant spasticity interfering with function, (2) selecting the muscle for injection, (3) determining the dosage, and (4) choosing the direction of the postinjection therapy.

Clinical range of motion is measured together with spasticity using the modified Tardieu scale (Boyd and Graham, 1999; Mackey, et al., 2004). This measure of spasticity is obtained when a joint is moved as fast as possible through its range of movement (V3 velocity) and the angle of "catch" elicited is measured using a goniometer. The difference between the angle of "catch" (R1) and the full passive range of movement (R2) reflects the potential range available in the joint if spasticity is eliminated.

Assessment of activity level requires careful observation of how spasticity and dystonia impact on the child's task performance. Videotaped assessments such as the Melbourne Assessment of Unilateral Upper Limb Function (Randall et al., 2001) and the Assisting Hand Assessment (Krumlinde-Sundholm et al., 2007) provide valuable information on a child's typical movement abilities. These observations are critical for (1) guiding muscle selection, (2) directing postinjection therapy, and (3) providing objective data measuring the change postinjection.

Goal Setting

The Canadian Occupational Performance Measure (COPM) (Law et al., 1994) is designed to detect change in a person's occupational performance. The COPM is an extremely useful tool for identifying and prioritizing goals pre- and postinjection of BoNT-A. The COPM responses can be transferred and scaled using the Goal Attainment Scaling (Kiresuk et al, 1994). This complementary approach enables goal identification, articulation, and measurement (Lowe et al., 2006; Wallen et al., 2007).

Intervention Postinjection of BoNT-A

Impairment Level: Stretching and Splinting

Active or passive manipulation of a muscle for 20 minutes immediately postinjection increases the efficacy of BoNT-A in the injected muscle and reduces diffusion to distant muscles (Minamoto et al., 2007). It is therefore important to provide immediate stretch to the child postinjection by applying a splint or encouraging active movement.

The general recommendation for *splint use* is for a minimum of 6 hours per night. This is based on evidence that contractures did not occur in children with cerebral palsy when lower limb muscles were stretched for more than 6 hours (Tardieu et al., 1988). However, evidence that static splinting maintains the mechanical-elastic properties of muscle is weak (Pin et al., 2006), with support for this intervention coming from animal studies (Williams, 1988; Williams et al., 1988) and limited evidence in the adult lower limb literature (Light et al., 1984; Steffen and Mollinger, 1995). The optimal splint design or position is currently unknown. However, day splinting using neoprene and Lycra garments is not recommended, with limited evidence for their efficacy (Corn et al., 2003; Knox, 2003; Nicholson et al., 2001) and the potential to reduce antagonist muscle movement.

Casting is clinically indicated when fixed contractures are present. This achieves a low-load prolonged duration muscle stretch. Typically, a serial program is implemented whereby a cast is reapplied every 3 to 7 days, gradually increasing the passive range of movement across a joint until the desired range is achieved. Three to four serial casts will usually be adequate to achieve the desired range of movement, and static splinting following the casting program is recommended. However, due to a lack of evidence for the efficacy of casting in this setting (Lannin et al., 2007), decisions and casting protocols are based on clinical experience.

Activity Level: Occupational Therapy

It is generally recommended that occupational therapy should commence 2 to 4 weeks following injection, with research supporting intensive bursts of movement-based training provided once or twice weekly for 2 to 3 months following injection.

However, the optimal program of occupational therapy has not been established, and the following discussion concerns the emerging trends in therapy after injection of BoNT-A.

Traditional upper limb occupational therapy practice involves a bimanual approach to training that is underpinned by several theoretical models (Chapparo and Ranka, 1997; Kielhofner, 1995; Law et al., 1997). Occupational therapists target the treatment of hand skills with specific task practice using a motor skill acquisition frame of reference (Kaplan and Bedell, 1999). This approach is well supported by recent advances in knowledge in the areas of neuroscience, basic mechanisms of hand function, and, more specifically, motor control and motor learning theories (Eliasson, 2005).

The practical application of a movement-based paediatric occupational therapy program, targeting activity level outcomes, should include the *following principles* based on a motor skill acquisition frame of reference (Kaplan and Bedell, 1999):

- Task analysis to identify if performance is limited by execution of movement or motor planning difficulties (i.e., sequencing of movements) (Steenbergen and Gordon, 2006; Steenbergen et al., 2007).
- Repetitive whole task practice of challenging, motivating, and purposeful activities (i.e., toys and games), carefully selected to facilitate development of goal-based skills and independence with task completion.
- Use modeling, physical assistance, verbal cues, or environmental adaptation to enable the child to understand the critical features of the task and the environment.
- Facilitate the children's learning and understanding of the role of their assisting hand (i.e., hemiplegic assisting hand) using active problem solving.
- Grading of physical or verbal assistance provided to complete tasks.
- Provide feedback focusing on the movement outcome, task, and environment rather than on the specific movement performance.
- Provide opportunities for the child to practice tasks in a range of contexts and environments.

Charles and Gordon (2006) have recently presented a similar protocol described as *Hand-Arm Bimanual Intensive Training* (HABIT), in which intensive practice of bimanual tasks is undertaken over a 2-week period. In this protocol, however, the therapist does not handle the child to facilitate movement or assist in task completion, but environmental adaptation is used. Specific movements required for task completion are also practiced repetitively and intensively using a protocol similar to behavioral shaping (Morris and Taub, 2001).

Constraint-induced movement therapy (CIMT) (Taub, et al., 1999) (see Chapters 30 and 31) combined with botulinum Neurotoxin A injection can be effective in providing intensive practice to young children with hemiplegia who do not spontaneously use their affected upper limb or have a significant developmental disregard. As the emerging evidence is as supportive of modified CIT as it is of CIT (Hoare et al., 2007), a modified protocol using a mitt and 2 hours of daily practice for 2 months is suggested. A bimanual training program should follow shortly after.

Goal-directed programs for children over the age of 5 years are aimed at maximizing the learning and performance of skills required for school and daily life that need to be considered. Goal-directed training is an activity-based approach to therapy aiming to improve a person's ability to engage in meaningful activities (Mastos et al., 2007). Programs are implemented using principles of motor learning (Schmidt and Lee, 1999) and are based on four components: (1) selection of a meaningful goal, (2) analysis of baseline performance, (3) intervention/practice regime, and (4) evaluation of outcome (Mastos et al., 2007).

Prior to injection of botulinum Neurotoxin A, the Canadian Occupational Performance Measure (Law et al., 1994) and Goal Attainment Scaling (Kiresuk et al., 1994) can be used to identify a meaningful goal for a child. The therapist must observe the child's baseline performance of the task to identify the specific areas of limitation. This process facilitates treatment planning and may also assist in determining appropriate muscles to be targeted for injection with BoNT-A. Following injection, the occupational therapy intervention focuses on specific and repetitive practice of the chosen task. The role of the therapist is to create a learning situation to develop active problem solving, exploration of alternative strategies, and repetitive practice.

Evidence-Based Practice

There is a growing body of high-quality research supporting the efficacy of upper limb occupational therapy intervention in children with cerebral palsy. More recent trials (Boyd, 2004; Greaves, 2004; Lowe et al., 2006; Russo et al., 2007; Wallen et al., 2007) evaluating the effects of BoNT-A and occupational therapy with occupational therapy alone have demonstrated positive gains on activity level outcomes in both the treatment and control groups.

Goal-directed training has been shown to be effective in attainment of meaningful goals and improved self-care and mobility as measured by the Pediatric Evaluation of Disability Inventory (Ahl et al., 2005; Ketelaar et al., 2001).

Discussion

BoNT-A is used to reduce spasticity and dystonia in affected muscles. This offers a window of opportunity to effect impairment and activity-based treatment strategies that can assist the child in upper limb functioning. Although specific regimes of upper limb therapy require further rigorous scientific evaluation, therapy postinjection targeting functional tasks identified by goal setting is gaining evidence of efficacy.

References

Ahl, L. E., Johansson, E., Granat, T., & Carlberg, E. B. (2005). Functional therapy for children with cerebral palsy: an ecological approach. Dev Med Child Neurol, 47(9), 613–619

Autti-Ramo, I., Larsen, A., Taimo, A., & von Wendt, L. (2001). Management of the upper limb with botulinum toxin type A in children with spastic type cerebral palsy and acquired brain injury: clinical implications. European Journal of Neurology, 8 Suppl 5, 136–144

Bax, M., Goldstein, M., Rosenbaum, P., Leviton, A., Paneth, N., Dan, B., et al. (2005). Proposed definition and classification of cerebral palsy, April 2005. Dev Med Child Neurol, 47(8), 571–576

Boyd, R. (2004). The central and peripheral effects of botulinum toxin A in children with cerebral palsy PhD dissertation, La Trobe University, Melbourne

Boyd, R. N., & Graham, H. K. (1999). Objective measurement of clinical finding in the use of botulinum toxin type A for the managment of children with cerebral palsy. Eur J Neurol, 6(Suppl. 4), S23–S35

Brin, M. F. (1997). Botulinum toxin: chemistry, pharmacology, toxicity, and immunology. Muscle Nerve Suppl, 6, S146–168

Chapparo, C., & Ranka, J. (1997). Occupational Performance Model (Australia) (Vol. Monograph 1). Sydney: OP Network - Total Print Control

Charles, J., & Gordon, A. M. (2006). Development of hand-arm bimanual intensive training (HABIT) for improving bimanual coordination in children with hemiplegic cerebral palsy. Dev Med Child Neurol, 48(11), 931–936

Corn, K., Imms, C., Timewell, G., Carter, C., Collins, L., Dubbeld, S., ,et al. (2003). Impact of second skin Lycra splinting on quality of upper limb movement in children. British Journal of Occupational Therapy., 66, 464–472

Eliasson, A. C. (2005). Improving the use of hands in daily activities: aspects of the treatment of children with cerebral palsy. Phys Occup Ther Pediatr 25(3), 37–60

Eliasson, A. C., Krumlinde-Sundholm, L., Rosblad, B., Beckung, E., Arner, M., Ohrvall, A. M., , et al. (2006). The Manual Ability Classification System (MACS) for children with cerebral palsy: scale development and evidence of validity and reliability. Dev Med Child Neurol 48(7), 549–554

Graham, H. K. (2000). Botulinum toxin A in cerebral palsy: functional outcomes.[comment]. Journal of Pediatrics, 137(3), 300–303

Greaves, S. (2004). The effect of botulinum toxin A injections on occupational therapy intervention outcomes for children with spastic hemiplegia., La Trobe University, Melbourne

Hoare, B. J., Wasiak, J., Imms, C., & Carey, L. (2007). Constraint-induced movement therapy in the treatment of the upper limb in children with hemiplegic cerebral palsy. Cochrane Database Syst Rev(2), CD004149

Jankovic, J., & Brin, M. F. (1997). Botulinum toxin: historical perspective and potential new indications. Muscle Nerve Suppl 6, S129–145

Kaplan, M. T., & Bedell, G. (1999). Motor skill acquisition frame of reference. In P. Kramer & J. Hinojosa (Eds.), Frames of Reference for Pediatric Occupational Therapy, (2nd ed., pp. 401–429). Baltimore: Williams and Wilkins

Ketelaar, M., Vermeer, A., Hart, H., van Petegem-van Beek, E., & Helders, P. J. (2001). Effects of a functional therapy program on motor abilities of children with cerebral palsy. Phys Ther, 81(9), 1534–1545

Kielhofner, G. (1995). A Model of Human Occupation. Theory and Application (2nd ed.). Baltimore: Williams and Wilkins

Kiresuk, T. J., Smith, J. E., & Cardillo, J. E. (1994). Goal Attainment Scaling: Applications, Theory and Measurement, Hillsdale, NJ: Lawrence Erlbaum

Knox, V. (2003). The use of Lycra garments in children with cerebral palsy: A report of a descriptive clinical trial. British Journal of Occupational Therapy., 66, 71–77

Krumlinde-Sundholm, L., Holmefur, M., Kottorp, A., & Eliasson, A. C. (2007). The Assisting Hand Assessment: current evidence of validity, reliability, and responsiveness to change. Dev Med Child Neurol, 49(4), 259–264

Lannin, N. A., Novak, I., & Cusick, A. (2007). A systematic review of upper extremity casting for children and adults with central nervous system motor disorders. Clin Rehabil, 21(11), 963–976

Law, M., Baptiste, S., Carswell, A., McColl, M. A., Polatajko, H., & Pollock, N. (1994). The Canadian Occupational Performance Measure. (2nd ed.). Toronto: Canadian Association of Occupational Therapists

Law, M., Stanton, S., Polatajko, H., Baptiste, S., Thompson-Franson, T., Kramer, C., et al. (1997). Enabling Occupation. An occupational therapy perspective. Ottawa: CAOT Publications

Light, K. E., Nuzik, S., Personius, W., & Barstrom, A. (1984). Low-load prolonged stretch vs. high-load brief stretch in treating knee contractures. Phys Ther, 64(3), 330–333

Lowe, K., Novak, I., & Cusick, A. (2006). Low-dose/high-concentration localized botulinum toxin A improves upper limb movement and function in children with hemiplegic cerebral palsy. Dev Med Child Neurol, 48(3), 170–175

Mackey, A. H., Walt, S. E., Lobb, G., & Stott, N. S. (2004). Intraobserver reliability of the modified Tardieu scale in the upper limb of children with hemiplegia. Dev Med Child Neurol, 46(4), 267–272

Mastos, M., Miller, K., Eliasson, A. C., & Imms, C. (2007). Goal-directed training: linking theories of treatment to clinical practice for improved functional activities in daily life. Clin Rehabil, 21(1), 47–55

Minamoto, V. B., Hulst, J. B., Lim, M., Peace, W. J., Bremner, S. N., Ward, S. R., , et al. (2007). Increased efficacy and decreased systemic-effects of botulinum toxin A injection after active or passive muscle manipulation. Dev Med Child Neurol, 49(12), 907–914

Morris, D. M., & Taub, E. (2001). Constraint-induced therapy approach to restoring function after neurological injury. Top Stroke Rehabil, 8(3), 16–30

Nicholson, J. H., Morton, R. E., Attfield, S., & Rennie, D. (2001). Assessment of upper-limb function and movement in children with cerebral palsy wearing Lycra garments. Developmental Medicine & Child Neurology, 43(6), 384–391

O'Brien, C. F. (1997). Injection techniques for botulinum toxin using electromyography and electrical stimulation. Muscle Nerve Suppl, 6, S176–180

Pin, T., Dyke, P., & Chan, M. (2006). The effectiveness of passive stretching in children with cerebral palsy. Dev Med Child Neurol, 48(10), 855–862

Randall, M., Carlin, J. B., Chondros, P., & Reddihough, D. (2001). Reliability of the Melbourne assessment of unilateral upper limb function. Developmental Medicine & Child Neurology, 43(11), 761–767

Reddihough, D. S., & Collins, K. J. (2003). The epidemiology and causes of cerebral palsy. Australian Journal of Physiotherapy, 49(1), 7–12

Russman, B. S., Tilton, A., & Gormley, M. E., Jr. (1997). Cerebral palsy: a rational approach to a treatment protocol, and the role of botulinum toxin in treatment. Muscle Nerve Suppl, 6, S181–193

Russo, R. N., Crotty, M., Miller, M. D., Murchland, S., Flett, P., & Haan, E. (2007). Upper-limb botulinum toxin A injection and occupational therapy in children with hemiplegic cerebral palsy identified from a population register: a single-blind, randomized, controlled trial. Pediatrics, 119(5), e1149–1158

Schmidt, R. A., & Lee, T. D. (1999). Motor control and learning: a behavioural emphasis, 2nd ed.. Champaign, IL: Human Kinetics Publishers

Steenbergen, B., & Gordon, A. M. (2006). Activity limitation in hemiplegic cerebral palsy: evidence for disorders in motor planning. Dev Med Child Neurol, 48(9), 780–783

Steenbergen, B., Verrel, J., & Gordon, A.M. (2007). Motor planning in congenital hemiplegia. Disabil Rehabil, 29(1), 13–23

Steffen, T. M., & Mollinger, L. A. (1995). Low-load, prolonged stretch in the treatment of knee flexion contractures in nursing home residents. Phys Ther, 75(10), 886–895; discussion 895–887

Taft, L. T. (1995). Cerebral Palsy. Pediatrics in Review, 16(11), 411–418; quiz 418

Tardieu, C., Lespargot, A., Tabary, C., & Bret, M. D. (1988). For how long must the soleus muscle be stretched each day to prevent contracture? Dev Med Child Neurol, 30(1), 3–10

Taub, E., Uswatte, G., & Pidikiti, R. (1999). Constraint-Induced Movement Therapy: a new family of techniques with broad application to physical rehabilitation--a clinical review. J Rehabil Res Dev, 36(3), 237–251

Wallen, M., O'Flaherty, S. J., & Waugh, M. C. (2007). Functional outcomes of intramuscular botulinum toxin type a and occupational therapy in the upper limbs of children with cerebral palsy: a randomized controlled trial. Arch Phys Med Rehabil, 88(1), 1–10

Williams, P. E. (1988). Effect of intermittent stretch on immobilised muscle. British Medical Journal., 47, 1014–1016

Williams, P. E., Catanese, T., Lucey, E.G., & Goldspink, G. (1988). The importance of stretch and contractile activity in the prevention of connective tissue accumulation in muscle. J Anat, 158, 109–114

Chapter 36
Pain Management: Multidisciplinary Back Schools and Future E-Health Interventions for Chronic Pain Sufferers

Miriam M.R. Vollenbroek-Hutten, Hermine J. Hermens, and Daniel Wever

After a couple of sessions the client became aware of his inadequate thoughts concerning pain and his inadequate behavior as a consequence.

Abstract Multidisciplinary interventions aiming at breaking the vicious circle of impaired functioning are effective for clients with chronic pain. However, because of the growing number of people with such complaints, these interventions cannot be provided totally on a face-to-face basis. Therefore, the possibilities of intervention in the client's daily environment professionally supervised through distance learning, that is, telemedicine, need to be considered.

Keywords Chronic pain • Feedback • Monitoring • Multidisciplinary rehabilitation programs • Telemedicine

Epidemiology

Musculoskeletal disorders constitute a major problem in the European Union. The overall prevalence of muscular pain affected by work is 17%. The reported 12-month prevalence of problems in the neck and upper limbs is in the range of 30.5% to 39.7% in people living in the Netherlands. Absence from work of 2 weeks or more caused by musculoskeletal disorders is about 53%. The costs for musculoskeletal disorders are estimated in European Union member states to be 0.5% and 2% of the gross national product. Moreover, pain complaints not related to work are a major and rapidly growing problem in Western industrialized countries. About 75 million Europeans (19%) complain of chronic pain (Breivik et al., 2006).

I. Söderback (ed.), *International Handbook of Occupational Therapy Interventions*,
DOI: 10.1007/978-0-387-75424-6_36, © Springer Science+Business Media, LLC 2010

Definition

Chronic pain is a complex disorder, the development and maintenance of which is influenced by biopsychosocial factors. This has resulted in wide recognition of the multidimensional approach, and varieties of multidisciplinary intervention have been developed. Among these, the *Multidisciplinary Roessingh Back School Rehabilitation Program* is the focus here. The program concerns interventions performed in client groups and focuses on the client's *self-management*. Clients need to learn to take responsibility for their situation and act on this when needed. Key elements in the intervention are exercise, training, and education. The number of people with chronic pain is still growing and, in the deficiency of available interventions, the restricted capacity of the health care system makes it impossible to offer all present and future clients with chronic pain face-to-face interventions. New, more effective, and more efficient ways of intervening need to be developed and implemented.

The provision of intervention in the client's home/work environment using ambulatory systems to monitor and provides feedback on inadequate behavior during everyday activities might be of potential value, which is exemplified by the myofeedback-based teletreatment services for feedback on muscle relaxation levels.

The interventions presented here are (1) the Multidisciplinary Roessingh Back-school Rehabilitation Program (RRP), and (2) the myofeedback-based teletreatment service (MYOTEL).

The Multidisciplinary Roessingh Back School Rehabilitation Program

Purpose

The RRP focuses on improving clients' health status by reducing their level of pain and disabilities and increasing functional capacity.

Method

Candidates for Intervention

The RRP is aimed at clients with specific low back pain for longer than 3 months and who experience disabilities in performing activities of daily living (ADL) and their work. These clients have developed a decreased-ability condition, that is, a vicious circle of back pain, inactivity due to back pain and fear, restricted performance of physical activities, and decreased physical capacity (Mayer et al., 1985).

   Inclusion criteria for the RRP are (1) ability to participate in daily activites for at least 3 days per week, (2) sufficient motivation, (3) ability to cooperate, and (4) trainable. Referral to the RRP follows a decision tree (van der Hulst et al., 2005; Vollenbroek-Hutten et al., 2004).

Setting

Clients with chronic low back pain are referred to the RRP program at a physical medicine and rehabilitation clinic by a general practitioner or specialist.

The Role of the Occupational Therapist

The occupational therapist (OT) is a member of the multidisciplinary rehabilitation team, which additionally consists of specialists in physical medicine and rehabilitation, physiotherapists, sport therapists, and, if needed, psychologists and dieticians.

   Rehabilitation team members perform assessments to screen clients suitable for RRP, goal setting, and evaluation. The OT and the physiotherapist conduct the interventions following the standard protocol on a weekly basis.

Results

Clinical Application

The RRP is based on the Swedish back school (Zachrisson-Forsell, 1980) and multi-dimensional pain programs (Fordyce et al., 1985). These interventions assume that clients with chronic low back pain develop a deconditioning syndrome. The aim of the RRP intervention is to influence health and perceived disabilities positively in the following ways:

* Enhancing clients' physical condition and learning how to balance their activity level with their capacity
* Providing insight into the mechanism important for the development and maintenance of back pain
* Teaching clients how to deal with pain and to take responsibility for their condition
* Stimulating and advising on ADL independence
* Integration into work
* Integration into movement and sports

Clients are treated in groups of up to eight participants each week for 7 weeks. The intervention includes the following features:

- Two hours of conditioning training, the purpose of which is to break through the vicious circle of deconditioning and focus on:
- Strength training of leg, back, and abdomen muscles using fitness apparatus. The training starts with two series of 10 movements at 60% of maximum force, and is built up to three series of 20 movements at 70% of maximum force.
- Cardiovascular (endurance) training on bicycle, rowing, or running ergometers. This training starts with 10 minutes at 65% to 80% of VO_2 max, depending on the client's baseline condition, and is built up gradually by 2 minutes per week to 20 minutes at the end of the program. Each session of conditional training consists of warming up, training, and cooling down. Clients also learn how to improve their condition in their own time, and are encouraged to do so.

- Half an hour of sports. During these sessions, attention is paid to:

  - Basic principles and elementary forms of sports aimed at teaching clients how to perform these sports activities ergonomically correctly.
  - Enhancing clients' experience that sports activity is a pleasant way to maintain condition.

- Half an hour of swimming. Swimming is considered to have a positive effect on health, on the premise that people need various forms of movement. Besides, as muscle tone decreases, many clients experience a decrease in pain during swimming, permitting an increase in condition.
- One-and-a-half hours of occupational therapy to create awareness of clients' level of physical functioning and their physical capacity, with the aim of bringing these two into balance. For this purpose, activities focus on giving insight into ergonomic principles, and practicing these principles in activities such as wrapping and unwrapping a bookcase and wallpapering, with feedback on how these are being done, with the aim of teaching clients to set their own effort limits.
- Four hours of physiotherapy to build up the client's activity level; improve muscle function; acquire awareness of posture while standing, sitting, and walking; and train while running, jumping, pushing, pulling, carrying, and cycling, as well as in sports and game activities.

During the sessions, clients act, experience, and get feedback on appropriate ways of performing the program for further application at home.

Following this program, clients with work-related deficits due to back pain may be offered individual occupational rehabilitation.

How the Interventions Eases Impairment, Activity Limitations, and Participation Restrictions

The RRP intervention focuses on teaching clients (1) to change behavior, especially thoughts that inhibit occupational performance; (2) self-management, such as taking responsibility for their own situation and acting on this in healthy ways;

(3) ergonomically correct performance of physical activities, sports, and work; and (4) increasing and maintaining physical condition to facilitate performance.

Evidence-Based Practice

The effects of multidisciplinary back school rehabilitation programs based on several systematic reviews and meta-analyses (van der Hulst et al., 2005) are good in some studies, but other studies report only moderate evidence of beneficial effects. However, the methodologic quality of the studies reviewed is often poor. Thus, the efficacy of multidisciplinary intervention for chronic low back pain in general is not yet clearly proven (van der Hulst et al., 2005). In a clinical trial, 30% to 50% of clients showed an improvement in disability level (Vollenbroek-Hutten et al., 2004).

The Myofeedback-Based Tele-Treatment Service - MYOTEL

Purpose

The MYOTEL focuses on improving clients' health status by reducing levels of pain and disability, increasing functional capacity, and improving work capacity.

Method

Candidates for the Intervention

The MYOTEL is intended for (1) clients with neck-and-shoulder disorders causing pain that restricts daily activities but still permits work, and (2) nonworking clients with chronic neck-shoulder complaints who want to reduce their disabilities. *Exclusion criteria* are general pain syndromes such as fibromyalgia, excessive overweight (body mass index >30), tumors, or severe deformities.

Setting

Referral to the MYOTEL program may be made by health professionals (general practitioner, neurologist, physiotherapist, rehabilitation physician, OT), or by clients themselves.

The MYOTEL program is conducted in the client's home or workplace environment.

The Role of the Occupational Therapist

The occupational therapist (OT) explains the aim and content of the intervention to clients in a face-to-face visit and teaches them how to relax taut muscles. Thereafter, the OT has a weekly consultative role to discuss progress, goal setting, and evaluation.

Results

Clinical Application

Theoretical Assumption

The MYOTEL is based on the assumption that clients with chronic pain have altered muscle activation patterns compared to asymptomatic controls (e.g., Nederhand et al., 2000). This is reflected especially in prolonged activation of muscles, that is, a decreased ability to relax after performing low dynamic, static, or mental tasks. The Cinderella hypothesis (Hägg, 1991) states that low levels of taut muscle may contribute seriously to the development and maintenance of chronic pain. Based on these findings, the MYOTEL focuses on creating awareness of this absence of sufficient muscle rest.

Technical Application

The ReTra equipment (Fig. 36.1) is used to measure raw electromyography (EMG) data from the trapezius muscle. These data are converted into percentages of relaxation time. The clients get auditory and vibratory feedback when relaxation time is insufficient (Hermens and Hutten, 2002).

The ReTra consists of (1) a harness with four incorporated surface electrodes that continuously measure surface electromyography (sEMG) from the trapezius muscle, (2) a portable unit that stores signals and processes functionality, and (3) a personal digital assistant (PDA) to provide continuous feedback to the client on the level of the taut muscle in the form of the EMG signals.

Client data are sent from the PDA (e.g., via GPRS) to a secure server. This is accessible to authorized health care professionals via a web portal, and is thus available all the time regardless of where the therapist is. The system enables the therapist to interpret the data both in real time and historically, permitting e-consultation.

The MYOTEL Intervention Program

As well as providing bio-data, clients keep a daily diary of their performed activities and the pain they experienced. At least once a week, but more often if needed, the OT and the client consult, face to face or by telephone.

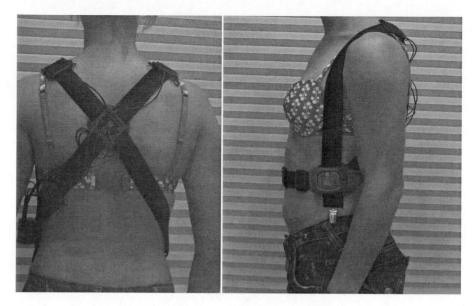

Fig. 36.1 The ReTra system worn by clients receiving the MYOTEL intervention. Left: Harness with incorporated dry surface electrodes. Right: Signal-processing, storage and vibration unit.

Material for this consultation is the therapist's study of the EMG data and the client's diary. The therapist identifies the problems seen in muscle patterns (relaxation and activation). Based on these data, together with the diary activities, events when the client experiences low levels of relative rest times (RRT) are identified.

Subsequently, therapist and client together seek solutions, and the client is taught appropriate skills and techniques to develop better functioning.

The week's progress is discussed: how clients learn to identify aspects relevant to their pain, plus the very important aspect of learning self-management. The consultation ends with new tasks and an appointment for next week.

Intervention normally ends after 4 weeks with a face-to-face visit. The MYOTEL program is presented in Fig. 36.2.

Evidence-Based Practice

Clients wear the harness with the surface electrodes (Fig. 36.1) during their performance of daily activities for 4 weeks. This gives very intensive and continuous *feedback* from tasks performed in their environment (Voerman et al., 2007a).

The program enables quick adaptation of client's behavior and shows the long-term effects of the intervention.

Hermens and Hutten (2002), investigated the processes underlying the feedback mechanisms, found that changes in the discomfort factor were especially associated with changes in catastrophic thoughts; reduction in disabilities was related to

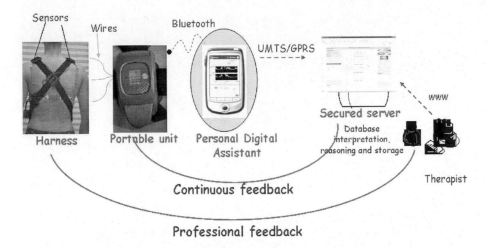

Fig. 36.2 Components, data transmission, and ways of feedback provision in the MYOTEL intervention.

decreased catastrophic thoughts about fear and avoidance of working. However, the percentage of explained variance was no more than 30% to 40%.

The myofeedback intervention has been evaluated in a number of studies (Hermens and Hutten, 2002; Huis in 't Veld et al., 2008; Voerman et al., 2006, 2007). The studies show that over the 4 weeks of the intervention the clients wore the equipment for at least 4 hours a day, 5 days per week. The results of a prognostic cohort study in 21 clients with work-related pain show that about 60% improved their pain/discomfort scores directly after myofeedback, and these were practically unaltered at 4-week follow-up. A remarkable finding is that 35% to 40% of the clients show a further improvement on pain/discomfort when the myofeedback had already ended (Hermens and Hutten, 2002). A prognostic cohort study in 14 clients with chronic whiplash disorders showed significant effects on pain and disabilities: 55% of the clients showed a clinically relevant reduction of pain and 36% of disabilities (Voerman et al., 2006). In a randomized clinical trial comparing myofeedback ($n = 41$) with ergonomic consultation ($n = 38$) for clients with work-related neck-shoulder pain in the Netherlands and Sweden (part of the NEW European project), 50% of the clients experienced a clinically relevant reduction in pain and disability, which persisted at a 6-month follow-up (Voerman et al., 2007). Myofeedback with remote data gathering and e-consultation is being tested in a cross-sectional study in 15 clients and 17 professionals to obtain insight into end-users' attitudes and self-efficacy regarding remote myofeedback intervention. Results showed that both clients and professionals expect the remote myofeedback intervention to be feasible. Attitudes were positive in 66% of the clients and 46% of the professionals. In addition, the majority of clients and professionals considered their self-efficacy sufficient for remote myofeedback intervention, and they expected at least the same effects as from the traditional intervention (Huis in 't Veld et al., 2007). A subsequent prognostic cohort study in 10 women with work-related pain showed that RRP is technically feasible. Eighty percent of clients reported a reduction in pain intensity and disability directly after RRP (Huis in 't Veld et al., 2008). Large randomized controlled trials are currently being run in four European countries (Netherlands, Germany, Belgium and Sweden) in the European MYOTEL project (www.myotel.eu).

Discussion

The most common interventions aimed at chronic pain disorders are multidisciplinary, of which the RRP program as outlined above is one. However, even with an indication tree for the decision on whether to intervene, the RRP is not effective for all clients. One explanation may be that not every client is inactive due to back pain and fear, and lowered physical capacity with, consequently, overloading. In Hasenbring's et al. (2001), model and in clinical practice, some clients lack fear but ignore the pain. These clients are probably much more helped by learning how to balance their activity patterns during the day than by physical reconditioning. Here, the present intervention including goal setting may probably be more effective. Another explanation why the intervention does not suit all clients might be that the skills learned in the rehabilitation program are too specific, occasioning problems with their generalization to daily life. This led to the notion that providing intervention in the client's daily environment by using ambulant monitoring and feedback systems could be effective. The telemedicine concept manifested in the MYOTEL service seems to be a good example. Results of the first evaluations indicate that this service is at least as effective as traditional interventions. In clients with chronic back pain, such an intervention should focus on activity levels. Recent research (van Weering, 2008) shows that although the overall activity levels of clients with chronic low-back pain do not differ from those of controls, their distribution of activities over the day differs significantly. An intervention in which the feedback is directed toward normalization of this disturbed activity pattern over the day might be very effective.

References

Breivik, H., Collett, B., Ventafridda, V., et al. (2006). Survey of chronic pain in Europe: prevalence, impact on daily life, and intervention. Eur J Pain, 10(4), 287–333.

Fordyce, W.E., Roberts, A.H., and Sternbach, R.A. (1985). The behavioral management of chronic pain: a response to critics. Pain, 22, 113–125.

Hägg, G.M. (1991). Static workload and occupational myalgia—a new explanation model. In: Anderson, P., Hobart, D., and Danoff, J., eds. Electromyographical Kinesiology (pp. 141–144). Amsterdam: Elsevier Science Publishers.

Hasenbring, M.I., Hallner, A.D., and Klasen, B. (2001). Psychologische Mechanismen im Prozess der Schmerzchronifizierung Unter- oder überbewertet? Schmerz, 15, 442–447.

Hermens, H.J., and Hutten, M.M.R. (2002). Muscle activation in chronic pain; its intervention using a new approach of myofeedback. Ind J Ergon, 30, 325–336.

Huis in't Veld, M.H.A., Voerman, G.E., Hermens, H.J., et al. (2007). The receptiveness toward N remotely supported myofeedback intervention. Telemed J E Health, 13(3), 293–301.

Huis in't Veld, R.M., Huijgen, B.C., Schaake, L., Hermens, H.J., Vollenbroek-Hutten, M.M., (2008). A staged approach evaluation of remotely supervised myo-feedback treatment (RSMT) in women with neck-shoulder pain due to computer work. Telemed J E Health. 14(6), 545–551.

Hulst, M., van der, Vollenbroek-Hutten, M.M.R., and Ijzerman, M.J. (2005). A systematic review of sociodemographic, physical and psychological predictors of (multidisciplinary or back school) intervention outcome for clients with chronic low back pain. Spine, 30(7), 813–825.

Mayer, T.G., Smith, S.S., Keeley, J., and Mooney, V. (1985). Quantification of lumbar function. Part 2: sagittal plane trunk strength in chronic low-back pain clients. Spine, 10(8), 765–72.

Nederhand, M.J., Ijzerman, M.J., Hermens, H.J., et al. (2000). Cervical muscle dysfunction in the chronic Whiplash Associated Disorder Grade II (WAD II). Spine, 25(15), 1938–1943.

van Weering, M.G.H., Vollenbroek-Hutten, M.M.R., Tönis, T.M. (2008). Daily physical activities in chronic lower back pain patients assessed with accelerometry. Eur J Pain (26) Epub ahed of print.

Voerman, G.E., Vollenbroek, M.M.R., and Hermens, H.J. (2006). Changes in pain, disability, and muscle activation patterns in chronic whiplash clients after ambulant myofeedback training. Clin J Pain, 22(7), 656–663.

Voerman, G.E., Sandsjö, L., Vollenbroek-Hutten, M.M.R., et al. (2007a). Changes in cognitive behavioural factors and muscle activation patterns after ambulant myofeedback training in work-related neck-shoulder complaints: Relations with pain and disability. J Occup Rehabil, 17(4), 593–609.

Voerman, G.E., Sandsjö, L., Vollenbroek-Hutten, M.M.R., et al. (2007b). Effects of ambulant myofeedback training and ergonomic counselling in female computer workers with work-related neck-shoulder complaints: a randomized controlled trial. J Occup Rehabil, 17(1), 137–152.

Vollenbroek-Hutten, M.M.R., Hermens, H.J., Wever, D., et al. (2004). Main and subgroup specific effects of a multidisciplinary rehabilitation program for clients with chronic low back pain. Clin Rehabil, 18(5), 566–580.

Zachrisson-Forsell, M. (1980). The Swedish back school. Physiotherapy, 66, 112–114.

Chapter 37
Pain Management: Functional Restoration for Chronic Low-Back-Pain Clients

Laura Stana, Anne Bouchez, Serge Fanello, and Isabelle Richard

Movement is not that dangerous, I can make it!

—Client

Abstract *Functional restoration* is a concept for intervention of low back pain that has been developed by Mayer et al. (1985). It relies on the concept that disability and participation restriction among clients with low back pain is the result of complex interactions among pain, physical deconditioning induced by inactivity, and psychosocial issues. The social cost, mainly indirect costs, induced by sick leave payments for chronic low back pain is high, and this has led to the development of multidisciplinary programs that include occupational therapy interventions.

Keywords Coping behavior • Ergonomics • Low back pain • Sick leave • Weight lifting

Definitions

Chronic low back pain is pain of the lumbar region lasting for more than 3 months.
   Functional restoration is the intervention program for nonspecific low back pain (i.e., infectious and tumor diseases are excluded) and other musculoskeletal diseases. The program is not aimed at reducing the level of pain, but rather focuses on physical reconditioning and coping strategies (Schonstein et al., 2003).

Background

Low back pain is a biopsychosocial issue. Treatments exclusively aimed at the biomedical aspects of low back pain, such as prescription of analgesic medicine, surgery, and corsets, are effective in the acute phase.

I. Söderback (ed.), *International Handbook of Occupational Therapy Interventions*,
DOI: 10.1007/978-0-387-75424-6_37, © Springer Science+Business Media, LLC 2010

363

Multidisciplinary functional restoration programs have been used in the chronic phase of low back pain since 1980s. Although differences among the various programs exist, they share a common framework, including (1) physical reconditioning, which is achieved by the clients' participation in intensive physical activities; (2) psychological counseling aimed at the development of coping mechanisms; and (3) modifications of the work environment (Poireaudeau et al., 2007; Schonstein et al., 2003).

Purpose

The objective of the functional restoration programs is that the clients return to work and resume social and leisure activities.

Method

Candidates for the Intervention

Functional restoration is indicated for clients suffering from chronic low back pain of nonspecific origin. Some programs are embedded in public policies aimed at reducing sick leave and enrolling only clients with work contracts (Loisel et al., 2003).

Epidemiology

The incidence of chronic low back pain in developed countries ranges between 60% and 90%. The prevalence is estimated at 5%. In the majority of cases (85–95%) pain and disability disappear within 3 months (Müllersdorf and Soderback, 2000).

Settings

The functional restoration programs are conducted by multidisciplinary teams and provided in rehabilitation outpatient facilities. They usually last for 3 to 5 weeks, and clients participate full time or part time.

Results

The Role of the Occupational Therapist

Occupational therapists (OTs) are responsible for the following:

- Assessments of activity limitations and participation restrictions using various available assessment instruments [e.g., Dallas pain questionnaire (Lawlis et al., 1989); Oswestry Low Back Pain Questionnaire (Fairbanks et al., 1980) or Capability to Perform Daily Occupations, an assessment adapted to occupational performances (Schult, 2002).
- Evaluation and retraining of activities directly related to work tasks, such as weight-lifting tasks. A client's ability to lift weights is measured using the progressive isoinertial lifting evaluation (PILE) (Mayer et al., 1988). The clients are required to lift blocks from the floor and place them on shelves at the level of the person's shoulder. The lifting capacity is measured by increasing the weight, starting with 5 kg (men) and 2.5 kg (women) and stepping up by 5-kg (men) and 2.5-kg (women) increments. The score is represented by the maximum weight that can be lifted.
- Investigation of the work tasks that are required by the clients to be performed during a workday. Based on the information, a training program is designed in which the client performs the work tasks in a simulated or real-life environment.
- Information on the benefits of physical activities. Clients often believe that reduction of performances of activities is necessary to treat their pain. The level of this restricting behavior is assessed by using the Fear-Avoidance Beliefs Questionnaire (FABQ) (Wadell et al., 1993).
- Thereafter, OTs and team members provide coherent information and demonstrate attitudes that promote the clients' active coping, aimed at decreasing clients' fear and avoidance of movements and increasing performances of daily activities and participation in social life.
- Counseling in which the client, relatives, coworkers, and managers participate to decide on possible modifications of the work environment. These interventions are individually performed at the workplace. They are directed to (1) physical aspects of the work environment, such as limiting weight lifting and the possible use of weight-lifting devices; and (2) management aspects of the work organization, such as possible cooperation between coworkers, and supervisors' attitude to the worker.

Clinical Application

Occupational Therapy Within a Multidisciplinary Pain Management Function Restoration Program

The programs are usually organized as intensive outpatient programs lasting 5 weeks with a full-time schedule. The interventions are performed in the rehabilitative setting, conducted in groups of five to 12 clients, or by individual counseling at the workplace.

The duration of the programs varies from 10 to more than 200 hours (Poireaudeau, 2007). The OT sessions account for approximately one third of all activities during the program.

The content of a functional restoration program includes the following:

- *Physiotherapy:* training of muscle flexibility, trunk muscle strengthening, and aerobic exercise for 1 to 3 hours per day
- *Sports activities:* for 1 to 6 hours per week
- *Occupational therapy:* clients perform weight-lifting tasks, or simulation of work tasks using, for example, gardening, bricklaying, for 1 to 2 hours per day
- *Psychological counseling:* performed in individual sessions or during group activities
- *Counseling:* during workplace visits

How the Intervention Eases Impairments, Activity Limitations, and Participation Restrictions

Functional restoration programs allow clients to "work in spite of pain" and thus resume performance of activities that help clients return to work.

Evidence-Based Practice

The functional restoration program has proved effective for (1) the main outcome measure of increasing participation of low back pain clients in returning to work; and (2) decreasing the number of days on sick leave (Jousset et al., 2004; Kaapa et al., 2006; Kool et al., 2007; Poireaudeau et al., 2007: Schonstein et al., 2003), and increasing the muscle endurance (Roche et al., 2007). These results are strongly dependent on the social security system of the country in which the program is conducted (Poireaudeau et al., 2007).

Discussion

The precise design of the functional restoration programs vary among rehabilitation clinics around the world. At present, there is restricted evidence for which intervention parts (Schonstein et al., 2003) or intensity (Roche et al., 2007) is required of the program to bring about a positive effect. Moreover, the cost-effectiveness of these programs also warrants further studies.

References

Fairbanks, J., Couper, J., Davies, J., and O'Brien, J. (1980). The Oswestry Low Back Pain Disability Questionnaire. Physiotherapy, 66, 271–273.

Jousset, N., Fanello, S., Bontoux, L., et al. (2004). Effects of functional restoration versus 3 hours per week physical therapy. A randomised controlled study. Spine, 29, 487–493.

Kaapa, E.H., Frantsi, K., Sarna, S., and Malmivaara, A. (2006). Multidisciplinary group rehabilitation versus individual physiotherapy for chronic non-specific low back pain. A randomized trial. Spine, 31, 371–376.

Kool, J., Bachmann, S., Oesch, P., et al. (2007). Function centered rehabilitation increase work days in clients with non-acute nonspecific low back pain: 1-year results from a randomised controlled trial. Arch Phys Med Rehabil, 88, 1089–1094.

Lawlis, G.F., Cuencas, R., Selby, D., and McCoy, C.E. (1989). The development of the Dallas Pain Questionnaire. An assessment of the impact of spinal pain on behavior. Spine, 14, 511–516.

Loisel, P., Durand, M.J., Diallo, B., Vachon, B., Charpentier, N., and Labelle, J. (2003). From evidence to community practice in work rehabilitation: the Quebec experience. Clin J Pain, 19(2), 105–113.

Mayer, T., Barnes, D., Kishino, N., et al. Progressive isoinertial lifting evaluation. I. (1988). A standardized protocol and normative database. Spine, 13, 993–997.

Mayer, T., Smith, S., Keeley, J., and Mooney, V. (1985). Quantification of lumbar function. Part 2: Sagittal plane trunk strength in chronic low-back pain patients. Spine, 10, 765–772.

Müllersdorf, M., and Soderback, I. (2000). Assessing health care needs. The actual state of self-percieved activity limitation and participation restrictions due to pain in a national-wide Swedish population. Int J Rehabil Res, 23, 201–207.

Poireaudeau, S., Rannou, F., and Revel, M. (2007). Functional restoration programs for low back pain. A systematic review. Ann Readapt Med Phys, 50, 425–429.

Roche, G., Ponthieux, A., Parot-Shinkel, E., et al. (2007). Comparison of a functional restoration program with active individual physical therapy for clients with chronic low back pain. A randomised controlled trial. Arch Phys Med Rehabil, 88, 1229–1235.

Schonstein, E., Kenny, D.T., Keeating, J., Koes, B.W. (2003). Work conditioning, work hardening and functional restoration for workers with back and neck pain. Cochrane Database Syst Rev, CD001822.

Schult, M.-L. (2002). Multidimensional assessment of people with chronic pain. A critical appraisal of the Person, Environment, Occupation Model. Monograph, Uppsala dissertations from the Faculty of Medicine, vol. 6, Uppsala University, Uppsala, Sweden.

Chapter 38
The Principles and Practice of Work and Ergonomics

Barbara A. Larson and Melaine T. Ellexson

The worker was experiencing wrist and hand pain. Once the tool was changed to an inline grip, his symptoms began to decrease.

Abstract Occupational rehabilitation programs address worker safety and productivity, using the organizing construct of participation, as defined by the International Classification of Functioning, Disability, and Health, as well as selected frames of reference that facilitate participation in work. Demographic and logistical factors of work-related musculoskeletal disorders, gender and age of onset, and epidemiology are identified. Clinical application and the role of the occupational therapist (OT) are examined in relation to the expected outcomes of an occupational rehabilitation program. Work as a performance area of occupation is discussed with an emphasis on worker function. Evidence related to work and ergonomics is presented from the standpoint of duration and cost, and worker quality of life.

Keywords Ergonomics • Human engineering • Occupational health • Task performance and analysis • Work

Definitions

Work: Productive or purposeful activities.

Task performance and analysis: The detailed examination of observable activity or behavior associated with the execution or completion of a required function or unit of work.

Occupational health: The promotion and maintenance of physical and mental health in the work environment.

Human engineering (ergonomics): The science of designing, building, or equipping mechanical devices or artificial environments for the anthropometric, physiologic, or psychological requirements of the people who will use them.

I. Söderback (ed.), *International Handbook of Occupational Therapy Interventions*,
DOI: 10.1007/978-0-387-75424-6_38, © Springer Science+Business Media, LLC 2010

Background

An occupational rehabilitation program addresses the needs of workers, while focusing on their ability to work safely and productively. The occupational therapist works in collaboration with the worker and other team members including case managers, employers, or selected agencies (AOTA, 2005).

The organizing construct, according to the International Classification of Functioning, Disability, and Health (ICF) as stated in Hemmingsson and Jonsson (2005), that a therapist uses participation in the intervention processes, here participation in work. This process is facilitated by the frame-works of the biomechanical approach (James, 2003), the occupational therapy practise framework (Schultz-Krohn and Pendelton, 2006) and the Person-environment-Occupation model (Law et al., 1996).

In the late 1970s and early 1980s, U.S. industry began to recognize its responsibility for active management and prevention of injury in the workplace (Ellexson, 1997; Jacobs and Baker, 2000). *Occupational rehabilitation* emerged as the umbrella term to describe programs that evolved to serve this worker population. Occupational rehabilitation encompasses work hardening, work conditioning, work rehabilitation, return to work, functional restoration, and other programs that rehabilitate the injured worker (Commission on Accreditation of Rehabilitation Facilities, 2008; Jacobs and Baker, 2000; King, 1998).

Purpose

The occupational therapist (OT) strives to enhance occupational performance, allowing the individual to engage in task completion, with the goal of full participation in work (American Occupational Therapy Association, 2002). Prevention strategies include ergonomic evaluation and design of the workplace, employee selection and screening, proactive injury management, and education and training of the work force (Larson and Ellexson, 2000; Saunders, and Stultz, 1998; Stein et al., 2006).

Job modifications, or reasonable accommodations, are considered if the worker is unable to perform essential job functions (Americans with Disabilities Act, 1990; Keilhofner, 2004). Modifying the workplace, and the tools and equipment used in the course of work activity, may aid an individual in compensating for the way tasks are completed.

Method

Demographics and Logistical Factors

Candidates for Occupational Rehabilitation

Diagnosis or disease categories include diseases of the nervous system, International Classification of Diseases (ICD) codes G00 to G09, and diseases of the musculoskeletal system and connective tissue, M00-M99 (ICD-10, 2007).

Gender and Common Age of Onset

According to the U.S. Bureau of Labor Statistics (BLS) 2007 data, "35 cases" with musculoskeletal disorders "per 10,000 full-time workers were days-away-from-work" and of these "men accounted for 64 percent of injuries and illnesses". Moreover, among all workplace injuries, 29 percent resulted in musculoskeletal disorders that requires time away from work (BLS, 2007).

Epidemiology

The U.S. Department of Labor (BLS, 2007), defines a musculoskeletal disorder (MSD) as an injury or disorder of the muscles, nerves, tendons, joints, cartilage, or spinal disks. The overall rate for all MSD cases was 39 per 10,000 workers in 2006 (BLS, 2007).

Settings

An occupational rehabilitation program may be provided in a hospital-based program, a freestanding program, a private or group practice, or in a work environment. Individuals are referred to these programs by physicians, insurance companies, workers' compensation agencies, case managers, employee health officers, or other health care providers dependent on local and national law (AOTA, 2005).

The Role of the Occupational Therapist in Applying the Intervention

The primary role of the occupational therapist (OT) is to provide services to individuals or populations with deficits, problems, or impairments in work performance (AOTA, 2005; Rice and Luster, 2002). The OT addresses factors that influence the participation in and performance of actual job tasks, including the worker's abilities, skills, neurobehavioral factors, physical health and fitness, cognition, and psychological and emotional well-being, and the environment in which the job exists (AOTA, 2005; Christiansen and Baum, 1997; Law, 2002).

Results

Outcomes of Occupational Rehabilitation

Clinical Application

Intervention planning for deficits or problems in the performance area of work is a multifaceted, complex process. The physical capacity of the worker as well as knowledge of the work tasks and routines, ergonomic stressors, tools and equipment, and other factors affecting the individual's ability to return to work must be identified

(AOTA, 2005; Haruko et al., 2006; King, 1998; Stein et al., 2006). A return-to-work program is interdisciplinary in nature, and often uses conditioning, work simulation, strengthening, and education to improve biomechanical, neuromuscular, cardiovascular, and psychosocial functions (CARF, 2008). Program effectiveness requires motivation and active participation by the worker (King, 1998).

Intervention that Directs the Worker to Function

Work is a performance area of occupation; it has specific activity demands and requires certain performance skills (AOTA, 2002). Deficits in body structure or body function limit the worker's ability to meet the activity demands of a given job (AOTA, 2002; World Health Organization, 2001). Changes in the worker's physical, psychological, or sociocultural status affect engagement in the occupation of work (Rice and Luster, 2002). The work capacity of the person is optimized through prevention, rehabilitation, education, and ergonomics (King, 1998; Larson and Ellexson, 2000). Future risk to the worker is minimized, while the individual's health and well-being are maximized through participation in work (Law, 2002).

Evidence-Based Practice

Workplace-based return-to-work interventions have been shown to have a positive impact on duration and costs of work disability, with weaker evidence supporting an increased quality of life for the workers (Franche, et al., 2005; MacEachen et al, 2006). Return to work was found to be more complex than managing physical function and included an individual's beliefs, roles, and the perceptions of others involved in the process (Christiansen and Baum, 1997; Law, 2002; MacEachen et al, 2006). Social and communication barriers were identified as negatively affecting return to work, while goodwill and trust were noted to play an important role in successful transition to work (MacEachen et al, 2006). While improved productivity through comprehensive ergonomic programming was supported in the literature, the data were reported to be the opinion of respected authorities and experts in the industry (Chiariello, 2003).

Discussion

While there is a need for stronger evidence in this area of practice, the resources available for occupational therapists are expanding. The Institute for Work and Health, an independent, nonprofit Canadian research organization (www.iwh.on. ca), provides evidenced-based information on interventions that enhance work performance, address injury and disability prevention, and facilitate successful return to work (Scheer, 2007).

Reimbursement for occupational rehabilitation services depends on the setting in which the service is provided. Payment sources include direct reimbursement, state or federal programs, or community agencies (AOTA, 2005).

References

American Occupational Therapy Association (AOTA). (2002). Occupational therapy practice framework: domain and process. Am J Occup Ther, 56, 609–639.

American Occupational Therapy Association (AOTA). (2005). Occupational therapy services in facilitating work performance. Am J Occup Ther, 59, 676–679.

Americans with Disabilities Act (ADA) of 1990, 42 U.S.C.A. § 12101 et seq. (West 1993).

Bureau of Labor Statistics (BLS). (2007). Nonfatal occupational injuries and illnesses requiring days away from work. http://www.bls.gov/iif/home.htm.

Chiariello, B. (2003). Does ergonomics improve productivity? An evidenced based analysis in Work Programs SIS Quarterly, 17 (4). American Occupational Therapy Association.

Christiansen, C., and Baum, C. (1997). Person-environment occupational performance—a conceptual model for practice. In: Christiansen, C., and Baum, C., eds. Occupational Therapy, Enabling Functioning and Well-Being (pp. 47–70). Thorofare, NJ: Slack.

Commission on Accreditation of Rehabilitation Facilities [CARF]. (2008). Medical Rehabilitation Standards Manual. Tuscon, AZ: CARF.

Ellexson, M.T. (1997). Job analysis and work-site assessment. In: Sanders, M.J., ed. Management of Cumulative Trauma Disorders (pp. 195–213). Boston: Butterworth.

Franche, R.-L., Cullen, K., Clarke, J., Irvin, E. Sinclair, S., and Frank J. (2005). Workplace-based return-to-work interventions: a systematic review of the quantitative literature. J Occup Rehabil, 15(4), 607–631.

Haruko, D., Page, J.J., and Wietlisbach, C.M. (2006). Work evaluation and work programs. In: Schultz-Krohn, W., and Pendelton, H., eds. Pedretti's Occupational Therapy for Physical Dysfunction (pp. 264–307). St. Louis, MO: Mosby.

Hemmingsson, H., and Jonsson, H. (2005). An occupational perspective on the concept of participation in the international classification of functioning, disability and health, some critical remarks. Am J Occup Ther, 59, 569–576.

International Statistical Classification of Diseases and Related Health Problems. 10th Revision (ICD-10). (2007). http://who.int/classifications/apps/icd/icd10online.

Jacobs, K., and Baker, N.A. (2000). Lesson 1. The History of Work-Related Therapy in Occupational Therapy (Self-Paced Clinical Course). Bethesda, MD: American Occupational Therapy Association.

James, A.B. (2003). Biomechanical frame of reference. In: Crepeau, E.B., Cohn, E.B., and Boyt Schell, B.A., eds. Willard and Spackman's Occupational Therapy (pp. 240–242). Philadelphia: Lippincott Williams & Wilkins.

Keilhofner, G. (2004). The Biomechanical Model in Conceptual Foundations of Occupational Therapy, 3rd ed. (pp. 79–93). Philadelphia: F.A. Davis.

King, P.M. (1998). Work hardening and work conditioning. In: King, P.M., ed. Sourcebook of Occupational Rehabilitation (pp. 257–273). New York: Plenum.

Law, M. (2002). Participation in the occupations of everyday life. Am J Occup Ther, 56, 640–649.

Law, M., Cooper, B.A., Strong, S., Stewart, D., and Rigby, P. (1996). The person-environment-occupation model. Can J Occup Ther, 63(1), 9–23.

Larson, B., and Ellexson, M. (2000). Blueprint for ergonomics. Work, 15, 107–112.

MacEachen, E. Clarke, J., Franche, R.-L., and Irvin, E. (2006). The process of return to work after injury: findings of a systematic review of qualitative studies. Scand J Work Environ Health, 32(4), 257–269.

Rice, V.J., and Luster, S. (2002). Restoring competence for the worker role. In: Trombley, C.A., and Radomski, M.V., Eds. Occupational Therapy for Physical Dysfunction, 5th ed. Baltimore, MD: Lippincott Williams & Wilkins.

Saunders, R.L., and Stultz, M.R. (1998). Education and training. In: King, P.M., Ed. Sourcebook of Occupational Rehabilitation (pp. 109–126). New York: Plenum.

Scheer, J. (2007). The institute for work and health: evidence for OT. OT Pract, 22, 23–24.

Schultz-Krohn, W., and Pendelton, H. (2006). Application of the occupational therapy practice framework to physical dysfunction. In: Schultz-Krohn, W., and Pendelton, H., Eds. Pedretti's Occupational Therapy for Physical Dysfunction (p. 38). St. Louis, MO: Mosby.

Stein, F., Soderback, I., Cutler, S.K., and Larson, B. (2006). Occupational Therapy and Ergonomics. London: Whurr.

World Health Organization (WHO). (2001). International Classification of Functioning, Disability and Health (ICF). Geneva, Switzerland: WHO.

Chapter 39
Reintegration to Work of People Suffering from Depression

Gabe de Vries and Aart H. Schene

Employees suffering from depressive disorder, treated by occupational therapy, increase their chances of going back to work again.

Abstract Employees suffering from depression have a high risk of becoming unemployed. A combination of treatment focused on depression and on work rehabilitation is effective. Occupational therapy and the Program for Mood Disorders at the Department of Psychiatry of the Academic Medical Centre in Amsterdam, The Netherlands, have developed three modules focused on work reintegration for clients suffering from depression. The modules have been investigated in a randomized controlled trial and seem to be effective in work reintegration.

Keywords Depression • Occupational rehabilitation • Work

Definitions

According to the *Diagnostic and Statistical Manual of Mental Disorders*, 4th edition, major depressive disorder (unipolar depression) "is influenced by both biological and environmental factors." It is characterized by the symptoms "depressed mood (such as feelings of sadness or emptiness), reduced interest in activities that used to be enjoyed, sleep disturbances, significant reduction in energy level, *cognitive impairments*, i.e., difficulty concentrating, holding a conversation, paying attention, or making decisions that used to be made fairly easily, suicidal thoughts or intentions" (American Psychiatric Association, 2000).

Work is a paid daily activity (Jacobs, 1991). *Work restarting* means that employees start working after a period of absenteeism caused by a depressive disorder.

I. Söderback (ed.), *International Handbook of Occupational Therapy Interventions*,   375
DOI: 10.1007/978-0-387-75424-6_39, © Springer Science + Business Media, LLC 2010

Background

Absenteeism from work is related to mental health problems in about 30% of cases. Of these, about one third are caused by mood disorders, especially depression (Schene et al., 2007). Depression causes absenteeism from work and, even more important, *presenteeism*, that is, loss of productivity while the employee is still at work but impaired by his or her mental health symptoms.

Work and depression have a complex relationship. Work-related problems can be one of the determinants of depression, while depression impairs work functioning and therefore contributes to problems or dysfunction in the work setting. The work burden plays a role in the pathogenesis of depression.

Work burden is determined by (1) the physical work load, that is, the *job strain*; (2) *psychological demands*, such as stress-factors at work; (3) the worker's *decision latitude* for organizing and take control over his or her work performances; and (4) available *social support* of colleagues, management, and the social support system around the worker (Bakker, 2003; Karasek and Theorell, 1990; Rasker et al., 2005).

A high work load in combination with a stressful home situation causes a higher risk of getting depressed (Croon et al., 2000). People with depression suffer more often from a lack of social support or are victims of bullying (de Roos and Sluiter, 2004). A self-perception of belonging to a lower status career and less capacity to fit into the work organization contributes to a higher risk of depression (de Roos and Sluiter, 2004).

In contrast, presenteeism may provoke problems at work caused by the following:

- *Cognitive limitations*, characterized by problems in concentrating on the work tasks, planning the performance of the work tasks, and limited capability to cope with complex stimuli.
- *Emotional restrictions cause* feelings of inferiority and guilt, and loss of interest and initiative. These symptoms create problems in executing daily activities at work, for example, accepting too much work while having difficulties in solving problems.
- *Social restrictions* are difficulties in dealing with colleagues, which are caused by a lower mood, introverted behavior, or social anxiety of the employee with a depression.

The interventions for the above problems are the following: (1) the focus for clients with *depression and work relationship problems* is on the clients' cognitive, emotional, and social restrictions; and (b) the focus for clients who are *restarting work* is on the issues of work load, capacity to organize, social support, and perspective of the client's role in the organization.

Purpose

The main purpose of the intervention is to enable clients to restart work as soon as possible and to function with more satisfaction. Being ready to restart work increases the chances of being employed, and clients suffering from depression who have restarted work report fewer symptoms of depression compared with clients who did not start working (de Vries et al., 2002).

Method

Candidates for the Intervention

The intervention is aimed at adult clients with depressive disorder, who are able to function in a work environment for a few hours a week. Excluded are clients with a psychotic depression or those who abuse alcohol or drugs.

Epidemiology

Mental disorders, particularly depression, are the most frequent source of occupational disability worldwide and are expected to increase. Employers are increasingly aware of the productivity costs associated with mental disorders and the importance of fostering a mentally healthy work force (Stuart, 2007). The total economic burden of depression in the year 2000 in the United States was $83.1 billion. Of this total, $26.1 billion was direct medical costs, $5.4 billion was suicide-related mortality costs, and $51.5 billion was workplace costs ($36.2 billion work absenteeism and $15.3 billion presenteeism) (Greenberg et al., 2003).

Depression was the third highest total cost of medical conditions studied that affected U.S. employees. Only hypertension and heart disease were more costly (Goetzel et al., 2004). For example, U.S. Air Force workers ($n = 209$) who reported depression symptoms were on sick leave significantly more days (2.0 days for any depression symptoms, 4.7 days for severe depression symptoms, vs. 0.15 days for no depression) (Planz, 2006).

Almost 4% of employed people of ages 25 to 64 had had an episode of depression in the previous year. Cross-sectional analysis indicates that these workers had high rates of reducing work activity because of a long-term health condition, having at least one mental health disability day in the past 2 weeks, and being absent from work in the past week. Thus depression was associated with reduced work activity (de Vries et al., 2002).

Settings

The intervention is developed to use in a psychiatric hospital, but can be used in a work setting or in a work-training center. The main condition is the ability of the client to work a few hours in his or her former work setting.

Professionals Involved into the Process of Restart Work

Most important is the *clients'* responsibility for restarting their work, reintegration at work, and performance of work tasks. Apart from health care services, other services are involved in the work restarting process. This rehabilitation approach combines care and work.

The *employer* is responsible for reintegration at the work setting. The *occupational physician* of the company is responsible to ascertain whether the client is able to return to work. The *general practitioner* is responsible for some aspects of health care and prevention. Referral to a psychiatrist also occurs. The *social worker* or alternative health care practitioners are cooperating with the employer and the occupational therapist (OT). The *OT* recommends to the client one of the interventions focused on work. The initial role of the OT is to coordinate the involved professionals and to administer the rehabilitation program.

A reintegration process succeeds only if the people involved have a common goal. In such a situation, it is important to know who is responsible for each part of the process. Furthermore, all involved professionals are informed about the client's progress and the results of each professional's contribution. All involved professionals should agree that the plan is appropriate for the client.

Results

Clinical Application

Analysis of Working Problems

This part of the intervention focuses on investigating the client's patterns of working and determine which work tasks cause problems. The intervention consists of five individual sessions over a 4-week period and includes the following:

The *register and intake session* gives the client the opportunity to express his or her attitudes about work and willingness to restart working. The OT explains the content, options, and goals of the occupational therapy intervention.

Work anamnesis intervention is a consultation with the client in which the OT systematically analyzes the clients education and work history. The client's coping with stressful situations is especially noted.

The *video observation* entails recording the client's performance of work tasks in a simulated work situation. These recordings are discussed with the client regarding his or her experiences of the current work load, relationships with colleagues, and the appropriateness of the work. The main goals are to analyze the problems in the present work situation, and to ascertain if there is an ineffective pattern to the way the client copes with stressful situations.

Depression and the Work Relationship

This part of the intervention focuses on investigating the patterns that cause stress in the working situation, and is directed at relieving the stress and giving the client an opportunity to take control over his or her working situation. This part takes about 6 months and consists of 20 group sessions, one each week; 10 individual sessions, one every second week; and three follow-up sessions over the course of half a year.

The *goals are* (1) reintegrating clients at work, (2) improving their ability to cope effectively with stress situations at work, (3) increasing their work satisfaction, and (4) preventing a new depressive episode.

In the *group sessions*, the OT presents themes such as working stress, capacities and incapacities, perfectionism, prevention, and conflicts at work. The clients' are given homework to do. Every group or individual session addresses (1) the work performance, (2) the patterns of coping behavior, (3) the home situation, and (4) the reintegration at work. Work performance is related to all aspects of functioning at work. Coping patterns are determined for each stressful situation. A work reintegration plan is created.

The *individual session* focuses on the client's personal and working situation regarding the progress of the interventions.

Restarting Work in Spite of Depression

This part of the intervention focuses on restarting work despite the clients' depressive disorder. It includes eight group sessions, four individual sessions, and one follow-up session. The clients need to be able to work for at least 2 hours a week in order to attend this part of the intervention. The client practices the new skills at the workplace.

The intervention assumption is that the remission of psychiatric symptoms will occur after restarting work. The intervention is based on the principle of individual placement support (IPS), meaning that the client should first work and then get training (Burns et al., 2008).

The intervention emphasizes the clients' ability to resume work through *adjustments of the work environment*, such as physical and psychological demands, decision latitude, and the social support of the coworkers and the employer. The adjustments are made on the basis of the client's experience at work and the effect of the depressive symptoms on the work capacity. The intervention also emphasizes the clients' participation in real or simulated work tasks.

The group meetings discuss issues relating to the clients' perceptions regarding the following:

- Cognitive, physical, and emotional aspects of the work.
- *The arrangement boundary*, that is, clients' opportunity to organize and arrange the work to enable them to do the work in the manner of their choosing.

- *The social support* provided by colleagues, their *personal perspectives, and* the clients' fitting into their work environment.
- The *home situation*, such as leisure time, chores, and responsibilities.

The Individual Sessions

The first session focuses on the client's specific problems. The second session is attended by the client and the employer, so that the employer can learn about the consequences of the depressive disorder for the work performance and information about the content of the intervention program. The client is asked to discuss with the employer his or her experience of the work load.

Evidence-Based Practice

The effectiveness of these occupational therapy modules has been evaluated in a randomized controlled trial (Schene et al., 2007). The results showed that the addition of occupational therapy to treatment (1) did not improve the outcome of the depressive disorder, (2) resulted in a reduction in sick-leave days during the first 18 months, (3) did not increase work stress, and (4) had a 75.5% probability of being more cost-effective than the treatment alone.

Nieuwenhuijsen et al. (2008), in a Cochrane review ($n = 2,556$) (one study concerned adjuvant occupational therapy), showed that "there is no evidence of an effect of medication alone, or psychological interventions or the combination of those with medication, on sickness absence of depressed workers."

Research with Web-based self-help interventions aimed at decreasing symptoms of depression, anxiety, and work-related stress (burnout) showed a statistically and clinically significant effect on symptoms of depression and anxiety. These effects were even more pronounced for participants with more severe baseline problems and for participants who completed the course. The effects on work-related stress and quality of life were less clear (van Straten et al., 2008).

Discussion

Depressive disorders have impact on absenteeism from work and the reduced work productivity of presenteeism. Interestingly, the epidemiologic aspects have been studied widely, while interventions to reduce the consequences are very limited.

The clinical experiences are that clients with minor or less severe depressive disorders are mostly able to continue working, albeit at a lower productivity level, but those clients with severe depressive disorders lose their jobs and never return to the workplace. Therefore, occupational therapy interventions have an additive value over regular treatments among those clients who have to reduce their working hours or stop working for a shorter period. Here it is important to refine occupational therapy interventions and evaluate the effectiveness in terms of absenteeism and presenteeism.

References

American Psychiatric Association. (2000). Diagnostic and Statistical Manual of Mental Disorders (DSM-IV-TR). Washington, DC: American Psychiatric Association. http://allpsych.com/disorders/mood/majordepression.html

Bakker, A.B. (2003). Working with Flow: How Dutch People can Create Their own Sources of Energy (Bevlogen aan het Werk: Hoe Nederland haar eigen energiebronnen kan creëren). In: Verhaar, K., ed. Sociale Verkenningen, Vol. 4: Waarden en Normen (pp. 119–141). Den Haag: Ministerie van SZW.

Burns T., Catty J., for the EQOLISE Group. (2008). IPS in Europe: The EQOLISE Trial. Psychiatr Rehabil J, 31(4), 313–317.

de Croon, E.M., Blonk, R.B.B., and Frings-Dresen, M.H.W. (2000). Stress in Professional Cargo Transport (Stress in het beroepsgoederenvervoer), Amsterdam: AMC Coronel instituut, report number 00-0.

de Roos, L., and Sluiter, J.K. (2004). Depression as Occupation Disease: Identifying Work Related Psychosocial Risks from Country Registration and a Systematic Literature Research. (Depressie als beroepsziekte: Identificatie van werkgebonden psychosociale risicofactoren uit de landelijke registratie en een systematisch literatuuronderzoek), Tijdschrift voor Bedrijfs en Verzekeringsgeneeskunde 12, 365–371.

de Vries, G. Kikkert, M.J., Schene, A.H., and Swinkels, J. (2002). Does a Work-Related Therapy Help Depressed Patients? Dutch Magazine of Occupational Therapy (Helpt arbeidshulpverlening bij patiënten met een depressie? Nederlands Tijdschrift voor Ergotherapie), 103–106.

Gilmour, H. and Patten, S.B. (2007). Depression and work impairment. Health Rep. 18(1), 9–22.

Goetzel R.Z., Long S.R., Ozminkowski R.J., Hawkins K., Wang S., and Lynch W. (2004). Health, absence, disability, and presenteeism cost estimates of certain physical and mental health conditions affecting U.S. employers. J Occup Environ Med, 46(4), 398–412.

Greenberg P.E., Kessler R.C., Birnbaum H.G., et al. (2003). The economic burden of depression in the United States: how did it change between 1990 and 2000? J Clin Psychiatry, 64(12), 1465–1475.

Jacobs, K. (1991). Occupational Therapy. Work-Related Programs and Assessments. Boston: Little, Brown.

Karasek, R., and Theorell, T. (1990). Health Work, Stress, Productivity and the Reconstruction of Working Life. New York: Basic Books.

Nieuwenhuijsen K., Bültmann U., Neumeyer-Gromen A., Verhoeven A.C., Verbeek J.H.A.M., and van der Feltz-Cornelis C.M. (2008). Interventions to improve occupational health in depressed people. Cochrane Database of Syst Rev (2):CD006237. doi: 10.1002/14651858. CD006237.pub2.

Pflanz, S.E., and Ogle, A.D. (2006). Job stress, depression, work performance, and perceptions of supervisors in military personnel. Military Medicine. 171(9), 861–865.

Rasker, P., Gaillard, A.W.K., Vliet, van G., and Vianen, M. (2005). Absence in the callcenter (Ziekteverzuim in contactcenters). Arbo Magazine, 4, 11–13.

Schene, A.H., Koeter, M.W.J., Kikkert, M.J., Swinkels, J.A., and McCrone, P. (2007). Adjuvant occupational therapy for work-related major depression works: randomized trial including economic evaluation. Psychol Med, 37, 351–362.

Stuart, H. (2007). Employment equity and mental disability. Curr Opin Psychiatry, 20(5), 486–490.

van Straten, A., Cuijpers, P., and Smits, N. (2008). Effectiveness of a Web-Based Self-Help Intervention for Symptoms of Depression, Anxiety, and Stress: Randomized Controlled Trial. FPP, Department of Clinical Psychology, Amsterdam, The Netherlands.

Chapter 40
Supported Employment for Individuals with Severe Mental Illness

Cynthia Z. Burton, Lea Vella, and Elizabeth W. Twamley

Far and away the best prize that life offers is the chance to work hard at work worth doing.

—Theodore Roosevelt, 1903

Abstract Occupational dysfunction is one of the most devastating and disabling consequences of severe mental illness. Supported employment (SE) is an evidence-based practice for assisting clients with severe mental illness to find and keep competitive jobs in the community. The key elements of SE include rapid, individualized job searching, job-based assessment, benefits counseling, time-unlimited job support, and integration of vocational and mental health services. Further, any client who wants to participate is eligible for SE services, and all services are based on the client's individual preferences.

Keywords Psychosis • Psychosocial intervention • Schizophrenia • Vocational rehabilitation

Definition and Background

Supported employment is a form of work rehabilitation that helps clients obtain competitive work (i.e., jobs that pay minimum wage or higher, that are available to any individual, regardless of disability status, and where disabled and nondisabled coworkers work together). The manualized form of supported employment, Individual Placement and Support (IPS), was developed by Becker and Drake (2003).

Supported employment programs provide clients with rapid, individualized job placement in competitive work. Placement is followed by on-the-job training as needed and ongoing, time-unlimited support from the employment specialist. Support can consist of any counseling, training, or coaching the client needs to keep the job. Assessment of the client is continuous and is based on experience in real-world jobs, rather than artificial settings. Supported employment programs are integrated within mental health care, such that the employment specialist is part of a multidisciplinary treatment team. As this is a community-based intervention, the employment specialist often conducts meetings in the client's setting of choice (e.g., library, career center, coffee shop, home) to focus on client strengths and rehabilitation rather than "patienthood." Work rehabilitation and employment can result in greater income, community integration, and improvement in symptom severity, increased self-esteem, and quality of life (Bond et al., 2001).

Supported employment is an evidence-based practice in psychiatric rehabilitation, with multiple randomized controlled trials and meta-analyses demonstrating its effectiveness over conventional vocational rehabilitation (Bond et al., 2001, 2004; Cook et al., 2005; Twamley et al., 2003).

Purpose

Supported employment focuses on improving the clients' occupational status.

Method

Candidates for the Intervention

Clients with psychiatric disabilities who want to return to work are good candidates for supported employment. Supported employment programs do not exclude clients for reasons of "work readiness," diagnosis, substance use history, legal history, or level of disability (Bond, 2004).

Epidemiology

Although most individuals with psychiatric illness want to work, employment rates are only 10% to 25% (Latimer et al., 2004). With the assistance of supported employment 51% to 55%, of clients who want to work can obtain jobs (Cook et al., 2005; Twamley et al., 2003).

Settings

Supported employment is most commonly used in outpatient psychiatric settings. Any client with a stated goal of working should be given supported employment.

The Role of the Occupational Therapist

The occupational therapist (OT), referred to in supported employment as the employment specialist, is responsible for delivering vocational services. The employment specialist typically has a bachelor's or master's degree and provides services to a caseload of 20 to 25 clients. In addition to the phases described above, the employment specialist may also provide transportation to interviews and attend interviews with the client, depending on the client's preference for disclosure.

Results

Clinical Application

Supported employment programs consist of the following phases: (1) initial assessment: discussion of the client's job skills, past employment experience, current employment goals and preferences, and benefits counseling; (2) job searching: collaborative effort to create a résumé, complete applications, and prepare for interviews; and (3) time-unlimited follow-up support: the employment specialist provides ongoing support as needed, and checks in regarding stressors, symptoms, or any problems at work.

How the Intervention Eases Impairments, Activity Restrictions, and Participation Restrictions

Severe mental illness is associated not only with psychiatric symptoms but also with cognitive impairment, including difficulty with attention, learning and memory, and problem solving. Employment specialists assist clients by helping them find jobs that are a good match for their energy level, their ability to cope with various job stressors, and their cognitive strengths. Once the client obtains a job, the employment specialist can help the client trouble-shoot symptom exacerbations and cognitive problems on the job. For example, the employment specialist might help a client who hears voices learn to ignore the voices in order to maintain attention on job tasks. The integrated nature of supported employment and mental-health-supported employment allows the employment specialist to work closely with other providers to help the client navigate medication adjustments or participate in other psychosocial treatment.

Evidence-Based Practice

The effectiveness of supported employment has been well established in the literature. Cook et al. (2005), in a multisite trial, found that supported employment resulted in greater placement in competitive work and greater earned income. In addition, a meta-analysis of 11 randomized controlled trials of vocational rehabilitation in schizophrenia and other psychotic disorders showed that 51% of supported-employment participants obtained competitive work, compared to only 18% of conventional vocational rehabilitation clients (Twamley et al., 2003). A 10-year follow-up study showed that one third of supported employment clients worked at least 5 years during the follow-up period (Salyers et al., 2004).

Discussion

Possible Criticism/Limitations

Despite numerous empirical studies of supported employment and the participants receiving services, few client predictors (e.g., diagnosis, age, gender, education level, co-occurring disorders) have been linked to better outcome. Thus, it is difficult to assess who would most benefit from a supported employment program. Although supported employment works best to help people with severe mental illness obtain competitive work, up to half of clients with severe mental illness do not work.

Common obstacles may include fear of losing disability benefits, comorbid medical illness, psychiatric symptom exacerbation, lack of motivation, or cognitive problems that interfere with job hunting. Among those who do work, job tenure is often brief (3 to 5 months) and unsatisfactory job endings are common (e.g., quitting or being fired without being hired elsewhere) (McGurk et al., 2005). Unskilled job placements are also common in supported employment programs, which may contribute to short tenure and job attrition.

Cost-Effectiveness

The annual cost of supported employment is $2000 to $4000 per client, which is similar to that of conventional vocational rehabilitation (Bond et al., 2001). A possible cost offset includes lower utilization of mental health services, such as day treatment among clients participating in supported employment (Bond et al., 2001).

Recommendations for Further Research

To improve the efficacy of supported employment programs, researchers are examining modifiable targets to enhance services. Current research efforts are aimed at augmenting supported employment with cognitive interventions to compensate for neuropsychological deficits commonly seen in severe mental illness (McGurk et al., 2007; Vauth et al., 2005; Wexler and Bell, 2005). Razzano et al. (2005) examined clinical factors that may affect employment among individuals with severe mental illness, and found that poor self-rated functioning, negative psychiatric symptoms, and recent hospitalization were associated with failure to obtain competitive work. These findings suggest that amelioration of negative symptom severity may increase the likelihood of job placement. Both cognitive remediation and psychiatric treatment will continue to be examined as interventions to improve vocational outcomes in individuals with severe mental illness.

References

Becker, D.R., and Drake, R.E. (2003). A Working Life for People with Severe Mental Illness. New York: Oxford University Press.

Bond, G. (2004). Supported employment: Evidence for an evidence-based practice. Psychiatr Rehabil J, 27(4), 345–359.

Bond, G., Becker, D., Drake, R., et al. (2001). Implementing supported employment as an evidence-based practice. Psychiatr Serv, 52(3), 313–321.

Bond, G., Salyers, M., Dincin, J., et al. (2007). A randomized controlled trial comparing two vocational models for persons with severe mental illness. J Consult Clin Psychol, 75(6), 968–982.

Cook, J., Leff, H., Blyler, C., et al. (2005). Results of a multisite randomized trial of supported employment interventions for individuals with severe mental illness. Arch Gen Psychiatry, 62(5), 505–512.

Latimer, E., Bush, P., Becker, D., Drake, R., and Bond, G. (2004). The cost of high-fidelity supported employment programs for people with severe mental illness. Psychiatr Serv, 55(4), 401–406

McGurk, S., Mueser, K., Feldmen, K., Wolfe, R., and Pascaris, A. (2007). Cognitive training for supported employment: 2–3 year outcomes of a randomized controlled trial. Am J Psychiatry, 164(3), 437–441.

McGurk, S., Mueser, K., and Pascaris, A. (2005). Cognitive training and supported employment for persons with severe mental illness: one-year results from a randomized controlled trial. Schizophr Bull, 31(4), 898–909.

Razzano, L., Cook, J., Burke-Miller, J., et al. (2005). Clinical factors associated with employment among people with severe mental illness: Findings from the employment intervention demonstration program. J Nerv Ment Disord, 193(11), 705–713.

Salyers, M.P., Becker, D.R., Drake, R.E., Torrey, W.C., and Wyzik, P.F. (2004). A ten-year follow-up of a supported employment program. Psychiatr Serv, 55(3), 302–308.

Twamley, E., Jeste, D., and Lehman, A. (2003). Vocational rehabilitation in schizophrenia and other psychotic disorders: A literature review and meta-analysis of randomized controlled trials. J Nerv Ment Disord, 191(8), 515–523.

Vauth, R., Corrigan, P.W., Clauss, M., et al. (2005). Cognitive strategies versus self-management skills as adjunct to vocational rehabilitation. Schizophr Bull, 31(1), 55–66.

Wexler, B., and Bell, M. (2005). Cognitive remediation and vocational rehabilitation for schizophrenia. Schizophr Bull, 31(4), 931–941.

Chapter 41
Individual Placement and Support: Helping People with Severe Mental Illness Get Real Jobs

Jonathan Garabette and Tom Burns

Individual Placement and Support (IPS) is the accepted evidence-based vocational rehabilitation intervention of choice in the United States, and there is now good evidence for its effectiveness in Europe.

Abstract Unemployment rates in people with severe mental illness (SMI) are historically extremely low. Traditional employment services use a "train and place" model, in which time is spent in secondary (sheltered) employment services before, if at all, attempting to obtain competitive employment. Individualized Placement and Support (IPS) is a method in which clients are helped to obtain competitive employment directly and then supported in these posts—a *"place and train" model.* IPS is the evidenced-based vocational rehabilitation program of choice in the United States, and there is now good evidence for it in Europe.

Keywords Mental disorders • Mentally ill persons • Schizophrenia • Supported employment • Vocational rehabilitation

Background

Prevocational training is traditionally the most widespread vocational rehabilitation model for people with severe mental illness. It consists of intensive preparation and sheltered work, prior to application for "competitive employment" (work in the community that anyone can apply for which pays at least the minimum wage). However, competitive employment is rarely obtained. Many clients either become stalled in the sheltered settings or are disengaged from the program (Bell et al., 1993; Drake et al., 1999).

    Supported employment, which emphasizes direct job placements, has been developed as an alternative model. The Individual Placement and Support (IPS) model is a specific, manually operated version, which increasingly replaces prevocational training. The Individually and Supported Model contains the following key features: (1) competitive employment as the goal; (2) clients are expected to obtain

I. Söderback (ed.), *International Handbook of Occupational Therapy Interventions,*
DOI: 10.1007/978-0-387-75424-6_41, © Springer Science + Business Media, LLC 2010

jobs directly, without lengthy preemployment training ("rapid job search"); (3) rehabilitation is treated as an integral component of mental health treatment rather than a separate service; (4) services are based on clients' preferences and choices; (5) assessment is continuous and based on real work experiences; and (6) follow-up support is continued indefinitely (Bond, 1998).

Purpose

The IPS program incorporates principles of supported employment and assertive community treatment. Key components are that it is (1) open to all with SMI, (2) a rapid job search is conducted based on the individual preferences of the client, (3) assessment is continuous, and (4) periods of unsuitable employment attempts are expected and viewed as a normal part of the process.

Method

Candidates for the Intervention

The IPS program has been developed specifically for people with *severe mental illness*. It is a community-based intervention, integrated into the community mental health team (CMHT). It combines the principles of supported employment with those of *assertive case management*. Zero-exclusion is a key principle, meaning that the program accepts any adult client with severe mental illness who wants to be in the program. No clients are screened out based on perceived job readiness, substance use, intellectual functioning, behavioral problems, or symptom severity.

Epidemiology

People living with severe mental illness (5 million people in the working-age population in Europe) have historically very high unemployment rates (61% to 85% across various settings), despite reports that the majority want to work (Crowther et al., 2001).

Settings

Clients are employed in any area of the primary labor market, depending on local availability and client suitability and preference. Regular meetings with a dedicated employment specialist occur in the community and at the client's place of work, and follow-up support is indefinite.

Results

The Role of the Occupational Therapist

Individual Placement and Support Program Staffing

The role of OTs in IPS is potentially controversial, as the program actively distances itself from traditional practices, which are regarded as overprotective and paternalistic. Staffing optimally consists of two IPS *employment specialists*, supervised by a *vocational coordinator* who manages referrals. While the vocational coordinator is expected to have a background in vocational rehabilitation, the employment specialists are not. Typically, they have no OT experience, though they are expected to have the ability to work with clients with severe mental illness. Their time should be spent exclusively as employment specialists, not involved in aspects of general case management usually expected of OTs in some traditional mental health rehabilitation settings.

Clinical Application

Administration

The IPS employment specialist actively searches for job opportunities that suit the client's interests and abilities and encourages rapid entry into the labor market. Once a client is employed, the employment specialist provides ongoing support to help maintain that employment. Assessment is continuous, and it is expected that clients may experience several jobs that prove unsuitable before settling in one.

Integrated within the client's treatment team, the employment specialist regularly consults other involved team members to ensure that vocational rehabilitation and mental health treatment are complementary (Latimer, 2001). The client should also be counseled regarding the possibilities of a "benefit trap" effect, in which there may be a perceived or real financial disincentive to work, due to loss of benefits.

Guidelines on the implementation and practice of IPS as set out by its originators are available (Becker and Drake, 1993), as is a fidelity scale to measure the degree to which an individual program conforms with the IPS model (Bond et al., 1997).

Therapeutic Principles of the Individual Placement and Support Program

Unlike prevocational training, IPS does not try actively to reduce clients' impairments but rather works around them. It compensates both for impairments and adverse symptoms that may have made it difficult for the client to find a job, and also helps clients maintain employment by finding jobs where their impairments are either not relevant or where adequate support is available (McGurk and Mueser, 2003).

Evidence-Based Practice

North American Evidence Base

The IPS program is now the evidence-based intervention of choice, and about 20 experimental and quasi-experimental studies have been published. Randomized controlled trials have demonstrated superior effectiveness for IPS against traditional services for vocational outcomes including finding employment, working competitively in the community, working more hours in a given month, and having higher earnings. A systematic review of 11 randomized controlled trials (RCTs) found that after a period of as short as 6 months, 30% of IPS clients were in competitive employment, compared to 6% of those who were receiving prevocational training. At 24 months, 15% of IPS clients were in employment, compared to 5% of the prevocational clients (Crowther et al., 2001).

Variance in efficacy has been linked with client factors such as (1) interest in finding a work (Macias et al., 2001), (2) differences in local labor markets, and (3) IPS model fidelity. The IPS principles of (1) integration of rehabilitation with mental health treatment, (2) employment specialists providing only employment services, and (3) the zero-exclusion criteria, show the highest correlations with employment rates, though not all fidelity components showed enough variance to be studied (Becker et al., 2001).

European Evidence Base

While IPS works well in North America, its efficacy cannot be automatically assumed in Europe, which has (1) a less work-oriented culture, (2) better welfare benefits (less financial incentive), and (3) more rigid labor markets (a barrier to employing those with severe mental illness). However, a recent RCT (Burns et al., 2007) of over 300 psychotic clients across six very different sites (in Bulgaria, England, Germany, Italy, the Netherlands, and Switzerland), found the following:

- The effect size of IPS was equal to North American trials (a doubling of employment rates), and showed a clear statistically significant relationship to local employment rates and a noticeable but not statistically significant impact of a benefit trap effect.
- IPS clients stayed longer in jobs (contrary to expectations).
- IPS clients showed reduced hospital admission rates. This was not demonstrated in the North American trials, and the fact may reflect better-integrated health care in Europe.

Discussion

The IPS program has demonstrated superior efficacy to standard services across a variety of settings and for a range of outcomes. In the U.S., it is the recommended evidence-based intervention for vocational rehabilitation, and its effectiveness in Europe has recently been demonstrated. The cost benefits of IPS vs. traditional vocational rehabilitation are still unclear, but the benefits of increased social inclusion from competitive employment are unequivocal (Morgan et al., 2007).

On balance, therefore, the evidence supports IPS as the vocational rehabilitation method of choice for severe mental illness. Further research and development should now be directed at identifying optimal methods to provide it.

References

Becker D.R., and Drake R.E. (1993). A Working Life: The Individual Placement and Support (IPS) Program. New Hampshire: Hampshire-Dartmouth Psychiatric Rehabilitation Research Center.

Becker, D.R., Smith, J., Tanzman, B., Drake, R.E., and Tremblay, T. (2001). Fidelity of supported employment programs and employment outcomes. Psychiatr Serv, 52(6), 834–836.

Bell, M.D., Milstein, R.M., and Lysaker, P.H. (1993). Pay as an incentive in work participation by clients with severe mental illness. Hosp Community Psychiatry, 44(7), 684–686.

Bond, G.R. (1998). Principles of the individual placement and support model: Empirical support. Psychiatr Rehabil J 22(1), 11–23.

Bond G., Becker D., Drake R., and Vogler K. (1997). A fidelity scale for the individual placement and support model of supported employment. Rehabilitation Counseling Bulletin. 40(4), 265–284.

Burns, T., Catty, J., Becker, T., et al. (2007). The effectiveness of supported employment for people with severe mental illness: a randomised controlled trial. Lancet, 370(9593), 1146–1152.

Crowther, R.E., Marshall, M., Bond, G. R., and Huxley, P. (2001). Helping people with severe mental illness to obtain work: systematic review. BMJ, 322(7280), 204–208.

Drake, R.E., McHugo, G.J., Bebout, R.R., et al. (1999). A randomized clinical trial of supported employment for inner-city clients with severe mental disorders. Arch Gen Psychiatry, 56(7), 627–633.

Latimer, E.A. (2001). Economic impacts of supported employment for persons with severe mental illness. Can J Psychiatry, 46(6), 496–505.

Macias C., DeCarlo L.T., Wang Q., Frey J., Barreira P. (2001). Work interest as a predictor of competitive employment: policy implications for psychiatric rehabilitation. Admin Policy Mental Health, 28(4), 279–297.

McGurk, S.R., and Mueser, K.T. (2003). Cognitive functioning and employment in severe mental illness. J Nerv Ment Dis, 191(12), 789–798.

Morgan, C., Burns, T., Fitzpatrick, R., Pinfold, V., and Priebe, S. (2007). Social exclusion and mental health: conceptual and methodological review. Br J Psychiatry, 191, 477–483.

Chapter 42
Conducting Transitional Strategies that Support Children with Special Needs in Assuming Adult Roles

Leonora Nel and Colette van der Westhuyzen

I'm so happy! I didn't believe this was ever possible. She earns a salary like any other person. Thank God. This is all because of this program.

—Client's parent

Abstract Transitional strategies are systematic interventions and procedures aimed at preparing learners with special needs for entry into the labor market and independent living. It is an individualized process, where occupational therapy interventions are carefully selected to enhance academic outcomes. The transition process moves from school-based prevocational training to job placement. The focus is on the valuable role of the occupational therapist (OT). This is of particular significance in countries where transition support has not been established.

Keywords Prevocational skills • Residential independence • Social integration • Supported employment • Transition • Vocational skills

Background and Definition

The quotation at the beginning of this chapter was from an interview with the mother of 20-year-old Johanna, who has severe cerebral palsy and spastic quadriplegia. Johanna underwent the occupation therapy-based prevocational training and transition support and now works as a kitchen assistant in a school hostel.

Access to equal work opportunities has become a major focus for youth services worldwide (UK Cabinet Office Strategy, 2007; US National Council on Disability, 2000). Young people with special needs due to disabilities are faced with numerous challenges. Therefore, they require specialized support to achieve successful transition to become adult workers (Burgstahler, 2003; Smart, 2004; Van Niekerk, 2007).

Transition is a habilitative strategy, and may include maintenance, preventative, or adaptive interventions aimed at changing the role of child to the role of adult.

I. Söderback (ed.), *International Handbook of Occupational Therapy Interventions*,
DOI: 10.1007/978-0-387-75424-6_42, © Springer Science+Business Media, LLC 2010

It covers the period between ages 16 and 25 years. Because an individual's ability to work forms an integral part of the adult's role, it is therefore the major focus of transition programs (U.S. Federal Government, 2004).

Transition outcomes are described in terms of employment, social and interpersonal networks, and role adaptation in the residential environment (Liu et al., 2007). It is an individualized process that starts in high school, where programming includes and emphasizes (1) work readiness, that is, prevocational preparation combined with vocational or work-specific preparation; and (2) social and life skills required for successful community integration. Transition further entails the commencement of ongoing supported employment, through which the individual gains access to meaningful work, and more importantly, is able to maintain it.

The outcome of transitional programs (Halpern, 1985) is the product of multi-disciplinary inputs, involving a range of professionals, such as educators, facilitators, medical professionals, physiotherapists, speech therapists, and adult rehabilitation service representatives, as well as the client's parents, employers, and others in the community (Wehman et al., 1985). Here, OTs have a knowledge base (Du Toit, 1991; Kielhofner, 2004) that is suitable for contributing to the transitional process as team members. Finally, the outcome of a transitional program is largely dependent on the client's motivation.

Purpose

Transitional programs are aimed at optimally developing clients' ability to efficiently perform tasks with specifically focus on work ability. The ultimate goal is successful integration into adult contexts.

Method

Candidates for the Intervention

Children with special needs who would benefit from rehabilitation services or would qualify for social support due to disability are candidates for this transitional intervention.

Epidemiology

All learners with special education needs will benefit from transition services, particularly those with more severe disabilities. Transition services are new in the South African context, and statistically significant data have not been gathered to establish reliable figures for the need for such services.

Settings

Referral for transitional program support usually occurs from (a) school-based support services that serve learners with special needs, or (2) health settings providing rehabilitation services. The occupational therapy transition service has a wide scope of interventions, such as health related, educational, social-emotional, or work related. This intervention may occur in a number of settings: school-based, community-based, or in the workplace.

The Role of the Occupational Therapist

In the process of supported employment, OTs acts as facilitators of vocational training and job placement. The OTs roles are that of a job coach. During the phase of prevocational preparation of the transitional process, the OTs focus on work and work behaviors, but all performance areas are systematically addressed to ensure that clients achieve optimal independence in their different adult roles.

Results

Clinical Application

Transitional programs entail a client-centered process where goal setting and intervention strategies are individualized. It is the product of thorough and ongoing assessment and problem solving.

An outline of the elements of supported employment applied to the OT's transition interventions is shown in Table 42.1 (Wehman et al., 1992).

The application of transitional strategies follows the occupational therapy process, and includes *assessments*, which are conducted by applying a holistic human development and function. It is wise to balance standardized, formal evaluations with clinical observations, work simulations, and collateral information gained from parents or caregivers or other members of the team. In the school setting the OT has access to comprehensive records covering background information, education, function, and multidisciplinary intervention.

The need for formal testing is often limited to the child's specific performance areas that have not been observed or addressed in previous interventions. The following functional areas are to be considered during the assessment process: (1) sensorimotor skills, (2) cognitive components, (3) cognitive integration, (4) psychosocial skills, (5) psychological performance components, and (6) adaptation in the performance areas of activities, work, and leisure (American Occupational Therapy Association Terminology Task Force, 1994). Information on performance

Table 42.1 Supported employment elements applied in occupational therapy transition strategies

Support element	Occupational therapy strategies
Consumer assessment (function, skills, interest)	Holistic assessment and analysis of all performance areas, components, and contexts.
Job development (job analysis and job matching, environmental adaptation and job modification)	Identify, generate, and negotiate appropriate in-service training positions. Apply principles of activity analysis, work simplification, and ergonomics to plan and implement structural or task adaptations, provide assistive technology, and ensure that both client and employer benefit.
Job placement	Therapeutic group work is used to train work-seeking behavior. Support (co-working and training) is given to achieve appropriate level of integration and performance when initialized into a job. Coworkers and employers are given support and training in strategies to effectively monitor and manage the client's work performance and integration. Regular on-site visits are performed to evaluate actual status.
Employer liaison, and job-site interventions (training, behavior management) with use of job retention strategies	Build professional relationships with employers, have regular feedback sessions, and offer therapeutic intervention to address or prevent problem areas identified by client, employer, job coach, or coworkers.
Individualized support	Coordinate and facilitate service delivered to address needs in all performance areas: health management, work, household management and independent living, transport and mobility, social integration, and leisure pursuits.

contexts is vital to ensure accurate and appropriate planning and programming for transition. The specific area of assessment of vocational skills should include aptitude tests, interest inventories, and prevocational readiness, which is best investigated through the use of work samples (Jacobs, 1991).

Planning of the transitional program should commence at the age of 14. Based on a critical analysis of the information gained during assessment, the therapist provides guidelines to the educational team regarding curricular components that would benefit the child's transition.

Occupational therapy program goals are objective stated and reasonable to attain during therapeutic sessions both in the school and in real community settings. It is recommended that individual intervention is limited, and preference be given to group work, as it supports the development of appropriate work behaviors in a therapeutic environment. Biannual review and reevaluation will be beneficial in ensuring that the process takes place smoothly and that appropriate goals are being pursued.

Prevocational Preparation

Education programs are enhanced by the OT providing the support and accommodations required by the learner's disability in the classroom, and also by including prevocational preparation in the form of task-centered therapeutic groups, marketable skills groups, and natural community and workplace experiences, with a specific focus on training prevocational skills (Jacobs, 1991).

The Youth Transition Program Model (Benz et al., 1999) provides an outline of how such a program should be constituted, with emphasis on the development of a good work ethic. It has been applied by Little People's School (Jacobs, 1991) and Pretoria School (Nel et al., 2007), which are examples of how the occupational therapy service complements the curriculum to achieve successful prevocational preparation.

How the Intervention Eases Impairments, Activity Limitations, and Participation Restrictions

Transitional strategies redefine disabled children's perspective on the future, moving them from the role of disabled person to empowered worker, thus being able to (1) engage in a variety of relationships, (2) contribute through service to the society, and (3) develop personal strengths and skills (Inman et al., 2007; Seyfarth et al., 1987; U.S. Federal Government, 2004).

Evidence-Based Practice

The success of transition strategies may be measured according to several parameters, such as, work, income, residential independence, personal satisfaction, and parent/caregiver satisfaction (Blackorby and Wagner, 1996). Very little evidence of OT-based prevocational training, vocational preparation, and transition in schools exists in the literature. The growing interest in this field of practice among school-based OTs, especially in developing countries, is indicative of the need for this service. New programs should be developed based on the successes of existing models, and allowing for adaptations relevant to the context (Mithaug, 1994) provides guidelines in this regard.

Discussion

The literature reflects lower than desired levels of success for persons who underwent transition support. However, personal communications verify the need for OTs to work with children living with disabilities. "There is a need to expand the focus in preparing learners for transition from school to the vocational environment" (Dr. Kitty Uys, personal communication, 2008). If this should become a reality, research that proves the evidence of transitional programs is greatly needed. This research may contribute to changing the attitude that vocational preparation and transition services are labor intensive and may be seen as a luxury.

References

American Occupational Therapy Association Terminology Task Force. (1994). Uniform terminology for occupational therapy. Am J Occup Ther, 48, 1047–1059.

Benz, M.R., Lindstrom, L., and Latta, T. (1999). Improving collaboration between schools and vocational rehabilitation: The youth transition program model. J Voc Rehabil, 13, 55–63.

Blackorby, J., and Wagner, M. (1996). Longitudinal post-school outcomes of youth with disabilities: findings from the national longitudinal transition study. Exceptional Children, 62, 399–413.

Burgstahler, S. (2003). DO-IT: Helping students with disabilities transition to college and careers. The National Center on Secondary Education and Transition (NCSET research to practice brief 2 (http://www.ncset.org/publications/viewdesc.asp?id=1168).

Du Toit, V. (1991). Patient volition and action in occupational therapy. Vona & Marie du Toit Foundation, Hillbrow, England.

Halpern, A.S. (1985) Transition: a look at the foundation. Exceptional Children, 51(6), 479–486.

Inman, J., McGurk, E., and Chadwick, J. (2007). Is vocational rehabilitation a transition to recovery? Br J Occup Ther, 70, 60–66.

Jacobs, K. (1991). Occupational Therapy Work-Related Programs and Assessments, 2nd ed. Boston/Toronto/London: Little, Brown.

Kielhofner, G. (2004). Conceptual Foundations of Occupational Therapy, 3rd ed. Philadelphia: F.A. Davis.

Liu, K.W.D., Hollis, V., Warren, S., and Williamson, D.L. (2007). Supported employment program processes and outcomes: experiences of people with schizophrenia. Am J Occup Ther, 61, 543–554.

Mithaug, D.E. (1994). Equity and Excellence in School-to-Work Transitions of Special Populations. University of California, Berkeley, CA, NCRVE Center Focus 6. (http://www.eric.ed.gov/ERICWebPortal/custom/portlets/recordDetails/detailmini.jsp?_nfpb=true&_&ERICExtSearch_SearchValue_0=ED372247&ERICExtSearch_SearchType_0=no).

Nel, L., van der Westhuyzen, C., and Uys, K. (2007). Introducing a school-to-work transition model for youth with disabilities in South Africa. Work, 29, 13–18.

Seyfarth, J., Hill, J.W., Orelove, F., McMillan, J., and Wehman, P. (1987). Factors influencing parents' vocational aspirations for their children with mental retardation. Mental Retard, 25, 375–362.

Smart, M. (2004). Transition planning and the needs of young people and their carers: the alumni project. Br J Spec Educ, 31, 128–137.

U.K. Cabinet Office Strategy. (2007). Improving the Life Chances of Disabled People: areas for more detailed analysis. (http://www.cabinetoffice.gov.uk/strategy/work_areas/disability/priority.aspx).

U.S. Federal Government. (2004). Individuals with Disabilities Education Improvement Act. (http://idea.ed.gov).

U.S. National Council on Disability. (2000). Transition and post-school outcomes for youth with disabilities: closing the gaps to post-secondary education and employment. (http://www.ncd.gov/newsroom/publications/2000/transition_11-01-00.htm).

Van Niekerk, M. (2007). Career exploration program for learners with special educational needs. Work, 29, 19–24.

Wehman, P., Kregel, J., and Barcus, J.M. (1985). From school to work: a vocational transition model for handicapped students. Exceptional Children, 52, 25–37.

Wehman, P., Sale, P., and Parent, W. (1992). Supported Employment. Strategies for Integration of Workers with Disabilities. Boston: Andover Medical Publishers.

Part IV
Interventions: The Occupational Therapist Enables for Recovery

Chapter 43
Interventions: The Occupational Therapist Enables Recovery

Recovery Interventions: Overview

Ingrid Söderback

Abstract This chapter surveys the occupational therapy interventions in which the occupational therapist (OT) enables the clients' activity, with the aim of resuming engagement in occupations. The OT's role is clarified. The interaction between the client and the activity is illustrated by two cases. Commonly used therapeutic media, such as arts and crafts, leisure and recreational activities, progressive relaxation, horticulture therapy, music therapy, complementary therapy with animals, and work-related activities, are discussed. Marie-Louise Huss's case illustrates how engagement in occupations brought meaning to the client's life and facilitated her recovery.

Keywords Dementia · Enabling occupation · Horticultural therapy · Life satisfaction · Meaningful occupations · Music therapy · Recreational activities · Therapeutic media.

Introduction

The Occupational Therapists' Role

The primary role of occupational therapists (OTs) (Fig. 43.1) is to arrange the environmental circumstances so that the clients can be gainfully occupied. In other words, the clients take part in an activity that not necessarily has a defined goal or is resulting in a product (Christiansen and Baum, 1997c). Here, the OT's work covers preparation and organization of the selected occupation or activity, and supplying the client with appropriate and necessary material and tools. A fundamental criterion is that clients' activity should fulfill their wishes and be chosen by them.

Enabling

The term *enabling* was first used by Christensen and Baum (1997). *Enabling interventions*, with recovery as the goal, are founded on the assumption that being

The occupational therapist

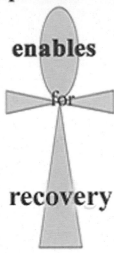

enables

for

recovery

Fig. 43.1 The occupational therapist's role in the occupational therapy interventions aimed at enabling activities that promote the client's feeling of recovery. The figure is a stylized Ankh-sign.

occupied (1) maintains the human being, (2) gives content to otherwise endless days of idleness and waiting for healing, (3) re-orientate leisure activities, (4) offers contact with other people, (5) eases solitude (Mosey, 1986), and (6) increases mastery and control of one's environment and the competence to handle it (Christensen, 1991).

Among these assumptions, Matuska et al. (2003) showed that 65 elderly people living in a community relieved their solitude through their participation in an occupational therapy wellness program. They increased their participation from 55% to 65% for three or more meaningful social and community activities per week.

Purpose

The purposes of interventions in which the OT enables the client to be occupied are (1) to fill the clients' time, so that they may experience meaning, involvement, and participation, and (2) to give purpose and opportunity to clients as they make choices regarding their activity. These factors contribute to clients' recovery, by enabling their engagement in activity, thus promoting good health and quality of life (Hammell, 2004). These purposes are "independent of whether a product is created or whether the activity gives visible results." The activity can be a step toward the client's renewed competence (Pedretti and Early, 2001).

The Case of the Group Members

This activity process without goals of producing a product is illustrated by the following case:

> Early in 1970, I was an OT in a long-stay geriatric hospital in Stockholm. I was responsible for a flexible (open) group of six to eight elderly clients, all of whom were about 80 years old. Except for one man, the clients were suffering from moderate-to-severe memory dysfunction. The clients were prescribed periods outside in the fresh air during the summer or changes of surroundings by visiting the winter garden for an hour, three times a week. The normal way of starting the intervention was that the aide placed the clients in their wheelchairs in a line. This precluded any conversation among the clients. I was frustrated by this, and sought some way of generating communication among them. I arranged the wheelchairs in a circle instead of a line. I started a game, a version of "Who's who?" in which the group has to guess what well-known figure one member is thinking of. In this version, Emma was to think of something particular. A knotted handkerchief was chucked to different group members. The ones who got the handkerchief had to guess what Emma was thinking of. After at least two rounds of this, the man without memory problems said: "Now you must tell us what you are thinking about, Emma", to which Emma replied: "I've forgotten."

At the next session the clients asked for the same game, suggesting that they felt meaning and implying that the group members' *activity* might have helped their recovery.

This case illustrates that the result of the game was unexpected and unimportant. The activity process was of main importance, the result less so. The clients' involvement in the game was clearly better than sitting in a line in their wheelchairs doing nothing. The game filled the participants' time for a while, and an OT has the professional knowledge of how to enable participation even among clients with severe memory impairments.

Characteristics of the Enabling Interventions

Interaction Between the Client and the Activity

The most prominent feature of the interventions where the OT enables clients' an activity is the *interaction between the client and the activity*. In addition, interactions between group members contribute to the recovery process (Pedretti and Early, 2001). The OT has a subordinated role during these sessions, in that *feedback from the activity and from other group members* can affect the clients' recovery. This is illustrated by the following case:

> Together with a colleague, I was a clinical lecturer for OT students doing practice at a Stockholm geriatric rehabilitation clinic. The OT's main work here was to investigate whether clients could be discharged to their homes. I was to demonstrate the assessment process to the students, and had a tape-recorder going during the sessions.
>
> Three clients, Elizabeth, Joanne, and Juliette, formed a group in the training kitchen. Following a stroke Elizabeth and Joanne had left-side paresis. Juliette's medical diagnosis was not established. The referring document stated that she might be in a deep depression or suffering from arteriosclerotic dementia. She had not said a word for several months.

The goal of the assessment session was to observe whether and how the three women communicated with each other and to investigate their motor and performances skills. The clients were asked to make coffee and bread and butter according to the Assessment of the Motor Process Skills (Fisher, 1993).

During the assessment session, Elizabeth and Joanne talked briefly in a few short sentences. When the coffee and bread and butter, were ready we all sat together at the table. The coffee was poured out. Then suddenly Juliette said: "Tastes good, this coffee."

Juliette's words were recorded evidence for the physician, who suddenly realized that Juliette had potential as a client in the 2-month rehabilitation program.

It seems that the process of making and drinking coffee triggered Juliette's recovery of speech! According to Ludwig (1993) such meaningful and planned tasks become therapeutic because the activity mediates between the client's inner and outer worlds. Moreover, such tasks help the client to achieve a sense of self.

The Form for the Interventions

The form for the interventions in which the OT enables activities is planned individual or group sessions. The main purposes are to facilitate clients' insight into their ability levels and their ability to express feelings (Stein and Roose, 2000). The OT's role is to organize and arrange the sessions (Schwartzberg, 1998), taking into consideration (1) the leadership style, (2) the structure of the group, (3) the number of group members, (4) the length and number of sessions, (5) selection of suitable tasks based on activity analysis and activity synthesis, (6) the tasks' degree of difficulty, (7) adaptation of the environment, and (8) clients' present functioning and ability that enables the client's to manage the chosen tasks (Kaplan, 1993; Stein and Roose, 2000).

The Therapeutic Media

Enabling recovery is the original form of the occupational therapy interventions often aimed at the elderly or at people with severe mental illness, who participate in day health services (see Chapter 44). These recovery interventions include steps to ensure the clients' activity that result in their being meaningfully occupied. Some of the therapeutic media used are as follows:

- *Arts and crafts*, which are used for providing the clients with a nonverbal form of communication, which gives them opportunities to express feelings and creative ideas (Macdonald, 1964; Stein and Roose, 2000).
- *Leisure activities* such as sports, sailing, rugby, or walking (Kratz and Soderback, 1998), as well as games, hobbies, and shopping.
- *Progressive relaxation therapy* (with or without a focus on music), which can be effective in lowering blood pressure, while qigong (eight sessions of 20 minutes) can benefit the psychological dimension of cardiac-disease sufferers (Hui et al., 2006).
- *Horticulture therapy*, which includes imagining nature, viewing nature, visiting a "healing garden," and gardening. Horticulture therapy may help recovery,

alleviate stress, increase well-being, promote participation in social life, and promote reemployment for people with mental or physical illness (Söderback et al., 2004). Martin et al. (2008) reported that spouses separated by illness (one partner lived at home, and the other partner in a nursing home) and who participated together in gardening activities experienced increased feelings of social participation and maintenance of their spouse role.

Gardening as a therapeutic medium is relevant for use among elderly people (see Chapter 46), dementia patients, those who are visually impaired, and those who have brain damage or depression.

- *Complementary therapy incorporating animals* is frequently used for children and adults with special needs such as autism and delayed psychosocial development. When animals are around, children use significantly more language and a greater social interaction occurs (Sams et al., 2006). Horseback-riding sessions for children at risk of poor school performance can positively affect their behavior (Kaiser et al., 2006). Mona Sams runs Mona's Ark in Troutville, Virginia, where she explores the value of using llamas, alpacas, ducks, rabbits, goats, and specially trained dogs as therapeutic facilitators. The animals become the client's friends, because they do not judge the client's challenges.

Sams states:

The purpose of incorporating animals [in the recovery intervention programs] is to reach clients who generally have not responded to traditional occupational therapeutic approaches.

Clients with cerebral palsy, developmental disabilities, including autism, Down syndrome, posttraumatic stress, visual impairments, and psychiatric disorders have all benefited from occupational therapy incorporating animals.

Individuals who are non-verbal often make the most significant improvement. Consistently they will begin non-verbal communication (sign language, picture exchange) and eventually speak to their animal friends. Working with persons who are non-verbal, often the speech pathologist will cotreat with the occupational therapist.

Llamas are especially therapeutic as they are curious, interactive, and pleasant to be visiting. The llamas will instinctively be responsive to people with special needs. They provide tremendous tactile input because of their wonderful fiber. Empowerment occurs when the clients get to a stage where they independently lead the llama. Compassion is consistently elicited by the llama, and this enables the therapy session to be effective and produce measurable positive change.

The clients attend the complementary therapy program on a weekly basis for a 45-minute session, and some attend two times weekly. Clients are evaluated and individual goals are established. Day programs for adults are seen on a small group basis.

The unique aspect of the approach is rather than the clients being transported to a farm, the farm comes to the clients.

Therapeutic activities:

Intervention goals incorporated in the sessions are training of:

- Fine motor skills: *grooming (with a metal comb), feeding, cutting carrots, attaching lead clamps on halters.*
- Bilateral coordination: *leading a llama through an obstacle course, cart driving with the llama.*

- Sensory stimulation/tolerances: *petting/stroking dogs and rabbits, brushing and grooming the llamas (using a circuit blower), throwing a tennis ball for the dog, riding the llama, carding and felting fiber from the animals.*
- Communication: *non-verbal communication with the animals using picture exchange or sign language (dogs can respond to signing), talking or reading to the animals, expressing feelings (clients with posttraumatic stress will often talk to the animals before they talk to staff).*
- Proprioceptive, vestibular functioning: *riding in the wagon with the Great Dane pulling and the child holds ropes from a harness, riding on the back of the llama, riding in llama cart, guiding llama through an 8-part obstacle course.*
- Psychological goals: *observing, responding, interpreting animal behaviors, adapting to natural consequences of behaviors toward animals. Developing nurturance and responsibility (feeding, caring, grooming another being, developing self-confidence, empowerment, when llama follows their lead, training for llama shows. Llama shows allow for cheering for peers, interacting with community at llama shows, receiving awards, and social interactions.*
- Functional task skills, *loading and unloading the animals and equipment at the settings, preparing for a llama show. Wet and dry felting animal fiber to make purposeful projects (e.g. wall hangings, pouches, cushions).*

(Sams, personal communication, 2008)

Some of the activities used for the recovery interventions are represented in this handbook:

- *Work- and task-related occupations* such as gardening (Söderback et al., 2004) (see chapter 46) and housework are frequently used.
- *Music therapy* is a multidimensional activity that addresses various human domains simultaneously" (see Chapter 47).
- In contrast to music therapy, *music in therapy* is used in hospitals for (1) movement relaxation therapy by creating a mood through the choice of music; (2) movement-balance therapy through client participation in rhythmic groups (Ferguson and Voll, 2004; Stein and Roose, 2000); and (3) singing as a part of aphasia therapy (Söderback, 1981) (see Chapter 48).
- *Recreational activities* such as visiting concerts, entertainments, film, stage plays, cafés and restaurants are employed in clinical practice. Such recreational activities were used in a stimulation program (see Chapter 45) among Alzheimer sufferers. Comparison with nonparticipants demonstrated a decrease in behavioral disturbances (Farina et al., 2006).

Occupation Brings Meaning to clients' Lives and a Feeling of Recovery

The activities used as therapeutic media for the enabling interventions aimed at the recovery of the activity process are presented in the case of Marie-Louise Huss (1978).

Marie-Louise's ability to do an activity is interpreted as giving meaning to her life, which to an outsider was a very troubled one. Here are Marie-Louise's own word (translated into English) about how she is able to continue living:

Looking back, I am mainly happy and surprised that I have managed so well in spite of everything. This is a tremendously useful view. When I run into difficulties nowadays, I take this view and it is strange how much smaller problems can seem (p. 153).

Marie-Louise was an enthusiastic person, 35-year-old person. She was living intensely in the here-and-now, interested in people, animals, literature, art, and experience. She was a drawing teacher with specialist studies in art and ethnology.

Marie-Louise's brain tumor made her unable to (1) swallow (she was fed through a tube into her stomach), (2) speak, (3) walk (she used a wheelchair), (4) use her right hand (due to paralysis), (5) breathe unaided (she was dependent on a cannula in her bronchus, a vacuum apparatus, plus the need assistants to help suck up phlegm, and (6) see the right side of her body.

Marie-Louise was first my colleague Gunilla Myrin's and then my professional responsibility during her 19-months visit to the Danderyd Hospital Rehabilitation Clinic, Stockholm. She visited the occupational therapy department nearly every weekday, some days twice, up to 4 hours per day until her death.

Marie-Louise spent much of this time typewriting. She got an ordinary typewriter 5 months after her tumor operation. It was hard for her to learn to write with her left hand and neglected visible sight. However, she was very glad to have the typewriter. It enabled her to communicate with her friends, to tell us about her will and desire to be occupied, which resulted in her book, Varit Väldigt Nära Döden (Been Very Close to Death), which was, published posthumously (Huss, 1978).

Her other main interests were painting and art therapy. She was in a special group educated by an art therapist. We planned an exhibition of Marie-Louise art, but it did not take place (Huss, 1978, p. 86, 163, 168, 172).

She completed much handicrafts work, such as sandpapering of prefabricated woodwork on a candle and a chopping-board, small mosaics, weaving on a narrow loom, cross-stitch embroidery on a cushion, enamel-work on plates, and textile printing of tablecloths. These activities enabled Marie-Louise to make gifts for her mother and friends, as well as articles for sale. Moreover, she participated in games and did jigsaw puzzles.

Our job as OTs was to enable Marie-Louise's activities by adjusting the tools, material, and performance of her various occupations. Thus, we adapted her wheelchair, and ergonomically and environmentally adapted her work space for the typewriter. For every session, we arranged the embroidery so that she could do it with one hand according to her actual level of adaptation, function, skills, and competence. Visits to exhibitions and museums were also arranged by us (Huss, 1978, p. 161).

The *outcome of the intervention* is expected to be the client's recovery. The term *recovery* is used here to emphasize the clients' healing process and increasing well-being. Christensen (1991) and Christensen and Baum (1997) observed that, even if not yet well understood, there are important relationships among occupation, health, and well-being. The underlying idea was that occupations influence health. Moreover, such recovery interventions reveal how clients, by activity, can experience joy and satisfaction, and can express a sense of their life's meaning (Clark and Larson, 1993).

The *effectiveness* of this type of interventions is sparsely documented in the literature. La Cour et al. (2005) showed that engagement of the terminally ill elderly in creative activities helped them to feel less isolated and more connected to life.

A year-long investigation of an occupational therapy program of 2 hours a day, 5 days a week for a group of patients with moderate-to-severe Alzheimer dementia showed that behavioral disorders improved appreciably (Baldelli et al., 2007).

Participants in psychoeducational groups valued the OT's careful enabling activities that had promoted optimal group structure, interaction among group members, adequate information, and a supportive milieu with limits on emotional disclosure (Cowls and Hale, 2005; see also Chapter 24).

References

Baldelli, M.V., Pradelli, J.M., Zucchi, P., Martini, B., Orsi, F., and Fabbo, A. (2007). Occupational therapy and dementia: the experience of an Alzheimer special care unit. Arch Gerontol Geriatr, 44(Suppl 1), 49–54.

Christensen, C. (1991). Occupational therapy. Intervention for life performance. In: Christensen, C., and Baum, C., eds. Occupational Therapy. Overcoming Human Performance Deficits (pp. 4–43, 49). Thorofare, NJ: Slack.

Christinsen, C., and Baum, C. (1997a). Occupational Therapy. Enabling Function and Well-Being. Thorofare, NJ: Slack.

Christensen, C., and Baum, C. (1997b). Understanding occupation. Definitions and concepts. In: Christensen, C., and Baum, C., eds. Occupational Therapy. Overcoming Human Performance Deficits (pp. 4). Thorofare, NJ: Slack.

Christensen, C., and Baum, C. (1997c). Glossary, In: Occupational Therapy. Overcoming Human Performance Deficits (pp. 591). Thorofare, NJ: Slack.

Clark, F., and Larson, E.A. (1993). Developing an academic discipline: the science of occupation. In: Hopkins, H.L., and Smith, H.D., eds. Willard and Spackman's Occupational Therapy (pp. 44–57). Philadelphia: Lippincott.

Cowls, J., and Hale, S. (2005). It's the activity that counts: What clients value in psycho-educational groups. Can J Occup Ther, 72(3), 176–182.

Farina, E., Mantovani, F., Fioravanti, R., et al. (2006). Efficacy of recreational and occupational activities associated to psychologic support in mild to moderate Alzheimer disease: a multi-center controlled study. Alzheimer Dis Assoc Disord, 20(4), 275–282.

Ferguson, S.L., and Voll, K.V. (2004). Burn pain and anxiety: the use of music relaxation during rehabilitation. J Burn Care Rehabil, 25(1), 8–14.

Fisher, A.G. (1993). The assessment of IADL motor skills: an application of many-faceted Rasch analysis. Am J Occup Ther, 47(4), 319–329.

Hammell, K.W. (2004). Dimensions of meaning in the occupations of daily life. Can J Occup Ther, 71(5), 296–305.

Hui, P.N., Wan, M., Chan, W.K., and Yung, P.M. (2006). An evaluation of two behavioral rehabilitation programs, qigong versus progressive relaxation, in improving the quality of life in cardiac patients. J Altern Complement Med, 12(4), 373–378.

Huss, M.-L. (1978). Varit Väldigt Nära Döden (Have Been Very Close to the Death) (in Swedish). Lund: Gustav and Ester Andersson.

Kaiser, L., Smith, K.A., Heleski, C,R., and Spence, L.J. (2006). Effects of a therapeutic riding program on at-risk and special education children. J Am Vet Med Assoc, 228(1), 46–52.

Kaplan, K.L. (1993). The directive group: short-term treatment for psychiatric patients with a minimal level of functioning. In: Fleming Cottrell, R.P., ed. Psychosocial Occupational Therapy. Proactive Approaches (pp. 99–107). US: The American Occupational Therapy Association.

Kratz, G., and Söderback, I. (1998). Wheelchair user's experience of nonadapted and adapted clothes during sailing, Quad rugby, or wheel walking. Paper presented at the American Congress of Rehabilitation Medicine, Seattle.

La Cour, K., Josephsson, S., and Luborsky, M. (2005). Creating connections to life during life-threatening illness: Creative activity experienced by elderly people and OTs. Scand J Occup Ther, 12(3), 98–100.

Ludwig, F.M. (1993). Gail Fidler. In Miller, R.J., and Waker, K.F., eds. Perspectives on Theory for the Practice of Occupational Therapy (pp. 17–40). Gaithersburg, MD: Aspen.

Macdonald, E.M. (1964). Occupational Therapy in Rehabilitation. A Handbook for Occupational Therapists, Students and Others Interested in This Aspect of Reablement. London: Baoööoère, Tindall and Cox.

Martin, L., Miranda, B., and Bean, M. (2008). An exploration of spousal separation and adaptation to long-term disability: Six elderly couples engaged in a horticultural programme. Occup Ther Int, 15(1), 45–55.

Matuska, K., Giles-Heinz, A., Flinn, N., Neighbor, M., and Bass-Haugen, J. (2003). Outcomes of a pilot occupational therapy wellness program for older adults. Am J Occup Ther, 57(2), 220–224.

Mosey, A.C. (1986). Psychosocial components of occupational therapy. In: Mosey, A.C., ed. Psychosocial Components of Occupational Therapy (pp. 16–18, 450–476). New York: Raven Press.

Pedretti, L.W., and Early, M.B. (2001). Occupational performance and models of practice for physical dysfunction. In: Pedretti, L.W., and Early, M.B. eds. Occupational Therapy. Practice Skills for Physical Dysfunction. London: Mosby.

Sams, M.J., Fortney, E.V., and Willenbring, S. (2006). Occupational therapy incorporating animals for children with autism: a pilot investigation. Am J Occup Ther, 60(3), 268–274.

Schwartzberg, S.L. (1998). Group process. In: Niestadt, M.E., and Crepeau, E.B., eds. Willard and Spackman's Occupational Therapy, 9th ed. (pp. 120–131). Philadelphia: Lippincott.

Söderback, I. (Editor, artist). (1981). Intellektuell Funktionsträning (IFT) –Träningsmaterial omkring 1000 sidor med papper och penna material. (Intellectual Functional Training (IFT). A training tool of about 1000 pages of paper and pen materiel) [Papper och penna material, indelat i sektioner; Perception, Spatial, Numerisk, Verbal förståelse, Verbalt flöde, Minne, Logik intellektuell förmåga. Cirka 1000 sidor. Paper and pen material, Sectorial divided into Perception, Spatial, Numerical, Verbal understanding, Verbal fluencies, Memory, Logical Intellectual functions. About 1,000 pages].

Söderback, I., Söderström, M., and Schälander, E. (2004). Horticulture therapy: The 'healing garden' and gardening in rehabilitation measures at Danderyd Hospital Rehabilitation Clinic, Sweden. Pediatr Rehabil, 7(4), 245–260.

Stein, F., and Roose, B. (2000). Pocket Guide to Treatment in Occupational Therapy. San Diego: Singular.

Chapter 44
Creating Opportunities for Participation Within and Beyond Mental Health Day Services

Wendy Bryant

Thinking about occupational alienation helped to make sense of people's experiences in mental health day services.

Abstract Mental health day services have been developed to bridge the gap between hospital services and community life. For people with long-term mental health problems, the occupational and social opportunities available within the day services can be used to support recovery and prevent relapse. When developed in collaboration with clients, these opportunities can overcome the experience of occupational alienation, characterized by meaninglessness, withdrawal, and boredom. Occupational alienation as a concept challenges occupational therapists (OTs) to design and adapt occupations that reflect personal and shared meanings, create a sense of ownership and belonging, and offer meaningful choices to clients.

Keywords Community mental health services • Participation

Background and Definition

This chapter explores how mental health day services can promote the recovery of people with long-term mental health problems, informed by the concept of occupational alienation.

Mental health day services have been established to (1) provide occupational and social opportunities for people, (2) offer a structure to the day, and (3) support networking with other people with mental health problems (Bryant et al., 2004, 2005).

Activities in day centers and hospitals have often reflected a tension between facilitation and support, as an overemphasis on safety and seclusion undermines efforts to promote recovery and provide meaningful occupational choices (Bates et al., 2006). Emphasis on recovery gives priority to the meanings that individual clients give to their experiences (Repper and Perkins, 2003). When occupations are perceived to be meaningless, it can be understood as occupational alienation, a risk factor contributing to occupational injustice (Townsend and Wilcock, 2004).

I. Söderback (ed.), *International Handbook of Occupational Therapy Interventions*,
DOI: 10.1007/978-0-387-75424-6_44, © Springer Science+Business Media, LLC 2010

Occupational therapy in the context of day services is concerned with restoring and maintaining skills and abilities that have been impaired or disrupted by the consequences of long-term mental health problems. This involves the creation of opportunities to engage in occupations that have been identified for their meaningfulness and relevance to everyday life.

Purpose

Mental health day services aim to promote, support, and facilitate the recovery of people with long-term mental health problems. Here, the concept of occupational alienation can be used to understand individual and collective experiences of meaningless occupations, withdrawal, and boredom (Bryant, 2008; Bryant et al., 2004, 2005).

Method

Candidates for the Intervention

Day services have been established to (1) provide occupational and social opportunities for people, (2) offer a structure to the day, and (3) support networking with other people with mental health problems, such as schizophrenia, mood disorders, and anxiety disorders (Bryant et al., 2004, 2005).

It is recognized that people with mental health problems experience social exclusion to a greater extent than other marginalized groups (Repper and Perkins, 2003). At times, this might be in the interests of public safety, when people are detained to prevent harm to themselves or others. However, the stigma of using mental health services extends beyond acute crises (Thornicroft, 2006). Promoting social inclusion has therefore involved challenging discrimination and prejudice, and developing services that make it easier to participate in community life (National Social Inclusion Programme, 2008). To achieve this, people who have survived mental health problems have suggested that research and service development involve them and draw on their direct experience of services (Beresford, 2005).

Epidemiology

Mental health problems are estimated to affect 12% of the world's population, with a disproportionate number of people experiencing additional problems, such as poverty. Despite the widespread experience of mental ill-health, within the developed and developing world significantly fewer health and social care resources are designated for people with mental health problems (World Health Organization, 2001a).

Settings

In the United Kingdom, social perspectives have become influential in how mental health services are designed and commissioned (Tew, 2005). The social model of disability identifies many factors that create disabilities beyond primary impairments, limiting activities and restricting participation (World Health Organization, 2001b). In the context of mental health problems, this means experiencing segregation and exclusion from community life because of powerful assumptions about a client's capacity, resulting in prejudice and discrimination (Sayce, 2000). Day services have been established to offer access to opportunities to be included in community life.

The Role of the Occupational Therapist

Historically, OTs have been key team members of day services, promoting an occupational and social focus alongside medical and psychological approaches (Farndale, 1961). In this setting, occupational therapy has evolved to facilitate recovery and reintegration into the community, supporting people in a safe and tolerant environment.

Knowledge of community life, which the client seeks to become part of, is an important aspect of occupational therapy. This knowledge can facilitate social integration and inclusion through the design, creation, and evaluation of occupations. This process should take place in collaboration with clients on an individual and collective basis, to overcome occupational alienation. Collaboration should be based on continuous and active engagement in meaningful occupation, dialogue, and power sharing.

Ongoing challenges posed by prejudice, ignorance, and fear about severe mental illness can severely limit occupational choices for clients. To achieve acceptance in the community, it is often necessary for clients to conceal their mental health problems (Thornicroft, 2006). However, occupational therapists can model nondiscriminatory practice by creating and developing opportunities for participation in mainstream community settings. Meaningful occupation can be the basis for creating safe and supportive relationships, and giving clients a sense of choice and control over their own recovery process. This sense of ownership and belonging is also facilitated by establishing repeated occupations, or habits or routines, in a social context such as the day services.

Results

Clinical Application

Engagement in Occupations

Combining an occupational and social perspective could be applied in different types of day services. Drop-in services, emphasizing social contact and support, offer people flexibility and choice in terms of whom they have social contact with, when they attend, and what they do. Alternatively, a person may be expected to turn up at a particular time in a particular place for a specific activity, for example an education class. From a distance, it could be assumed that clients would be more occupationally alienated and socially excluded if they were sitting alone in a drop-in session, doing nothing and not speaking with anyone (Fig. 44.1).

Conversely, an individual attending a class to improve basic literacy and numeracy skills might be assumed to be engaged in a meaningful occupation and to be socially integrated. In some instances, this might not be true, and so these assumptions have to be questioned. Occupational therapists have to recognize the interpretations they impose on clients' experiences. Collaborative work will expose the validity of these interpretations.

Content of the Occupational Therapy

Increased awareness of occupational alienation will offer a way of understanding why people appear to be bored, disengaged, or uninterested, and how to respond by

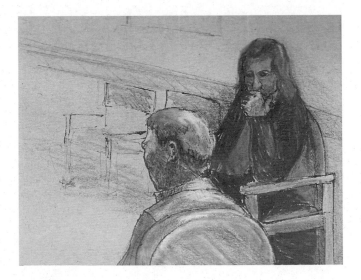

Fig. 44.1 Sitting alone.

adapting or creating occupational opportunities for individuals, groups, and communities. Occupational alienation describes the combined experiences of meaninglessness, withdrawal, and boredom. In response, the occupational therapist could consider meaningfulness, belonging, and occupational choice:

- *Meaningfulness* is a personal perspective, and often changing (Hasselkus, 2002). Thus there is potential for people to be occupationally and socially alienated in every session or setting. Recognizing this through an increased awareness of occupational alienation can enhance the work undertaken by clients and OTs to promote engagement and recovery.
- A person might find that what they are doing is meaningless because of their own mental state. In this situation, it is important to *design occupational opportunities* in collaboration with clients, to identify what could be meaningful and what could transform their internal sense of alienation. Safety, in terms of the physical, social, and emotional environment, is vitally important to support this process.
- *Belonging:* Clients might be withdrawn and occupationally alienated because the opportunities offered within day services are not meaningful to them. They cannot develop a sense of belonging to the sessions, or a sense of ownership over the process and products of their activities within the services. By focusing on what people do, it is possible to foster a sense of belonging through occupation, supporting relationships and any attitudinal changes in shared experiences (Fig. 44.2). There is a risk that these experiences may not always be positive, which is why the social aspect is important. The sense of belonging can be achieved through people accepting who you are, and equally, recognizing and accepting what you do. These issues of acceptance and recognition are important for the final issue of occupational alienation.

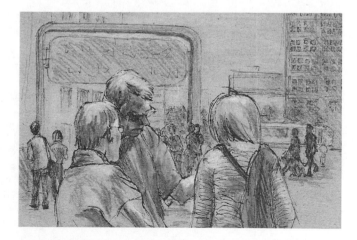

Fig. 44.2 Shared experiences.

- *Making occupational choices:* Being able to make realistic, informed choices requires a client-centered approach (Sumsion, 2007). A *dialogue*, based on the *occupations performed* as much as on conversations, should take place to facilitate this process. Locating this dialogue in a social context, for example a group, will help clients perceive what can be achieved through occupation not only through their own participation, but also through observing that of others.

Evidence-Based Practice

Living in a Glasshouse

The recent emphasis on social inclusion has generated a review of day services in the United Kingdom. Traditionally therapeutic and supportive functions have been combined within the services, alongside monitoring progress (Catty et al., 2005a).

Attendance has been encouraged on a session basis, following in-patient treatment, or to prevent admission. The social environment of day services has been valued by clients, but the extent to which social aspects are given priority over therapeutic functions depends on the organizational priorities (Catty et al., 2005a). Social contact and support is emphasized more in day services provided by social care and non-governmental organizations, in contrast to the time-limited treatment offered in health care settings. However, repeated evaluation has not distinguished significant differences for long-term clients (Carter, 1981; Catty et al., 2005b; Jones, 1972).

The OTs need to give equal consideration to the social and occupational aspects of recovery, regardless of organizational priorities. This is supported by the research of Townsend et al. (2000), Rebeiro et al. (2001), and Bryant et al. (2004), and the principles of occupational justice and injustice, in particular the occupational risk factor of occupational alienation (Bryant, 2008; Wilcock, 2006).

The research that informed this approach involved 39 mental health day clients in four focus groups (Bryant et al., 2004). They were asked to share and discuss their experiences in the day services, so that the services could be developed and improved. The research was conducted by an independent team of three OTs. Clients highlighted their experiences of feeling separate and unconnected, of being prevented from supporting each other, and of being rejected by the wider community because of their mental health problems. The metaphor of the glasshouse for day services suggested the potential for fostering vulnerability and dependency, while offering shelter from the wider world (Fig. 44.3). Within the glasshouse, what people did was restricted and highly visible from the outside. Thus there were tensions between shelter and segregation, safety and dependency, and visibility and invisibility. These tensions resulted in organizational efforts to control occupational opportunities and the social environment. It was suggested that the concept of occupational alienation offered a way of understanding and working with these tensions, and allowing clients more control and choice.

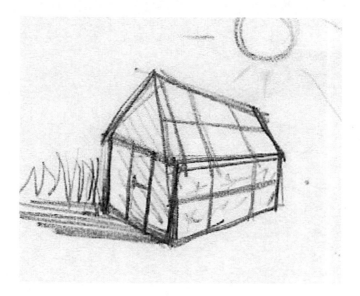

Fig. 44.3 Living in a glass house.

Discussion

Clients have emphasized the importance of having meaningful occupational opportunities in a safe and social environment, to which they felt they belonged. The importance of belonging in terms of mental health and well-being has been supported in the work of OTs (Rebeiro et al., 2001; Wilcock, 2006). The social dimension, beyond medical and psychological approaches, has been emphasized in strategies to overcome social exclusion (National Social Inclusion Programme, 2008). However, there has been an emphasis on integration into mainstream social resources, possibly at the expense of social networks for support between clients. Considering occupational alienation incorporates the social dimension, but also emphasizes the importance of what people do and the right to participate in meaningful occupation, not only to safeguard health and well-being but also to achieve social integration. It also raises questions about how the meaningfulness of occupations is judged and by whom, and the necessity for ongoing critical dialogue.

In the research informing this chapter, clients had positive experiences of day services, and it is suggested that increased awareness of occupational alienation would, in many instances, confirm and illuminate good practice as well as inform service development. In particular it would enable occupational and social aspects to be considered as equal to, if not more important than, medical and psychological aspects. This has been identified as being important beyond occupational therapy, for example by Sayce (2000). Working from the experiences of clients and staff, future research could develop understanding of how occupational therapy and theory can inform and facilitate the recovery process in community mental health settings such as day services. In particular, it would be useful to explore the tension between seeking social integration and sustaining a safe place for clients to recover. It is important to develop a greater understanding of how people judge what is a *meaningful* occupation and what is a *meaningless* occupation, and who makes that judgment and with what implications. The experiences of clients suggests that occupational alienation may be intrinsic to the experience of mental health problems at certain stages, especially in the context of risk management and the restriction of occupational choices for safety reasons. Reflecting on and exploring these, issues in depth will enhance practice and thus the client experience.

References

Bates, P., Gee, H., Klingel, U., and Lippmann, W. (2006). Moving to inclusion. National Social Inclusion Programme. http://www.socialinclusion.org.uk/publications/Movingtoinclusion.pdf.

Beresford, P. (2005). Social approaches to madness and distress: user perspectives and user knowledges. In: Tew, J., ed. Social Perspectives in Mental Health (pp. 13–31). London: Jessica Kingsley.

Bryant, W. (2008). Occupational, social and intrapersonal alienation explored in the community. In: McKay, E.A., Craik, C., Lim, K.H., and Richards, G., eds. Advancing Occupational Therapy in Mental Health Practice (pp. 89–102). Oxford: Blackwell.

Bryant, W., Craik, C., and McKay, E.A. (2004). Living in a glass house: exploring occupational alienation. Can J Occup Ther, 5(71), 282–289.

Bryant, W., Craik, C., and McKay, E.A. (2005). Perspectives of day and accommodation services for people with enduring mental illness. J Mental Health, 14(2), 109–120.

Carter, J. (1981). Day Services for Adults. National Day Care Survey. London: George Allen and Unwin.

Catty, J., Goddard, K., and Burns, T. (2005a). Social services and health services day care in mental health: the social networks and care needs of their users. Int J Social Psychiatry, 51(1), 23–34.

Catty, J., Goddard, K., and Burns, T. (2005b). Social services and health services day care in mental health: do they differ? Int J Social Psychiatry, 51(2), 151–161.

Farndale, J. (1961). The Day Hospital Movement in Great Britain. Oxford: Pergamon.

Hasselkus, B. (2002). The Meaning of Everyday Occupation. Thorofare, NJ: Slack.

Jones, K. (1972). A History of the Mental Health Services. London: Routledge and Kegan Paul.

National Social Inclusion Programme. (2008). From Segregation to Inclusion: Where Are We Now? A Review of Progress Towards the Implementation of the Mental Health Day Services Commissioning Guidance. London: Department of Health.

Rebeiro, K., Day, D., Semeniuk, B., O'Brien, C., and Wilson, B. (2001). Northern initiative for social action: an occupation-based mental health program. Am J Occup Ther, 55(5), 493–500.

Repper, J., and Perkins, R. (2003). Social Inclusion and Recovery. Edinburgh: Balliere Tindall.

Sayce, L. (2000). From Psychiatric Patient to Citizen. Overcoming Discrimination and Social Exclusion. Basingstoke: Macmillan.

Sumsion, T. (2007). Client-Centred Practice in Occupational Therapy, 2nd ed. Edinburgh: Churchill Livingstone Elsevier.

Tew, J., ed. (2005). Social Perspectives in Mental Health. London: Jessica Kingsley.

Thornicroft, G. (2006). Shunned: Discrimination Against People with Mental Illness. Oxford: Oxford University Press.

Townsend, E., Birch, D., Langley, J., and Langille, L. (2000). Participatory research in a mental health clubhouse. Occup Ther J Res, 20(1), 18–43.

Townsend, E., and Wilcock, A. (2004). Occupational justice. In: Christiansen, C., and Townsend, E., eds. Introduction to Occupation. The Art and Science of Living (pp. 243–273). Englewood Cliffs, NJ: Prentice Hall.

Wilcock, A. (2006). An Occupational Perspective of Health, 2nd ed. Thorofare, NJ: Slack.

World Health Organization. (2001a). Mental Health: New Understanding, New Hope. Geneva: WHO.

World Health Organization. (2001b). The International Classification of Function. Geneva: WHO.

Chapter 45
Conducting an Intervention Program Mediated by Recreational Activities and Socialization in Groups for Clients with Alzheimer's Disease

Elisabetta Farina and Fabiana Villanelli

Our research group has demonstrated behavioral, cognitive, and functional gains in outpatients with Alzheimer's disease who participated in interventions mediated by recreational and occupational activities.

Abstract Interventions with recreational activities (games and art therapies) are frequently offered to people with dementia in nursing homes or day-care centers. Our group has demonstrated behavioral and, to a lesser extent, cognitive and functional gains in patients treated with recreational-occupational activities when compared to patients undergoing other kinds of cognitive treatment or to controls receiving only routine care. Patients recruited from the Alzheimer Assessment Unit of our center were divided into groups of four clients. The training involved fifteen 3-hour sessions.

Treatment comprised an orientation task, recreational activities (conversation, music listening, party games, collage, and games with balls, clubs, cones, and hopping) and occupational activities of daily living (setting and clearing the table, preparing tea or coffee, washing hands and dishes). Caregivers received educational and psychological support.

While our studies clearly have some limitations (above all the lack of randomization), we have found that the literature, coupled with our findings, supports the notion that a group activity program, based mainly on recreational and occupational activities, can achieve improvement in Alzheimer's disease patients, above all behaviorally.

Keywords Alzheimer's disease • Recreational therapy

Background and Definitions

Interventions mediated by recreational activities, such as games and art therapies involving music, dance, and art, are frequently offered to people with dementia and are useful to ameliorate mood and avoid social isolation in nursing homes or day-care centers.

I. Söderback (ed.), *International Handbook of Occupational Therapy Interventions*,   423
DOI: 10.1007/978-0-387-75424-6_45, © Springer Science+Business Media, LLC 2010

The primary purposes of using recreational activities, according to the guidelines of American Therapeutic Recreation Association (ATRA) (2008), are to restore, remediate, or rehabilitate function in order to improve functioning and independence, and reduce or eliminate the effects of illness or disability.

Activity is a basic human need expressed in leisure and work pursuits. Unfortunately, dementia leads to boredom and isolation due to a low rate of activity participation, resulting in agitated or passive behaviors, and functional loss.

Recreational services enable recreational resources aimed at improving clients' health and well-being (Fitzsimmons, 2003). Despite their wide use, few controlled studies demonstrate the efficacy of interventions mediated by recreational activities that decrease behavioral problems, improve mood, and increase socialization (Gerber et al., 1991; Karlsson et al., 1988; Rovner et al., 1996).

Teri et al. (1992) and Teri (1994), have developed a protocol that is based on behavior psychotherapy and includes interventions aimed at increasing clients' participation in pleasant activities. This protocol improves clients' and caregivers' mood.

Purpose

The aims of interventions mediated by recreational, personal, and interpersonal activities of daily living (ADL), in which outpatients with Alzheimer's disease participate, are (1) to support the maintenance of ADL, (2) to improve the clients' well-being, (3) to reduce behavioral disturbances, and (4) to favor socialization.

Methods

Candidates for the Intervention

Clients can participate in the intervention program mediated by recreational activities and socialization in a group when the *inclusion criteria* are (1) a diagnosis of Alzheimer's disease [according to the National Institute of Neurological and Communicative Disorders and Stroke and the Alzheimer Disease and Related Disorders Association (now known as the Alzheimer's Association (NINCDS-ADRDA)] (McKhann et al., 1984), (2) with or without associated cerebrovascular lesions, and (3) mild or moderate cognitive impairment between 0.5 and 2 on the clinical dementia rating (CDR) assessment (Hughes and Berg, 1982).

Clients are ineligible for participation when the *exclusion criteria* are (1) memory dysfunction (Mini-Mental State Examination [MMSE] score less than 15) (Folstein et al., 1975), (2) severe aphasia (token test score less than 20) (Spinnler and Tognoni, 1987), (3) severe auditory or visual loss, or (4) overt behavioral disturbances (delusions, hallucinations, agitation).

Epidemiology

Alzheimer's disease usually affects elderly people of both sexes; however, female gender represents a risk factor for the disease.

Settings

Our typical referral method entails recruiting clients from the Alzheimer Assessment Unit of S. Maria Nascente, Clinical Research Center, Don Gnocchi Foundation, Italy. They are then treated and periodically tested in the center's day hospital.

The Role of the Occupational Therapist in Applying the Intervention

Ideally, the interventions using recreational activities and socialization in a group should preferably be administered by an occupational therapist (OT) who is a member of a multidisciplinary team (Teri et al., 2003). The prerequisites for OTs to conduct a successful intervention program are (1) close interaction between clients and OTs (Wood et al., 2005), (2) an attractive environment, and (3) the presence of enough staff.

Results

Clinical Application

Program Organization

All clients have a support interview with a psychologist at the beginning and at the end of the program. Caregivers have the same type of interview at the beginning, in the middle, and at the end of the program. The clients follow a standardized short educational program with a rehabilitation therapist. This procedure ensures psychological support both to the client and caregiver to face the disease and to give the caregiver useful ways of interacting with the client positively. General principles and strategies to cope with memory and behavioral disturbances, to support the clients with their ADL, and to make the home environment safer are included.

Mediated Activities

The intervention program is mediated using the following:

1. *Recreational activities*, such as conversation, music listening, party games (bingo, dominoes, Scrabble, Snakes and Ladders, stick games), collage, poster creation, and games with balls, clubs, cones, and hopping.
2. *Activities of daily living*, such as setting and clearing the table, preparing tea or coffee, washing hands and dishes (Farina et al., 2006a).

Use of these activities should be individualized to (1) match the clients' functional skills (level of dementia) and interests, and (2) provide appropriate stimulation and enrichment, thus mobilizing the available cognitive resources and support fulfillment of the performance of the chosen activity without clients experiencing frustration.

Administration of the Intervention Program

Clients participate in groups of four in the intervention program mediated by *recreational activities and socialization in a group*. The group constellations are organized according to the client's sex (either same sex or two males and two females) and the severity of dementia.

The program involves fifteen 3-hour sessions. The sessions are preceded by a meal together, enabling all participants to socialize and create a lively atmosphere. Sessions are carried out according to the following schedule:

Weeks 1–4: Three days per week, one session per day
Week 5: Two days per week, one session per day.
Week 6: One day per week, one session.

Each session includes the following:

- An *orientation* task conducted for about 10 minutes. Spatial and temporal orientation is trained, and each member is encouraged to introduce him- or herself to other participants. The orientation training follows the principles described in the literature (Olazara et al., 2004; Spector et al., 2003). Two reality-orientation boards, one for time and one for place, assist the participants.
- *Reinforcement of spatiotemporal parameters* is applied for the whole session using the boards.
- Later, *recreational-occupational activities* are performed for about 50 minutes.
- *Occupational activities* follow for about 1 hour. These activities include step identification, verbal prompting, and modeling, used to assist participants in recreational activities and ADL.
- Finally, members of the group are involved in other *recreational activities* for about an hour.

Environment

Sessions are performed in a large room with a kitchen area, including cooking equipment and eating utensils, tables and chairs, and all the material necessary for the recreational and occupational activities.

How the Intervention Eases Impairments, Activity Limitations, and Participation Restrictions

The recreational activities and socialization intervention allow restoration of interpersonal interaction, ease social isolation, and decrease behavioral disturbances. Participation in pleasant activities improves the client's well-being, and occupational activities favor the maintenance of residual independence in everyday life.

Evidence-Based Practice

Cognitive and functional gains (Zanetti et al., 1997) and improvement in behavior have been found in clients with dementia who have participated in the recreational and occupational activities (Farina et al., 2002) associated with psychotherapy for clients and caregivers (Farina et al., 2006a). The clients belonging to the recreational group showed a significant improvement in behavior. When comparing baseline with posttraining condition, clients displayed a substantial reduction in disruptive behavior, and a tendency to a general reduction in behavioral symptoms compared to controls. This reduction was mirrored by a significant reduction in caregiver reaction to behavioral disturbances (Farina et al., 2006b).

Discussion

Clients with Alzheimer's disease who participate in a group activity program, mainly based on recreational and occupational activities improved their *functional behavior* (Farina et al., 2006; Martichuski et al., 1996; Rovner et al., 1996) and, briefly (less than 6 months), their *cognitive function* (Farina et al., 2006a).

However, long-term reinforcement programs have lasting effects (Metitieri et al., 2001; Orrell et al., 2005; Spector et al., 2000; Zanetti et al., 1995). The necessity for long-term interventions to maintain positive effects raises the problem of costs. However, the program is based on group sessions, allowing savings in personnel resources compared to individual techniques. Moreover, relatives and caregivers assisting clients at home can be trained to conduct this type of intervention to reinforce and prolong the benefits.

References

American Therapeutic Recreation Association (ATRA) (2008). Definition statement. http://atra-online.com/cms/

Farina, E., Fioravanti, R., Chiavari, L., et al. (2002). Comparing two programs of cognitive training in Alzheimer's disease: a pilot study. Acta Neurol Scand, 105(5), 365–371.

Farina, E., Mantovani, F., Fioravanti, R., et al. (2006a). Evaluating two group programmes of cognitive training in mild to moderate Alzheimer's disease: is there any difference between a "global" stimulation and a "cognitive-specific" one? Aging Ment Health, 10(3), 1–8.

Farina, E., Mantovani, F., Fioravanti, R., et al. (2006b). Efficacy of recreational and occupational activities associated to psychologic support in mild to moderate Alzheimer disease: a multicenter controlled study. Alzheimer Dis Assoc Disord, 20(4), 275–282.

Fitzsimmons, S. (2003). Dementia Practice Guidelines for Recreation Therapy. Alexandria, VA: American Therapeutic Recreation Association (ATRA), 2003.

Folstein, M.F., Folstein, F.E., and Mchugh, P.R. (1975). Mini mental state: a practical method for grading the cognitive state of clients for clinician. J Psychiatr Res, 12, 189–198.

Gerber, G.J., Prince, P.N., Snider, H.G., Atchinson, K., Dubois, L., and Kilgour, J.A. (1991). Group activity and cognitive improvement among clients with Alzheimer's disease. Hosp Community Psychiatry, 42, 843–845.

Hughes, C.P., and Berg, L. (1982). A new clinical scale fort the staging of dementia. Br J Psychiatry, 140, 566–572.

Karlsson, I., Brane, G., Melin, E., Nyth, A.I., and Rybo, E. (1988). Effects of environmental stimulation on biochemical and psychological variables in dementia. Acta Psychiatr Scand, 77, 207–213.

Martichuski, D.K., Bell, P.A., and Badshaw, B. (1996). Including small group activities in large special care units. J Appl Gerontol, 15, 224–237.

McKhann, G., Drachman, D., Folstein, M., Katzman, R., Price, D., and Stadlan, E. (1984). Clinical diagnosis of Alzheimer's disease: report of National Institute of Neurological and Communicative Disorders and Stroke and the Alzheimer Disease and Related Disorders Association (now known as the Alzheimer's Association, (NINCDS-ADRDA) Work group under the auspices of Department of Health and Human Services Task Force on Alzheimer's disease. Neurology, 34, 934–944.

Metitieri, T., Zanetti, O., Geroldi, C., et al. (2001). Reality orientation therapy to delay outcomes of progression in clients with dementia. A retrospective study. Clin Rehabil, 15(5), 471–478.

Olazaràn, J., Muñiz, R., Reisberg, B., et al. (2004). Benefits of cognitive-motor intervention in MCI and mild to moderate Alzheimer disease. Neurology, 63(12), 2348–2353.

Orrell, M., Spector, A., Thorgrimsen, L., and Woods, B. (2005). A pilot study examining the effectiveness of maintenance cognitive stimulation therapy (MCST) for people with dementia. Int J Geriatr Psychiatry, 20(5), 446–451.

Rovner, B.W., Steel, C.D., Shmuely, Y., and Folstein, M.F. (1996). A randomized trial of dementia care in nursing homes. J Am Geriatr Soc, 44, 7–13.

Spector, A., Orrel, M., Davies, S., and Woods, B. (2000). Reality orientation for dementia. Cochrane Database Syst Rev, 4, CD001119. Review update in Cochrane Database Syst Rev, 3, CD001119.

Spector, A., Thorgrimsen, L., Woods, B., et al. (2003). Efficacy of an evidence-based cognitive stimulation therapy programme for people with dementia: randomised controlled trial. Br J Psychiatry, 183, 248–254.

Spinnler, H., and Tognoni, G. (1987). Standardizzazione e taratura italiana di test neurospicologici Ital. J Neurol Sci, 6(suppl), 35–38.

Teri, L. (1994). Behavioral intervention of depression in clients with dementia. Alzheimer Dis Assoc Disord, 8(suppl 3), 66–74.

Teri, L., Truax, P., Logsdon, R., Uamoto, J., Zarit, S., and Vitaliano, P.P. (1992). Assessment of behavioral problems in dementia: the Revised Memory and Behavior Problem Checklist. Psychol Aging, 7, 627–631.

Teri, L., Gibbons, L.E., McCurry, S.M., Logsdon, R.G., Buchner, D.M., Barlow, W.E., Kokull, V.A., LaCroix, A.S., McCormick, W., and Larson, E.B. (2003). Exercise plus behavioral management in patients with Alzheimer disease: A randomized Controlled trail. 15(290), 2015–2022.

Wood, W., Harris, S., Snider, M., et al. (2005). Activity situations on an Alzheimer's disease special care unit and resident environmental interactions, time use, and affect. Am J Alzheimers Dis Other Demen, 20, 105–116.

Zanetti, O., Binetti, G., Magni, E., Rozzini, L., Bianchetti, A., and Trabucchi, M. (1997). Procedural memory stimulation in Alzheimer's disease: impact of a training programme. Acta Neurol Scand, 95, 152–157.

Zanetti, O., Frisoni, G.B., De Leo, D., Dello Buono, M., Bianchetti, A., and Trabucchi, M. (1995). Reality orientation therapy in Alzheimer disease: useful or not? A controlled study. Alzheimer Dis Assoc Disord, 9(3), 132–138.

Chapter 46
Horticultural Therapy for the Cognitive Functioning of Elderly People with Dementia

Midori Yasukawa

Horticultural therapy using a periodic and effective method may improve cognitive and psychosocial functioning of elderly people with dementia.

Abstract Horticultural therapy is an intervention using a set of recreational activities that include the beneficial effect of plants and nature for the prevention or treatment of illness. The intervention is not limited either by the client's age or illness. The aim is to improve the patients' quality of life (QOL) (Fukushima et al. 2005). This cost-effective therapy has advantages at the community level compared with other therapies.

This chapter discusses the benefits of using horticultural therapy with a focus on cognitive function among elderly people with dementia.

Keywords Cognitive function • Dementia • Horticultural therapy • MMSE (Mini–Mental State Examination) • Quality of life (QOL)

Background

In developed countries there is a rapidly increasing occurrence of dementia in the elderly. Dementia is normally treated with drugs that offer temporal symptomatic control of cognitive decline and have demonstrated efficacy for patients with mild to moderate dementia, although some drugs have some deteriorating effects. The nonpharmacologic interventions are alternative therapies that include bright light therapy, exercise and behavior management techniques, validation therapy (i.e., improvement of communication), psychotherapeutic intervention, art therapy, music therapy, occupational therapy, and horticultural therapy.

Among these therapies, horticultural therapy is aimed at improving the patients' cognitive function and thus their quality of live. It encourages patients to use their five senses in activities such as basking in the sun, feeling the wind blow, and hearing the song of birds and the sound of water flowing. This therapy is low-cost.

I. Söderback (ed.), *International Handbook of Occupational Therapy Interventions*,
DOI: 10.1007/978-0-387-75424-6_46, © Springer Science+Business Media, LLC 2010

Horticultural therapy has been applied in many countries, such as Australia, Germany, Korea, New Zealand, the United States; and Sweden (Söderback et al., 2004). The patients have physical and mental impairments due to illness or injury. Some hospitals and health care centers have applied horticultural therapy for bedridden patients and those with a history of depression and lack of self-esteem (Lee et al., 2008a). It has also been used for the rehabilitation of prisoners (Lee et al., 2008b).

In Japan, the keeping of house plants and private gardens is a popular recreational activity, and the traditional arts of *bonsai* (potted plants) and Buddhist rock gardens attest to a long history of the application of gardening for maintaining the balance between physical and mental health. Currently, approximately 40% of the population of Japan is engaged in recreational (for no financial gain) horticultural activities (Matsuo, E. 2002).

Horticultural therapy in Japan was developed in 1980 because of a growing elderly population and an insufficient system of care for patients with dementia. These factors caused the patients' reduced self-control and social abilities that could be the reason of many cases of depression. This issue encouraged the development of new therapies that followed a more holistic approach, addressing both physical and mental aspects of dementia. Among these therapies horticultural therapy seems to be very suitable for Japanese patients who feel inclined to horticulture, as many do. This therapy (1) is tailored to the patients' needs and ability; (2) has clear goals for the patient; (3) emphasizes gardening activities; (4) is conducted by health care professionals, such as horticultural therapists or medical/health and welfare experts; and (5) focuses on improving health and welfare. This therapeutic approach has been studied in the elderly who have participated in horticultural therapy during the past 10 years (Yasukawa, 2002).

This chapter describes the application of horticultural therapy for elderly people with dementia as an additional occupational therapy intervention.

Purpose

Horticultural therapy entails people interacting with plants, in this case to improve the cognitive function of elderly patients with dementia or with mental or physical disabilities. The main purpose of horticultural therapy is to provide these patients with graded and carefully designed gardening activities. The interactive idea of horticultural therapy is presented in Fig. 46.1 (Yasukawa, 2002).

Horticultural therapy can also be used as an educational tool that provides children with the knowledge of basic horticultural techniques and awareness of the health care issues regarding the elderly (Tennessen and Lalli, 1997).

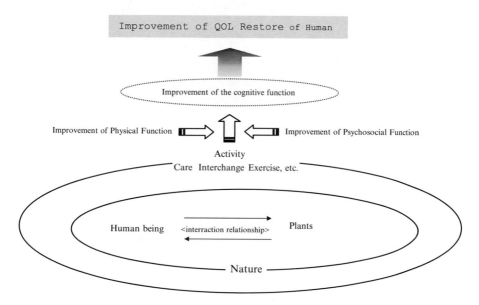

Fig. 46.1 The process of development of human welfare and improvement of quality of life using horticulture therapy.

Method

Candidates for the Intervention

Horticultural therapy is applicable for a wide range of patients suffering from stroke, traumatic brain injury, developmental and mental disorders, dementia, or depression. The patients participating in horticultural therapy in this chapter are presented in Table 46.1.

In Japan, horticultural therapy is favorably used by senior citizens who prefer a home-based activity and live in group homes. Traditionally, adult children will take care of the health of their elderly parents. However, the increasing number of working women prevents many families from taking care of their elderly family members at home (Okamoto et al., 1998). Some reports show that dementia-affected elderly people who are admitted to hospitals or nursing homes quickly develop more advanced dementia symptoms (Motonaga and Asada, 2002; Shimamura et al., 1998; Tanaka and Kato, 2007), with a decrease in cognitive function along with socially inappropriate behavior. The most common problematic behaviors among people with dementia are delusion, refusal of care, and verbal abuse (Tanaka and Kato, 2007).

Table 46.1 Patients participating in the horticultural therapy presented in this chapter

Group	Patient	Age	Sex	Previous profession	Physical function				Physical condition / Present medical record					Conversation ability	Experience in gardening and agricultural activities
					Walking	Eye sight	Hearing	Paralysis	Hyper-tension	Diabetic	Hyper-lipemia	Heart disease	Other		
GH-S: (n = 9)	A	85	Male	Office worker	Δ* 2	Δ* 5			×		×		Gout, glaucoma		No
	B	85	Female	Unclear	Δ* 2				×	×					Yes
	C	80	Female	Unclear					×				Osteoporosis, Spinal disease		Yes
	D	90	Female	Enterpreneur	Δ* 2	Δ* 4	Δ						Brain Apoplexy		Yes
	E	92	Female	Farmer	Δ* 2		Δ		×			×	Malignant tumor		Yes
	F	87	Female	Kimono-maker			Δ		×				Malignant tumor, abdominal and aortic aneurysm		Yes
	G	71	Female	Office worker									Brain apoplexy		No
	H	80	Female	Enterpreneur	Δ* 2	Δ			×			×			Yes
	I	76	Female	Restaurant worker	Δ* 2	Δ			×				Brain apoplexy, brain atherosclerosis		Yes

GH-T: (n = 12)										
J	90	Male	Organization worker	Δ*2	Δ			×		Δ
K	76	Male	Unclear	Δ*2			×	×	Prostatomegaly	Δ
L	82	Male	Farmer		Δ	×				
M	90	Male	Civil servant			×				
N	86	Male	Enterpreneur	Δ*2	Δ			×	Malignant tumor	Δ
O	97	Male	Farmer		Δ		×			Δ
P	81	Female	Farmer				×			
Q	88	Female	Enterpreneur	×*1						
R	84	Female	Farmer	Δ*2		×				
S	85	Female	Teacher		Δ	×	×			
T	80	Female	Part timer			×				
U	88	Female	Farmer		Δ	×				

Δ little disorder; × disorder; *1 using wheelchair; *2 uses a cane; *3 dyschromatopsia; *4 nearsighted; *5 uses a hearing aid.

The symptoms of dementia can act as a barrier to communication, creating frustration and disruptive behaviors, particularly for long-term care residents (Moniz-Cook et al., 2003), because of three factors: neurogenic causation (Foundas et al., 1995), psychogenic causation (Pietrukowic and Johnson, 1991), and deterioration of physical condition (Horowitz, 1997).

Epidemiology

In Japan, the numbers of demented elderly are expected to increase from 2,480,000 in 2002 to 4,990,000 in 2025 (Japan Ministry of Health, Labor, and Welfare, 2006).

Setting

Patients with dementia who participate in horticulture therapy in Japan live in group homes, nursing homes, long-term care facilities, long-term medical treatment hospitals, and centers for disabled people.

The Role of the Horticultural Therapist

The horticultural therapist acts as *a teacher, a guide,* and *a facilitator* for the patients in the horticulture sessions (Table 46.2), and *an advisor* for the other staff. Through interviews the therapy content is adapted to the individual patients' condition.

Prior to each therapy session, the horticultural therapist conducts relaxing activities and mild gymnastics. These activities are also repeated after the sessions and before the patients return to their wards. The therapy sessions end with a

Table 46.2 The therapist's role during a therapy session and its purposes

Session time	Activity	Purpose
Before	Interview	Obtain information on the physical and mental condition of patients
	Relaxing gymnastic	Warming up of body before activity
During	Horticultural activity	Teach basic techniques in horticulture
		Assist the patients' activities during therapy
After	Relaxing gymnastic	Cooling down and relaxing after horticultural session
	Interview	Obtain information on the patients' feelings about the session
		Encourage patients to increase their self-esteem
		Provide some direction in life for patients

discussion of the patients' perception about the value of participating. This part of the therapy sessions is aimed at increasing the patients' self-esteem.

The role of the staff is to assist the horticultural therapist and to help the patients to carry out a therapy session. The staff is responsible for maintaining the continuity of the session and for recording additional information about the patients' physical and psychosocial condition during the therapy sessions.

Results

Clinical Application

The horticultural therapy program was carried out for 3 months, with 12 sessions each week (Table 46.3). Prior to a horticultural therapy session, information on the patients' physical and psychosocial conditions is gathered by the horticultural therapist. This information is combined with weather data, such as air temperature and humidity. This information is used to decide where to hold the session—outdoors or indoors. In hot weather, rain, or high humidity, the horticultural therapy is carried out indoors in order to prevent any negative effects on the patients. The therapy session is facilitated by using a specially designed mobile gardening cart for outdoor (Fig. 46.2) and indoor use (Fig. 46.3).

The Horticultural Therapy Sessions

The therapeutic sessions are performed in the following way:

*   Prior to a session, the patient's physical and mental condition is investigated and a short interview is carried out with the aim of determining the present mood of the patient (Fig. 46.4).
*   The activities that will be carried out during the session are carefully explained.
*   The patients perform five minutes of relaxing gymnastics and sing a song accompanied by some music (Fig. 46.5).
*   The patients work in groups of three or four, together performing a horticulture task. In addition, each patient performs an individual horticulture task (Fig. 46.6). Examples of tasks performed during therapy sessions are (1) artistic activities, such as flower pressing (Fig. 46.7); (2) picking flowers; or (3) pick vegetables, and cooking and eating them.
*   A discussion is held at the end of every session, during which the therapists and the patients share their feelings about the session and their expectations for the next one (Fig. 46.8).
*   After the session, the staff meets to plan the next session.

Table 46.3 Program for horticultural therapy

Session	Contents	Allocate time (hour)	Temp.°C/ Humid.%
1	□ Opening remarks □ Planting sunflowers □ Group planting of summer flowers in a round planter	1.5	28/28
2	□ Observing the sunflowers □ Planting white radish sprouts □ Group planting of summer flowers (flower "Ya-tai") □ Care for group planting in a round planter	1.5	28/28
3	□ Observing the sunflowers □ Planting qing-geng-cai □ Observing the white radish sprouts □ Care for group planting in a round planter and flower "Ya-tai"	1.25	28/38
4	□ Harvesting and tasting the white radish sprouts □ Hydroponic cultivation of pothos □ Care for group planting in a round planter and flower "Ya-tai"	1.25	32/36
5	□ Replant the qing-geng cai □ Plant the radish □ Care for group planting in a round planter and flower "Ya-tai"	1.25	30/34
6	□ Observing the sunflowers □ Observing water cultured pothos □ Replanting the radish □ Care for group planting in a round planter and flower "Ya-tai"	1.25	24/40
7	□ Observing and thin out the radish □ Caring for group planting in a round planter and flower "Ya-tai" □ Make pressed flowers	1.5	24/40
8	□ Replanting the pothos □ Observe and care the radish □ Care for group planting in a round planter and flower "Ya-tai"	1.5	24/40
9	□ Observing sunflowers □ Lay out the pressed flowers □ Care for group planting in a round planter and flower "Ya-tai"	1.5	28/35
10	□ Making framed pressed flowers–1 □ Care for group planting in a round planter and flower "Ya-tai"	1.5	24/50
11	□ Making frame for the pressed flowers–2 □ Care for group planting in a round planter and flower "Ya-tai"	1.5	18/68
12	□ Harvesting the radish and qing-geng cai □ Care for group planting in a round planter and flower "Ya-tai" □ Framed pressed flower show □ Taking a ceremonial photograph □ Tasting party □ Closing address	1.25	18/53

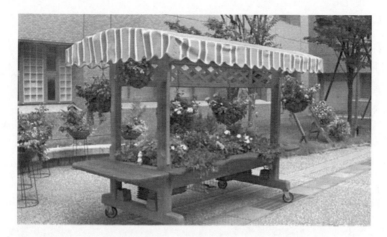

Fig. 46.2 Outdoor horticultural therapy group session using a mobile garden, Hana-Ya-tai.

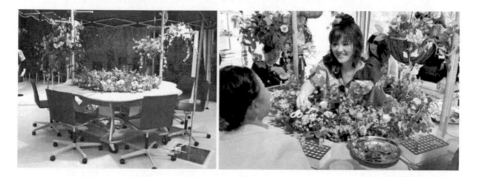

Fig. 46.3 A: Indoor horticultural therapy setting. B: Walk-in garden.

How the Intervention Eases Dementia

Horticultural therapy encourages elderly people with dementia to participate in physical activities. These easy exercises performed in contact with nature may stimulate movements, cardiac activities, and brain frontal lobe activities. In addition, the interaction with other group members and the experience of doing horticulture activities are expected to stimulate memory and basic psychosocial functions.

Evidence-Based Practice

Horticulture therapy significantly (p <.05) (Fig. 46.9) influenced the cognitive function of patients with dementia (Table 46.1), as demonstrated by the results of

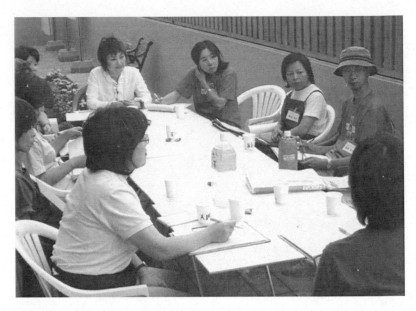

Fig. 46.4 Meeting of therapist and staff before and after session discussing and exchanging ideas and information.

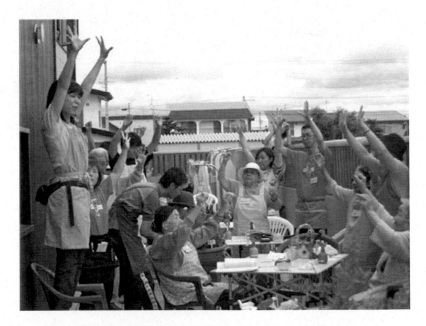

Fig. 46.5 Relaxing gymnastic activities before and after horticultural therapy sessions.

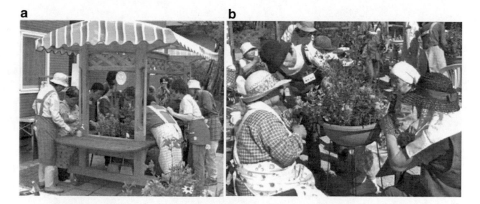

Fig. 46.6 A,B: Participants in horticultural therapy taking care of plants.

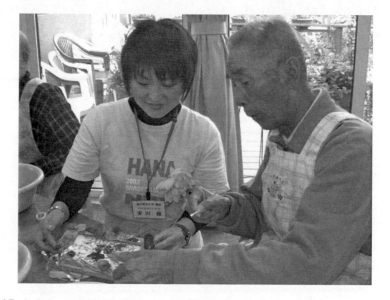

Fig. 46.7 Artistic activity of making pressed flowers from therapy garden.

the Mini–Mental State Examination (MMSE) (Folstein et al., 1975); the scores were 16.9 ± 4.3 before participation and 18.9 ± 4.2 after participation) (Yasukawa, unpublished data). These result were similar to the results for schizophrenia patients (Minei et. al., 2008).

In the interviews, the patients experienced improvement in communication, affect display, expression, spontaneity, activity, interest in communication exchange, and role behavior that contributed to normalization of family relationships and life rhythm adjustment. These results agree with Neuberger's (2008) statement that

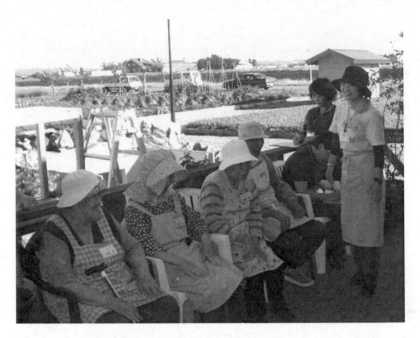

Fig. 46.8 Information exchange between therapists and participants after horticultural therapy sessions.

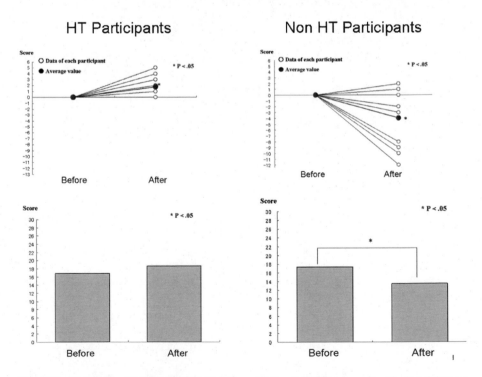

Fig. 46.9 Changes on the Mini–Mental State Examination (MMSE) score of horticultural therapy participants compared to nonparticipants.

horticultural therapy positively influences recovery, communicational skills, and body functioning.

Conclusion

The elderly patients with dementia who practiced horticultural therapy showed increased cognitive ability. Key factors for successful cognitive improvement are the contact with growing plants and the interaction among the participating patients and staff that generates patients' improved quality of life (Yasukawa, 2003).

There is an increased interest in a holistic approach to medical treatment. Here, horticultural therapy offers a combination of medical, environmental-friendly, and artistic approach that benefits the development of new values and the culture of modern society (Mooney and Milstein, 1994).

Acknowledgments This study funded by Japan Society for the Promotion of Scientific Research (JSPS) the   Grant-in Aid for Scientific Research KAKENHI (B2 15390678). http://www.jsps. go.jp/english/e-grants/grants.html. The results of this study were presented at the 2003 International Conference on Alzheimer's Disease and Related Disorders (ICAD).

References

Folstein, M., Fostein, S.E., McHugh, P.R. (1975). Mini–Mental state: a practical method for grading the cognitive state of patients for the clinician. J Psychiatr Res, 12(3), 189–198.

Foundas, A.L., Macauley, B.L., Raymer, A.M., Maher, L.M., Heilman, K.M., and Gonzalez Rothi, L.J. (1995). Ecological implications of limb apraxia: evidence from mealtime behavior. J Int Neuropsychol Soc, 1, 62–66.

Fukushima, T., Nagahata, K., Ishibashi, N., Takahashi, Y., and Moriyama, M. (2005). Quality of life from the viewpoint of patients with dementia in Japan: nurturing through an acceptance of dementia by patients, their families and care professionals. Health Social Care Community, 13, 30–37.

Horowitz, A. (1997). The relationship between vision impairment and the assessment of disruptive behaviors among nursing home residents. Gerontologist, 37, 620–628.

Japan Ministry of Health, Labour, and Welfare. 2006. Kongou no koreika no shinten: 2025 nen no chokoureishakaizo [Advance of aging in the future: Super Aging Society in 2025.]

Matsuo, E. (2002). Jiyujikan Design Kyokai. Leisure Hakusho (in Japanese). Humanity in Horiculture - Healing and Pleasure. International Society for Horticultual Sceine. Acta Horticulturae R Home Page. http://www.actahort.org/members/showpdf?booknrarnr=790_3.

Lee, S., Kim, M.S. and Suh, J.K. (2008a). Effects of horticultural therapy of self-esteem and depression of battered women at a shelter in Korea. Proceedings of the Eight International People-Plant Symposium on Exploring Therapeutic Powers of Flowers, Greenery, and Nature. Acta Horticulturae, 790, 139–142.

Lee, S.M., Suh, J.K. and Lee, S. (2008b). Horticultural therapy in a jail: correctional care for anger. Proceedings of the Eight International People-Plant Symposium on Exploring Therapeutic Powers of Flowers, Greenery, and Nature. Acta Horticulturae, 790, 109–114.

Minie, T., Kiyuna, T., Tanaka, M., and Takaesu, Y. (2008). Horticultural therapy for the aged with chronic schizophrenia. Proceedings of the Eight International People-Plant Symposium on Exploring Therapeutic Powers of Flowers, Greenery, and Nature. Acta Horticulturae, 790, 63–66.

Moniz-Cook, M., Stokes, G., and Agar, S. (2003). Difficult behaviour and dementia in nursing homes: five cases of psychosocial intervention. Clin Psychol Psychother, 10, 197–208.

Mooney, P.F., and Milstein, S.L. (1994). Assessing the benefits of a therapeutic horticulture program for seniors in intermediate care, In: Francis, M., Lindsey, P., and Rice, J.S., eds. The Healing Dimensions of People-Plant Relations (pp. 173–194). Davis, CA: University of California Center for Design Research.

Neuberger, K. (2008). Some therapeutic aspects of gardening in psychiatry. Proceedings of the Eight International People–Plant Symposium on Exploring Therapeutic Powers of Flowers, Greenery, and Nature. Acta Horticulturae, 790, 83–90.

Okamoto, E., Murashima, S., and Saito, E. (1998). Effectiveness of day care service for elderly patients with dementia and their caregivers as observed by assessment of nursing-home inpatients comparison of days with and without day care services. Jpn J Public Health, 45, 1152–1161 (in Japanese).

Pietrukowicz, M.E., and Johnson, M.M.S. (1991). Using life histories to individualize nursing home staff attitudes toward residents. Gerontologist, 31, 102–106.

Shimamura, K., Takatsuka, N., Inaba, R., Iwata, H., Yoshida, H. (1998). Environmental factors possibly associated with onset of senile dementia. (In Japanese). 45 (3) 203–212.

Söderback, I., Söderström, M., and Schälander, E. (2004). Horticulture therapy: the "healing garden" and gardening in rehabilitation measures at Danderyd Hospital Rehabilitation Clinic, Sweden. Pediatr Rehabili, 7(4), 245–260.

Tanaka, M., and Kato, T. (2007). A cross-sectional survey of nursing-home inpatients with dementia or physical disability in patients' assessments. Ehime Univ Faculty Educ Bull, 54, 43–49.

Tennessen, D.J., and Lalli, V.A. (1997). Horticulture intergenerational learning as therapy, a New Project Publication for 4H clubs and local geriatric programs. HortScience, 32, 427–558.

Yasukawa, M. (2002) A study of the effectiveness of horticultural therapy in the care of elderly people: Validation of effects on mental and physical functions and social functions. Doctoral thesis of Kyushu University Graduate School of Bio-resource and Bio-environmental Sciences.

Yasukawa, M. (2003) Horticultural Therapy: Complimentary and Alternative Medicine that makes use of Characteristics of plants. (In Japanese). In: Sumitani, S., ed. An Introduction to Studies on Integrated Approaches to the Environment and Welfare (pp. 181–195). Tokyo.

Chapter 47
Medical Music Therapy: Evidence-Based Principles and Practices

Cheryl Dileo and Joke Bradt

> *Music therapy offers many possibilities for clients who are experiencing a range of health problems. In the words of a client, "Music therapy helps me to feel like a whole person again."*

Abstract Because of its flexibility, versatility, and utility with a wide range of clients and clinical issues, as well as its acceptability by clients and the documentation of its effectiveness, music therapy will undoubtedly continue to grow as a viable approach in all facets of health care. As has been realized throughout the ages, music is an indispensable part of the human experience and an essential component to achieving quality of life.

Keywords Behavioral discipline • Complementary therapy • Music therapy • Psychotherapy • Sensory art therapies

Definition

Music is a multidimensional phenomenon, capable of addressing various human domains simultaneously. The American Music Therapy Association (2005) defines music therapy as "the clinical and evidence-based use of music interventions to accomplish individualized goals within a therapeutic relationship by a credentialed professional who has completed an approved music therapy program."

In contrast, other music practices in hospitals implemented by medical personnel (e.g., using prerecorded music to enhance mood) or by professional musicians (e.g., using live music for entertainment) do not comprise the necessary components of music therapy (Dileo and Bradt, 2007; Dileo and Reuer, 2007).

Music therapy is always involves the following:

- A credentialed professional music therapist
- A process that includes individualized assessment, intervention, and evaluation
- The use of the range of experiences possible within music
- A relationship between therapist and client that develops through the music

I. Söderback (ed.), *International Handbook of Occupational Therapy Interventions*,
DOI: 10.1007/978-0-387-75424-6_47, © Springer Science+Business Media, LLC 2010

Background

Although the therapeutic properties of music have been acknowledged since the beginning of recorded history, the scientific discipline of music therapy did not emerge until after World War I, when musicians visited veterans' hospitals to perform for military personnel who were experiencing battle-related physical and emotional traumas. The positive and sometimes dramatic responses to music observed among patients led to the hospitals' hiring of musicians and to the need for specialized training for musicians to implement this work. The first university music therapy training program was established in 1944, and the National Association for Music Therapy was created in 1950 (Dileo and Reuer, 2007).

Purpose

Music therapy is used to improve, maintain, remediate, or prevent one or more of the clinical issues in clients, as specified in their needs for habilitation or rehabilitation.

Method

Candidates for the Music Therapy Intervention

Typically, clients are referred to music therapy based on criteria established by the music therapist as well as the facility's expectations of music therapy's contribution to intervention (Magee and Wheeler, 2006).

Settings

Music therapists work both individually and in groups in a wide range of clinical settings with persons who experience various psychological, physical, cognitive, social, financial, or spiritual problems.

The Role of the Music Therapist

Music therapists are trained to systematically effect nonmusical outcomes in all of the human domains (physiologic, psychological, cognitive, social, spiritual, and behavioral).

In the United States music therapists may enter the field at the bachelor's level after completion of a rigorous, standardized curriculum in music and music therapy; the biological, behavioral, and social sciences; and an extended internship and the successful passing of the national board-certification examination (administered by the independent Certification Board for Music Therapy). Master's degrees and a full PhD program in music therapy are available and strongly encouraged (Dileo and Reuer, 2007).

Results

Clinical Application

Music is capable of affecting the various human domains simultaneously. When used by a credentialed music therapist within the context of a trusting, therapeutic relationship, its outcomes may be well documented. Several systematic reviews and meta-analyses show the effect of music therapy among clients with the diagnoses of heart diseases (Bradt and Dileo, (2009), cancer (Dileo et al., 2008), schizophrenia (Gold, et al., 2008a), autism (Gold, et al., 2008b), depression (Maratos, et.al., 2008) or dementia (Vink, et al., 2008) and among clients who is near their end of life (Bradt and Dileo, 2008b) or living with acquired brain damage (Bradt, et al., 2008). Further music therapy is used for anxiety reduction before operation (Dileo and Bradt, 2008) and in mechanically ventilated clients (Dileo, et al., 2008). Evidence of the many potential outcomes of music therapy intervention continues to accumulate in various areas of human functioning. Promising results have been noted for music therapy's effects on physiologic parameters, mood, depression, and pain, as well as in reducing agitation in clients with dementia. Preliminary data on the cost-effectiveness of music therapy interventions indicate decreases in pain medication and in the length of stay in intensive care units.

The Process of Music Therapy

Assessments

The music therapy process begins with a detailed assessment process that identifies the client's needs, musical preferences and relationship to music, medical and social history, ability to communicate, and physical, cognitive, and emotional capabilities (Dilco and Reuer, 2007). This information is collected from the client, the family, the client's records, and standardized measures or specially designed music therapy assessment instruments. In addition, the music therapist may engage the client in music to observe his or her capabilities and responses directly. It is not unusual for the latter assessment strategy to reveal information about the client that cannot be gleaned from other sources.

Goal Setting

Based on assessment results, a decision is made as to whether music therapy may be of potential benefit to the client. If so, specific physical, psychological, cognitive, social, spiritual, or behavioral goals are identified, and music therapy interventions best suited to meet these goals are planned (this may also be done in collaboration with the client's intervention team, where relevant). Evaluation of the client's progress toward the established goals is ongoing throughout intervention and documented in the client's records. A final summary of progress is documented at the termination of music therapy services (Dileo and Reuer, 2007).

Intervention

Music therapy interventions comprise a wide range of possible experiences within music and may be categorized as follows: (1) receptive, (2) creative, or (3) re-creative, or a combination of these categories; within these approaches all types, styles, and genres of music may be utilized.

In receptive approaches, the client "receives" music passively by listening or by having music vibrations applied directly to the body ("vibroacoustic therapy") (Wigram and Dileo, 1997). The music used may be pre-composed, specially composed by the client or therapist, or may be created spontaneously by the therapist (e.g., matched to physiologic parameters of the client).

Receptive approaches include, but are not limited to, music listening, song choices, music and imagery, music visualization, music-assisted relaxation, lyric analysis, and music therapy entrainment. Music is selected by the therapist according to its inherent qualities and structural elements along with its intended therapeutic purposes. The client's preference for and familiarity with the music are also factors in its selection; consideration is given to the evocative potential of the music in stimulating memories, associations, and images inconsistent with therapeutic goals (Dileo and Reuer, 2007). When using receptive approaches, the therapist often processes the client's reaction to the music verbally.

In *creative approaches*, the client improvises or creates music or songs spontaneously using voice or musical instruments, or purposefully composes music or songs alone or with the therapist.

In *re-creative approaches*, the client performs previously composed music on an instrument, sings pre-composed songs, conducts music, or learns to play an instrument. In combined approaches, music therapy is used in conjunction with non–music therapy approaches, with the assumption that music will enhance the effectiveness of the method used.

Combined approaches may include, for example, music and meditation, music and hypnosis, music and touch/massage, music and movement, and music and other arts experiences. In all music therapy approaches, the client needs no musical skills or previous musical training, as the therapist is able to facilitate the client's engagement in music using specialized methods (Dileo and Reuer, 2007).

The Use of Music Therapy to Address Clinical Goals

For clients with *impaired physical functioning*, active participation in music-making, such as playing instruments, requires purposeful and coordinated movements and may provide specific activation of small and large muscle groups, thereby enhancing strength, functional movement, appropriate body alignment, bilateral coordination, and breath control (Magee and Wheeler, 2006). In addition, auditory rhythmic stimulation may provide for the cuing and structuring of movement and walking (Thaut, 2000).

In a similar manner, listening to client-preferred, sedative music may *affect physiologic parameters*, such as heart rate, blood pressure, and respiration, and there is some evidence of its influence on stress hormones, immune function, and biochemical phenomena (Dileo and Bradt, 2005). The therapist may improvise music to match a physiologic parameter of the client (e.g., respiration rate). Once matched and sustained for a short period, the therapist gradually decreases the pulse of the music to encourage a slowing down of the breath (Dileo and Reuer, 2007).

The therapist may also improvise music according to the specific details of a client's *report of pain* using the process of music therapy entrainment (Dileo and Bradt, 1999). Music may serve as the focal point during a painful procedure, or the therapist and client may chant or sing together to decrease accelerated respiration.

The use of music therapy to *reduce physiologic arousal* is a common practice. Music itself may serve as the relaxation agent, with the client passively listening to music performed live by the therapist or through prerecorded music. Additional relaxation techniques may be combined with the music, including progressive muscle relaxation, autogenic suggestions, breathing techniques, and visual imagery (Dileo and Bradt, 2007; Dileo and Reuer, 2007).

Music therapy may be used to *enhance social and psychological functioning* as well as *quality of life* in a variety of ways. Listening to live or recorded music may improve mood and decrease depression for a range of clients. Playing an instrument or creating an original song may improve self-esteem and provide for an alternate means of expression. Listening to and discussing lyrics of specially selected songs with a music therapist may facilitate self-awareness and personal insight. Improvising music or performing in a group may strengthen connectedness with others and facilitate the acquisition of social skills.

Music therapy may be used to *stimulate cognitive functioning* in clients suffering from a variety of conditions. For example, hearing and singing songs may evoke memories, promote attention to the task at hand, increase orientation to time and place, and enhance abstract thinking (Magee and Wheeler, 2006).

Clients' *spiritual and existential needs* may be supported through music therapy approaches that involve singing hymns, writing songs that provide messages of encouragement and hope, and discussing song lyrics relevant to spiritual issues.

In addition, music therapy may provide comfort to clients and their families by *facilitating relationship completion* and support for the transition (Dileo and Parker, 2005).

Lastly, music therapy may be used to *encourage behavioral changes* in clients, for example, providing the motivation to engage in and comply with intervention. This is attributable to its effects on other aforementioned domains, such as reducing pain, decreasing depression, etc.

Discussion

Music therapists may contribute greatly to the interdisciplinary team because of the range of clinical issues that they may address using this intervention modality. Because of the inherent pleasure and enjoyment associated with music engagement, clients often demonstrate less resistance to music therapy, and client capabilities not obvious in other intervention areas are often observed. This client information is often considered valuable by the intervention team.

Music therapists may serve as consultants to occupational therapists or they may develop ways of combining their areas of expertise to the benefit of the clients they serve. For example, music and occupational therapists may co-design interventions aimed at enhancing a client's fine motor skills using adapted musical instruments.

References

American Music Therapy Association. (2005). http://www.musictherapy.org

Bradt, J., and Dileo, C. (2009, in press). Music for people with coronary heart disease review. The Cochrane Database of Systematic Reviews, Issue 2, CE 006577.

Bradt, J., and Dileo, C. (2008). Music therapy for symptom relief and support in end-of-life care [Protocol]. Cochrane Pain, Palliative Care and Support Group. Cochrane Database of Systematic Reviews, 2. Art. No.: CD007169. DOI: 10.1002/14651858.CD007169.

Bradt, J., Magee, W.L., Dileo, C., Wheeler, B., and McGilloway, E. (2008). Music therapy for acquired brain injury [Protocol]. Cochrane Stroke Group, Cochrane Database of Systematic Reviews, Issue 1.

Dileo, C., and Bradt, J. (1999). Entrainment, resonance and pain-related suffering. In: Dileo, C., ed. Music Therapy and Medicine: Theoretical and Clinical Applications (pp. 181–188). Silver Spring, MD: American Music Therapy Association.

Dileo, C., and Bradt, J. (2005). Medical Music Therapy: A Meta-Analysis and Agenda for Future Research. Cherry Hill, NJ: Jeffrey Books.

Dileo, C., and Bradt, J. (2007). Music therapy: applications to stress management. In: Lehrer, P., and Woolfolk, R., eds. Principles and Practice of Stress Management, 3rd ed. New York: Guilford.

Dileo, C., and Bradt, J. (2008). Music for Preoperative Anxiety. [Protocol] Cochrane Anaesthesia Group, Cochrane Database of Systematic Reviews, 1.

Dileo, C., Bradt, J., and Grocke, D. (2008a). Music for anxiety reduction in mechanically ventilated clients [Protocol]. Cochrane Anaesthesia Group, Cochrane Database of Systematic Reviews, 1.

Dileo, C., Bradt, J., Grocke, D., and Magill, L. (2008b). Music interventions for improving psychological and physical outcomes in cancer clients [Protocol]. The Cochrane Gynaecological Cancer Group, Cochrane Database of Systematic Reviews, 1.

Dileo, C., and Parker, C. (2005). Final moments: the use of song in relationship completion. In: Dileo, C., and Loewy, J., eds. Music Therapy at the End of Life. Cherry Hill, NJ: Jeffrey Books.

Dileo, C., and Reuer, B. (2007). Applications of music therapy in the continuum of care for the cardiac client. In: Vogel, J., and Krucoff, M., eds. Integrative Cardiology (pp. 281–303). New York: McGraw-Hill.

Gold, C., Heldal, T.O., Dahle, T., Wigram, T. (2008a). Music therapy for schizophrenia or schizophrenia-like illnesses [Systematic Review]. Cochrane Schizophrenia Group Cochrane Database of Systematic Reviews. 1, 2008.

Gold, C., Wigram, T., and Elefant, C. (2008b). Music therapy for autistic spectrum disorder [Systematic Review]. Cochrane Developmental, Psychosocial and Learning Problems Group Cochrane Database of Systematic Reviews. 1.

Magee, W., and Wheeler, B. (2006). Music therapy for clients with traumatic brain injury. In: Murrey, G.J., ed. Alternative Therapies in the Intervention of Brain Injury and Neurobehavioral Disorders: A Practical Guide (pp. 51–74). Binghamton, NY: Haworth.

Maratos, A.S., Gold, C., Wang, X., and Crawford, M.J. (2008). Music therapy for depression [Systematic Review]. Cochrane Depression, Anxiety and Neurosis Group Cochrane Database of Systematic Reviews. 1.

Thaut, M.H. (2000). A Scientific Model of Music in Therapy and Medicine. San Antonio, TX: IMR.

Vink, A.C., Birks, J.S., Bruinsma, M.S., and Scholten, R.J.P.M. (2008). Music therapy for people with dementia [Systematic Review]. Cochrane Dementia and Cognitive Improvement Group Cochrane Database of Systematic Reviews. 1.

Wigram, T., and Dileo, C. (1997). Music Vibration and Health. Cherry Hill, NJ: Jeffrey Books.

Chapter 48
Music as a Resource for Health and Well-Being

Norma Daykin and Leslie Bunt

Abstract This chapter explores the use of music as a resource for health. Drawing on Bruscia's 1998 distinction between music *in* therapy and music *as* therapy, current evidence regarding the contribution of music to a range of outcomes, including physiologic, psychological, clinical and social impacts, is outlined.

The chapter identifies key issues for practitioners to consider when using music. These include the background and experience of clients, the importance of facilitation skills, and the need to cope with the sometimes powerful emotional responses to music.

Finally, the chapter highlights the need for further research into the ways in which music can contribute to treatment, rehabilitation, and quality of life in a wide range of settings.

Keywords Health • Music • Music therapy • Quality of life

Background

Music can be a resource for health and well-being in a range of settings, and there are many ways in which music can contribute to treatment and rehabilitation. There are key issues, challenges, and considerations for practice in using music therapeutically.

Music has been used to enhance health and well-being for centuries. Up until the second half of the 20th century, music was used mainly in hospitals as an entertaining diversion, as an aid to convalescence, and as a morale-booster (Bunt, 1994). During the past 50 years there has been growing recognition of the clinical benefits of music, including listening and playing, in a wide variety of health care settings. These benefits have mostly been explored within professional music-therapy literature. However, the purpose of this chapter is to identify the broad uses of music in health care.

I. Söderback (ed.), *International Handbook of Occupational Therapy Interventions*,
DOI: 10.1007/978-0-387-75424-6_48, © Springer Science+Business Media, LLC 2010

Purpose

Recorded music and live music performance can be used in a variety of ways to contribute to prevention and rehabilitation for children and adults with a wide range of conditions. Music can do the following:

- Create a *relaxing and calming atmosphere.*
- Be a form of *physical activity; music making* supports both individual and group treatment plans.
- *Offer emotional and psychological* support.
- *Enhance motivation.*
- Provide *opportunities for enjoyment and social interaction.*
- Help clients *cope with chronic or challenging conditions.*

Method

Candidates for the Intervention

Music can benefit a wide range of clients of all ages, both genders, and different socioeconomic backgrounds.

Settings Where Music Is Used

Diverse musical approaches are adopted in many health and social care settings including primary care, preschool nurseries, hospitals, hospices, residential care homes, community day centers for adults with physical disabilities and sensory impairments, prisons, special schools, and mainstream schools. Music therapy is well established in a number of health care areas, particularly child and adult mental-health and learning disabilities services (Bunt and Hoskyns, 2002). Music is also increasingly used in other disciplines such as cancer care (Daykin et al., 2006).

Result

Clinical Application

The Contribution of Music

Bruscia (1998) distinguishes between music *in* therapy and music *as* therapy. We can regard music *in* therapy and music *as* therapy as two poles on a continuum, with different professionals contributing to the range of musical activities in between.

Music in therapy exists in a variety of settings, as many professionals might use music to enhance quality of life and create an atmosphere conducive to healing and rehabilitation. For example, rhythm can be used to structure and organize activity, helping people with physical disabilities to improve control over their movements. Playing instruments and singing can offer alternative means of communication for people with impairments. Music can help to reduce depression and anxiety relating to a wide range of conditions, boosting self-esteem and facilitating expression of a range of emotions. Listening to music and taking part in music-making can facilitate exploration and cathartic release as well as providing opportunities for reflection, reminiscence, and self-awareness. Further, music can offer patients and clients a valuable resource for creating meaning in their lives, and helping them to make sense of their situation. Finally, music can enhance communication between professionals and patients and among individuals, significant others, and families.

Music as an adjunctive therapy, supporting a range of treatment objectives, can be a therapy in its own right. In *music as therapy,* music is the agent of therapeutic change and practitioners rely on specialist knowledge of psychotherapeutic approaches and music-therapy techniques.

Evidence-Based Practice

Evidence of clinical effects of music was reviewed by Staricoff (2004). Music was found to reduce anxiety and depression as well as improve physiologic indicators such as blood pressure in a number of fields including cancer care and cardiovascular care. Research also identified clinical impacts of music in neonatal care, including reduced length of hospital stay.

Music may help to reduce stress during medical screening or diagnosis. Further, improvements in psychological variables relating to pain, and reduced use of medication to reduce pain after surgery, were associated with music. The review found support for particular types of music, including classical and meditative types, and it found that live music, when appropriate, has more significant benefits than recorded music. The use of familiar tunes may be helpful in areas such as mental health care, although it is important that patients can exercise choice and control over this aspect of their environment.

Recent clinical studies have associated music therapy interventions with improved communication in participants with autistic spectrum disorder (Gold et al., 2006) as well as improved mental state in patients with schizophrenia (Gold et al., 2005).

Discussion

Research has shown that music can offer a wide range of benefits in health care settings, from environmental enhancement to clinical benefits and therapeutic outcomes. To benefit from music, participants do not need to have any particular knowledge, and even taking part in music making does not require any kind of instrumental ability, provided the session leader has the appropriate facilitation skills. However, participants' views about music may be influenced by previous experience, such as education, which may not always be positive (Daykin et al., 2007). When music is used to facilitate expression and communication, it can evoke powerful emotional responses in participants. Those leading these activities require sensitivity as well as appropriate knowledge and skill to ensure that these responses are not negative for clients.

While clinical studies have identified outcomes for music therapy, further research is needed on the benefits and risks of music activity more broadly defined. Research is also needed to understand the roles and contributions of the different professional groups that currently make use of music as a resource for health and well-being in health care settings.

References

Bruscia, K. (1998). Defining Music Therapy, 2nd ed. Gilsum, NH: Barcelona Publications.

Bunt, L. (1994). Music Therapy: An Art Beyond Words. London: Routledge.

Bunt, L., and Hoskyns, S., eds. (2002). The Handbook of Music Therapy. Hove: Brunner-Routledge.

Daykin, N., Bunt, L., and McClean, S. (2006). Music and healing in cancer care: a survey of supportive care providers. Arts Psychother, 33, 402–413.

Daykin, N., McClean, S., and Bunt, L. (2007). Creativity, identity and healing: participants' accounts of music therapy in cancer care. Health: An Interdisciplinary Journal for the Social Study of Health, Illness and Medicine, 11(3), 349–370.

Gold, C., Heldal, T.O., Dahle, T., and Wigram, T. (2005). Music therapy for schizophrenia or schizophrenia-like illnesses. Cochrane Database of Systematic Reviews, 2, CD004025. DOI: 10.1002/14651858.CD004025.pub2.

Gold, C., Wigram, T., and Elefant, C. (2006). Music therapy for autistic spectrum disorder. Cochrane Database of Systematic Reviews, 2, CD004381. DOI: 10.1002/14651858. CD004381.pub2.

Staricoff, R. (2004). Arts in Health: A Review of the Medical Literature. London: Arts Council England, Research Report 36.

Part V
Interventions: The Occupational Therapist Promotes Health and Wellness

Chapter 49
Introduction

Ingrid Söderback

Abstract This part of the handbook contains chapters that exemplify the occupational therapy interventions in which the occupational therapists (OTs) promote health and wellness (Fig. 49.1) The chapters contain descriptions of the interventions that are aimed at preventing (1) accidents at home among older people, (2) accidents at work and workplaces, and (3) traffic accidents among drivers with functional impairments. In Chapter 50, Avlund and Vass discuss the general divisions, definitions, and aims of preventive interventions. This part of the Handbook also includes Shannon's important report on how the clients' motivation to change behavior will be enhanced by use of a specific consultative method.

Keywords Behavior • Health • Motivation • Older people • Prevention • Road-users • Workers

I. Söderback (ed.), *International Handbook of Occupational Therapy Interventions*,
DOI: 10.1007/978-0-387-75424-6_49, © Springer Science+Business Media, LLC 2010

459

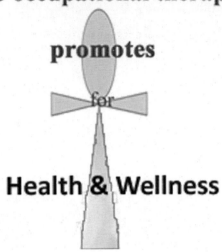

The occupational therapist

promotes

Health & Wellness

Fig. 49.1 The occupational therapist 's role as promoter for the clients' health and wellness by using consultative methods that prevent ill health, impairments, and disabilities. The figure is a stylized Ankh-sign.

Chapter 50
Preventive Interventions: Overview

Kirsten Avlund and Mikkel Vass

Prevention and health promotion are key issues for
maintaining good health and function as prerequisites
for a good life in old age.

Abstract Prevention in old age is most appropriately defined by referring to prevention of impairments, activity limitations, and inability to participate in social activities. Thus, *primary prevention* strives to prevent activity limitation and non-participation (e.g., guidance on possibilities of refitting the home to prevent falls). *Secondary prevention* focuses on discovering early signs of activity limitations and taking urgent and relevant steps to prevent the disablement process from spiraling or to restore daily activities (e.g., encouragement of exercise to prevent pains related to osteoarthritis in knees and hips). *Tertiary prevention* aims to avoid further decline in cases where impairment, activity limitations, and nonparticipation are irreversible (e.g., information on well-functioning transport schemes for disabled people to enjoy interpersonal and other social relations).

Keywords Health promotion • Older people • Prevention

Background

It is well known that "prevention is better than cure" (Rose, 1992). Through the years, the concept of prevention has aimed to stop disease from arising. Thus, it is no surprise that prevention has always been closely connected with medical thinking and its frame of reference. The World Health Organization originally based its definition of health on the absence of illness, but in recent decades, the definition has changed radically. The organization's 1998 Ottawa Charter on Health Promotion (1986) brought the concept of *health promotion* to the fore, and health is today seen more as the basis for achieving a good quality of life than as the purpose of life. In addition to the personal desires of avoiding serious diseases or disabilities, health promotion has also come to encompass social, cultural, environmental, and other external aspects. For this reason, when using the concept prevention, we must clearly define what we want to prevent.

I. Söderback (ed.), *International Handbook of Occupational Therapy Interventions,*
DOI: 10.1007/978-0-387-75424-6_50, © Springer Science+Business Media, LLC 2010

In practice, health promotion and illness prevention are often difficult to separate. In short, *prevention* deals with avoiding or removing threats to general health, while *health promotion* also strives to improve health, impairments, activities, and social participation by, for instance, giving people the spirit and joy that come from being engaged in everyday activities.

Prevention and health promotion are therefore closely linked, and the term *prevention* is used here in a broad sense, including health promotion. Consequently, it is not sufficient to incorporate only health promotion in preventive interventions. If, for instance, preventive activities can avert a risk situation, the risk must be recognized and the necessary offers extended. However, at the same time, professional activities should be designed based on the client's physical and mental resources.

Definitions

Traditionally, *prevention* is divided into primary, secondary, and tertiary prevention, defined as follows (Naidoo and Wills, 2000):

- Primary prevention aims to avoid diseases.
- Secondary prevention focuses on tracking and treating diseases in their early stages.
- Tertiary prevention centers on preventing relapses or aggravation of existing diseases.

In the elderly, it often proves difficult to distinguish clearly among these three levels, since, for example, secondary and tertiary prevention of diseases may actually be primary prevention of activity limitation and nonparticipation.

In this context, it is therefore more appropriate to limit the definitions of prevention/*health promotion* as follows:

- *Primary prevention* strives to prevent activity limitation and nonparticipation.
- *Secondary prevention* focuses on discovering early signs of activity limitations and taking urgent, relevant steps to prevent the disablement process from spiraling or to restore daily activities.
- *Tertiary prevention* aims to avoid further decline in cases where impairment, activity limitations, and nonparticipation are irreversible.

Examples of Primary Prevention Aimed at the Elderly

- Suggestion of annual influenza vaccination in the autumn to avoid infections (focus is on health) (Ljubuncic et al., 2008).
- Advice and guidance on individual physical activity aimed at strengthening muscles, tendons, and balancing ability to avoid falls and possible fractures (focus is on impairment) (Singh, 2002).

- Advice on daily intake of vitamin D and calcium to reduce the risk of weakened bones and malnutrition and to strengthen muscles (focus is on impairment) (Binkley, 2007).
- Guidance on possibilities of improving or refitting the home to prevent falls (focus is on activity limitation) (Tinetti et al., 1994; see Chapters 51 and 52).
- Information on possibilities for social and physical activity in the community (focus is on activity limitation and participation) (Cohen-Mansfield et al., 2004).
- Arranging social activities in the community (focus is on participation).

Examples of Secondary Prevention Aimed at the Elderly

- Blood pressure measurements and other regular control measures among people with diabetes to prevent late complications such as reduced vision or cardiovascular complications and defective renal function (focus is on health) (Gill, 2002).
- Early treatment of uncomplicated urinary tract infections to prevent spells of confusion and falls due to dehydration (focus is on health).
- Offer and encouragement of exercise to prevent pains related to osteoarthritis in knees and hips (focus is on impairment and activity limitation).
- Guidance in use of compensatory strategies in daily activities for persons with early signs of decline (focus is on activity limitation and participation).
- Suggestions of, for instance, contacting day centers, pensioners' clubs, or volunteers for involuntary socially isolated people (focus is on participation).

Examples of Tertiary Prevention Aimed at the Elderly

- Offers of rehabilitation and training of impairments after illness (focus is on impairment and activity limitation) (Jette et al., 1999).
- Information on well-functioning transportation options and help for disabled people to enjoy interpersonal and other social relations (focus is on participation).

Discussion

There is burgeoning evidence supporting a diverse array of multidimensional home- and center-based programs for prevention of functional decline, disability, and falls (Beswick et al., 2008; Campbell and Robertson, 2006; Gill et al., 2002, 2004; Stuck et al., 2002). The premise for the assessment is a multidimensional approach, including health, social, and mental factors, and multidimensional interdisciplinary follow-up. However, it is possible to prevent numerous diseases and consequences of disease by a variety of interventions on a healthy life style, such as physical training (Singh, 2002).

Conclusion

This chapter has described examples of preventive and health promotion strategies among older adults. Health promotion and prevention are important lifelong.

This part V of the Handbook gives examples of prevention of traffic accidents (also see Chapter 53) and work-related impairments (also see Chapters 54 to 56). Finally, the special consultative technique of motivational interviewing is aimed at encouraging clients to take responsibility for their health behavior, with the intention of avoiding disease and disability in general (also see Chapter 57).

References

Beswick, A.D., Rees, K., Dieppe, P., et al. (2008). Complex interventions to improve physical function and maintain independent living in elderly people: a systematic review and metaanalysis. Lancet, 371, 725–735.

Binkley, N. (2007). Does low vitamin D status contribute to "age-related" morbidity? J Bone Miner Res, 22, 55–58.

Campbell, A.J., and Robertson, M.C. (2006). Implementation of multifactorial interventions for fall and fracture prevention. Age Ageing, 35(Suppl 2), 60–64.

Cohen-Mansfield, J., Marx, M.S., Biddison, J.R., and Guralnik, J.M. (2004). Socio-environmental exercise preferences among older adults. Prev Med, 38, 804–811.

Gill, T.M. (2002). Geriatric medicine: It's more than caring for old people. Am J Med, 113, 85–90.

Gill, T.M., Baker, D.I., Gottschalk, M., Peduzzi, P.N., Allore, H., and Byers, A. (2002). A program to prevent functional decline I physically frail, elderly persons who live at home. N Engl J Med, 347, 1068–1074.

Gill, T.M., Baker, D.I., Gottschalk, M., Peduzzi, P.N., Allore, H., and Van Ness, P.H. (2004). A prehabilitation program for the prevention of functional decline: Effect on higher-level physical function. Arch Phys Med Rehabil, 85, 1043–1049.

Jette, A.M., Lachman, M., Giorgetti, M.M., et al. (1999). Exercise—it's never too late: The strong-for-life program. Am J Public Health, 89, 66–72.

Ljubuncic, P., Globerson, A., and Reznick, A.Z. (2008). Evidence-based roads to the promotion of health in old age. J Nutr Health Aging, 12, 139–143.

Naidoo, J., and Wills, J. (2000). Health Promotion. Foundations for Practice. London: Baillière Tindall.

Ottawa Charter on Health Promotion. (1986). First International Conference on Health Promotion, Ottawa, Canada. http://www.api.or.at/akis/download/whodoc/ottawa%20charter.pdf.

Rose, G. (1992). The Strategy of Preventive Medicine. Oxford: Oxford University Press.

Singh, M.A.F. (2002). Exercise comes of age: Rationale and recommendations for a geriatric exercise prescription. J Gerontol Med Sci, 57A, M262–M282.

Stuck, A.E., Egger, M., Hammer, A., et al. (2002). Home visits to prevent nursing home admission and functional decline in elderly people: Systematic review and meta-regression analysis. JAMA, 287, 1022–1028.

Tinetti, M.A., O'Neill, E.F, Ryan, N.D. et al. (1994). A multifactorial intervention to reduce the risk of falling among elderly people living in the community. N Engl J Med, 331, 821–827.

Chapter 51
Preventing Falls in the Elderly Using "Stepping On": A Group-Based Education Program

Lindy Clemson

I feel more confident and I'm going out more.

—Marie, a client

It's made me more aware, just so much more aware. Of the buses, of my place. Of making it brighter inside, getting rid of leaves outside, of everything.

—Roleena, a client

What you have done is focus on our abilities. No one else has done that.

—Nancy, a client

I have had some near falls but you have a quicker recovery and your muscles don't collapse.

—Herbert, a client

Abstract *Stepping On* is a multifaceted falls-prevention program for the community-residing elderly. The programs are held in local community venues and run for seven 2-hour weekly sessions, with a follow-up home visit contact and a 3- month booster session. About 30% of older people who fall lose their self-confidence and start to go out less often. Inactivity leads to social isolation and loss of muscle strength and balance, increasing the risk of falling. Stepping On aims to break that cycle, engaging people is a range of relevant fall preventive strategies. Stepping On content draws on current evidence for falls prevention. The program has been proven to reduce falls. A detailed manual is available to enable occupational therapists to run the program.

Keywords Accidental falls • Fall prevention • Home and community safety • Self-efficacy • Small group work

I. Söderback (ed.), *International Handbook of Occupational Therapy Interventions*,
DOI: 10.1007/978-0-387-75424-6_51, © Springer Science+Business Media, LLC 2010

Background

The Stepping On program was developed by occupational therapists in 2003, building on earlier work in falls prevention. The manual evolved by incorporating information from content experts, literature reviews, and the views of our older participants. The research team, led by an occupational therapist, provides evidence of its effectiveness.

Definition

A multifaceted approach to falls prevention is based on current and emerging evidence.

The conceptual basis of the Stepping On program is as follows:

- It incorporates a *decision-making model* (Janis and Mann, 1977) used to explore barriers and options. The model has been operationalized into a list of five prompts to elicit reflection and prompt discussion (Clemson and Swann, 2008).
- It applies Bandura's (1977, 1986) *social cognitive theory* on the influences of self-efficacy and skill mastery. It uses mastery experiences and positive reframing to encourage adaptation and action.
- It uses *adult learning principles* (Egger et al., 1990) to help participants self-manage their risk of falls. This aspect of the program recognizes that the older adult has the capacity for learning and change. A variety of learning strategies include storytelling, brainstorming, and problem solving.
- It uses the *group process* as a learning environment. This enables the participants to draw on "knowledge from outside the group in order to process it within, and subsequently use it outside" (Jacques, 2000). A sense of ownership of strategies is fostered, and sharing occurs in a trusting environment.

Purpose

The purpose of this program is as follows:

- Managing falls and reducing the risk of falling.
- Maintaining safety at home and in the community.
- Building confidence in negotiating the environment and in other fall risk situation.

Method

Candidates for the Intervention

The program is targeted to community-residing elderly people who are around 70 years of age and over and who have had a fall or are fearful of falling. People who have a cognitive impairment and those who are homebound, mobile only on a walker, or in a wheelchair are excluded. Typically, there are more women in the groups than men, which reflect the demographic of the aging population. Our research supports specific benefit for men who have fallen (Clemson et al., 2004), so we encourage inclusion of both genders.

Epidemiology

Falls are a common and serious problem for older people. Some 30% to 35% of persons who are age 70 or older fall each year (O'Loughlin et al., 1993). Injurious falls are a leading cause of hospitalization and can lead to social isolation and premature institutionalization (Tinetti and Williams, 1997). Risk factors for falls include poor balance, reduced lower leg strength, poor vision, chronic disorders, and sleep disturbances (O'Loughlin et al., 1993). Fear of falling is also a common occurrence, with a reported incidence of 30% to 70% (Vellas et al., 1997) and increasing with age. It is more prevalent in those who report multiple falls, poorer health, or unsteady balance (Lack, 2005). Fear of falling itself can lead to restricted activity and decreased quality of life (Vellas et al., 1997). As falls are multifactorial, it makes sense to conduct multidimensional interventions. Core interventions known to have an impact supported by meta-analyses are exercise and environmental adaptation (Clemson et al., 2008; Gillespie et al.,2005).

Settings

Venues chosen should be in an accessible place in the community, situated near public transportation.

Preventing Strategies

People who have experienced a fall are at much higher risk of falling again. Recruitment aims to reach those people in the community who are beginning to fall and to invite them to register for the program.

The kinds of strategies found to be useful (Clemson et al., 2007) include the following:

- *Mailings* to older members of sporting and other clubs that are known to include larger numbers of seniors.
- *Mailings* to medical practitioners.
- A *newspaper article* with a picture of a local resident who has graduated from the Stepping On program, commenting about how he is more independent or feels safer getting out and about.
- *Brochures* to former participants to share with their peers.
- Information directed at local medical practitioners, elderly care community teams, and physiotherapists, who may be useful sources of referral.

Results

The Role of the Occupational Therapist in Applying the Intervention

The program is facilitated by a health professional experienced in group-work and in working with the elderly. Occupational therapists (OTs) are ideal to fill this role (Peterson and Clemson, 2008). A focus is on boosting follow through with safety behaviors by targeting those behaviors that have the most impact on reducing risk and reinforcing their application to the individual's home and community setting. The facilitator requires the capacity to engage the participants in reflection, problem solving, and behavioral change strategies. The program is suited to health professionals who work within a paradigm of enablement and empowerment (Townsend and Whiteford, 2005). An occupational therapist is required as an expert for the home environment sessions, various behavioral segments, and community safety segments.

Clinical Application

Stepping On is a community-based program (Clemson and Swann, 2008) that uses a small-group learning environment to improve fall self-efficacy, encourage behavioral change, and reduce the risk of falling.

In contrast to other prescriptive approaches, Stepping On enables the elderly to take control and explore different coping behaviors and safety strategies in their everyday lives.

The program is multifaceted and draws on evidence-based practice. At its core is a set of home-based balance and strength exercises known to be effective in fall prevention (Campbell et al., 1997). Other strategies include environmental and behavioral home safety, community safety, coping with visual loss, and regular visual screening and medication management.

Stepping On runs for seven 2-hour sessions with a follow-up home visit contact and a booster 3-month session Table 51.1. A team of content experts who are skilled in relevant aspects of falls prevention introduce key content areas. For example, we include a physiotherapist to teach the exercises in the initial stages of the program and a mobility officer from the Guide Dogs Association to introduce the strategies for coping with low vision. Information is shared and reinforced within the context of the group. Each session provides time for reflection and sharing accomplishments and ends in planning action and homework for the next week. The balance and strength training is practiced or reviewed each week, and one session includes a community mastery experience during which community mobility and discrete skills (e.g., negotiating grass or curb ramps) are practiced.

Table 51.1 Overview of stepping on, reducing falls and building confidence: a community-based prevention program (from Clemson et al., 2004)

Session 1: Introduction, Overview, and Risk Appraisal
Building trust, overview of program aims, sharing fall experiences, choosing what to cover, and introducing the balance and strength exercises.

Session 2: The Exercises and Moving About Safely
Review and practice exercises, explore the barriers and benefits of exercise, moving about safely, such as chairs and steps, learning not to panic after a fall.

Session 3: Home Hazards
Identify hazards in and about the home and problem-solving solutions.

Session 4: Community Safety and Footwear
Generate strategies to get around in the local community and reduce the risk of falling. Learn about the features of a safe shoe and identify clothing hazards.

Session 5: Vision and Falls, Vitamin D, and Hip Protectors
Recognize the influence of vision on risk of falling. Review strategies to reduce risk of falling from visual dysfunction. Identify the importance of vitamin D, sunlight, and calcium to protect from fall injury. Introduce the benefits of hip protectors for those fearful of hip fracture. Identify behavioural sleep alternatives to taking sedatives.

Session 6: Medication Management and Mobility Mastery Experiences
Identify medication risks and falls. Explore strategies to reduce risk of falls from medication side effects or misuse. Review of exercises, with opportunity for questions and upgrading. Review and further explore strategies for getting out in the local community safely. Or, for some participants, practice safe mobility techniques learnt during the program, in a nearby outdoor location. Identify strategies to assist in safely using buses.

Session 7: Review and Plan Ahead
Express personal accomplishments from the past 7 weeks and reflect on the scope of things learned. Review anything requested. Finish any segment not adequately completed. Determine safety strategies to protect against bag snatching. Identify strategies to assist in safely using trains. Time for farewells and closure.

Follow-up home visit: To support follow though of fall-prevention strategies and activities and to assist with home adaptations and modifications if required.

Three-month booster session: Review achievements and how to keep it going.

Evidence-Based Practice

The program was evaluated using a randomized trial (Clemson et al., 2004). The trial involved 310 community residents aged [370] years who had a fall in the previous 12 months or were concerned about falling. The primary outcome measure was falls, ascertained by using a monthly calendar for each participant. Results showed that after 14 months the intervention group had reduced falls by 31% ($p = .025$). There were better outcomes for those in the program in that they maintained their confidence in the more mobile activities of daily living (ADL) tasks (Mobility Efficacy Scale [MES], $p = .042$) used more protective behaviors (Fall Behavioral Scale for Older People [FaB], $p = 0.024$). They maintained their physical activity levels to a greater degree compared to the controls, though the difference in this latter finding did not reach significance.

Discussion

Stepping On is an effective program that is a viable option to include in a community fall prevention strategy. It builds individual capacity, enabling the elderly to reduce their risk of falling and regain their confidence. Follow-up support has been found to be an essential element of the program.

Further work is being done to explore the implementation and sustainability of programs like Stepping On within community services. Clemson is currently leading a team of researchers at the University of Sydney in a study to explore the implementation and sustainability of Stepping On with minority groups.

References

Bandura, A. (1977). Self-efficacy: toward a unifying theory of behavioural change. Psychol Rev, 84, 191–215.

Bandura, A. (1986). Social Foundations of Thought and Action: A Social Cognitive Theory. Englewood Cliffs, NJ: Prentice-Hall.

Campbell, A.J., Robertson, M.C., Gardner, M.M., Norton, R.N., Tilyard, M.W., and Buchner, D.M. (1997). Randomised controlled trial of a general practice programme of home based exercise to prevent falls in elderly women. Br Med J, 315(25), 1065–1069.

Clemson, L., Cumming, R.G., Kendig, H., Swann, M., Heard, R., and Taylor, K. (2004). The effectiveness of a community-based program for reducing the incidence of falls among the elderly: a randomized trial. J Am Geriatr Soc, 52(9), 1487–1494.

Clemson, L., MacKenzie, L., Ballinger, C., Close, J., and Cumming, R.G. (2008). Environmental interventions to prevent falls in community dwelling older people: a meta-analysis of randomized trials. J Aging Health, 20(8), 954–971.

Clemson, L., and Swann, M. (2008). Stepping On: Building Confidence and Reducing Falls. A Community Based Program for Older People, 2nd ed. Camperdown, Australia: Sydney University Press. info@sup.usyd.edu.au.

Clemson, L., Taylor, K., Cumming, R.G., Kendig, H., and Swann, M. (2007). Recruiting older participants to a randomized trial of a community-based falls prevention program. Australas J Ageing, 26(1), 35–39.

Egger, G., Spark, R., and Lawson, J. (1990). Health Promotion Strategies and Methods. Sydney: McGrath-Mill.

Gillespie, L.D., Gillespie, W.J., Robertson, M.C., Lamb, S.E., Cumming, R.G., and Rowe, B.H. (2005). Interventions for preventing falls in elderly people (Cochrane Review). Cochrane Database of Systematic Reviews . Art. No.: CD000340. DOI: 10.1002/14651858.CD000340.

Jacques, D. (2000). Learning in Groups: A Handbook for Improving Group Work, 3rd ed. London: Kogan Page.

Janis, I.L., and Mann, L. (1977). Decision Making: A Psychological Analysis of Conflict, Choice, and Commitment. New York: Macmillan.

Lack, H.W. (2005). Incidence and risk factors for developing fear of falling in older adults. Public Health Nursing, 22(1), 45–52.

O'Loughlin, J.L., Robitaille, Y., Boivin, J.-F., and Suissa, S. (1993). Incidence of and risk factors for falls and injurious falls among the community-dwelling elderly. Am J Epidemiol, 137(3), 342–354.

Peterson, L., and Clemson, L. (2008). Understanding the role of occupational therapy in fall prevention for community dwelling older adults. OT Pract, 13(3), CE1–8.

Tinetti, M.E., and Williams, C.S. (1997). Falls, injuries due to falls, and the risk of admission to a nursing home. N Engl J Med, 337(18), 1279–1284.

Townsend, E., and Whiteford, G. (2005). A participatory occupational justice framework. Population-based processes of practice. In: Kronenberg, F., Algado, S., and Poollard, N., eds. Occupational Therapy Without Borders. Learning from the Spirit of Survivors (pp. 210–226). London: Churchill Livingstone.

Vellas, B.J., Wayne, S.J., Romero, L.J., Baumgartner, R.N., and Garry, P.J. (1997). Fear of falling and restriction of mobility in elderly fallers. Age Ageing, 26(3), 189–193.

Chapter 52
Preventive Home Visits to the Elderly and Education of Home Visitors

Kirsten Avlund and Mikkel Vass

A brief, manageable, and ongoing educational intervention of professionals making preventive home visits is feasible and improves older people's functional mobility and reduces the need for institutional living.

Abstract Functional decline can be prevented in older home dwelling people through education of preventive home visitors and local general practitioners. Education was based on simple messages and professional routines respecting local health care cultures. Education must be ongoing, and 80-year-olds benefit more than 75-year-olds. There may be gender differences for beneficial effects, and organizational factors may be of importance. The number and regularity of visits are of importance, and if it is the same visitor each time, he or she can establish good rapport during the visits.

Keywords Education • Effectiveness study • Older people • Preventive home visits

Definitions and Background

The aging demography of many welfare societies highlights the need to prevent disability in later life. In professional health care education and clinical practice, little attention has been given to geriatrics and interdisciplinary care, but there is ample opportunity to improve interventions among older persons through educational programs (Gill, 2005).

Proactive assessment schemes give primary health care providers new opportunities to enhance active life expectancy (Beswick et al., 2008). Preventive home visit programs for community-dwelling older adults seem to reduce disability (Huss et al., 2008).

Preventive home visits constitute a *dynamic* process aiming at establishing *relations* that, within the framework of the community and senior citizen policies, allow the elderly to preserve or improve the long-term possibilities of leading a good,

I. Söderback (ed.), *International Handbook of Occupational Therapy Interventions*,
DOI: 10.1007/978-0-387-75424-6_52, © Springer Science+Business Media, LLC 2010

independent life without disability, postponing the need for any help (Vass et al., 2006, 2007a).

The content of preventive home visits should encompass the following:

- Trustful contact
- Structured interview
- Overall assessment
- Agreements and management plans
- Follow-up

The key elements of assessment are as follows:

- Functional ability
- Mobility
- Medication
- Nutrition
- Mental problems
- Falls
- Incontinence
- Social isolation
- Hearing, vision, and chiropody
- Social events
- Moving
- Bereavement

A preventive home visitation program was established in Denmark by legislation in 1998 (Danish Ministry of Social Affairs, 1995). Municipalities are obliged to offer preventive home visits twice a year to all home-dwelling citizens 75 years and older. Visits do not comprise a health check. The act aims at supporting personnel resources, networking, and social support. Hospital, general practice, and community services are all fully tax financed in Denmark.

Purpose

The aim of preventive home visits is to prevent or delay the onset of impairments and activity limitations, and to sustain social participation. The aim of education of preventive home visitors is to optimize the preventive home visits, so that larger proportions of older people may obtain enhanced life expectancy.

Besides attaining concrete offers of assistance and support, the elderly who are visited by preventive staff gain confidence in the public sector's ability to assist if the need should later arise, which creates a sense of security in their daily lives. If they live alone or have small network of family or friends, or have none, the visit also gives them the important message that they are not forgotten. The approach to each individual also enables local authorities to establish contact with people with whom they would otherwise not be in touch.

Method

Candidates for the Intervention

Educational programs for staff in Danish municipalities are not routinely offered. Home visitors have different professional backgrounds and are mainly nurses, occupational therapists, and physiotherapists. Some municipalities also employ especially trained social workers in the program.

Epidemiology

After 10 years of a national program offering free preventive home visits to the home-dwelling elderly, approximately 60% of the targeted population accepts and receives the visits; the percentage increases with increasing age. The program is a part of the home care system in 40% of the municipalities, and in another 40% it is a separate section under the social municipality department. Fourteen percent choose to let the program be a separate section in relation to different groupings of elderly based on frailty. Less than 50% of municipalities have made specific guidelines and quality assurance indicators, and more than the half have systematically used the visits to collect information on community needs and desires of the elderly, which is used for administrative and political purposes.

   Almost all municipalities contact the targeted group of elderly by letter, and continue to inform them regularly and at least yearly about the possibility of a home visit.

Settings

Preventive home visits are offered as part of routine primary care in Danish municipalities. All persons aged 75 and older are offered two preventive home visits per year. Beginning in 2005, the elderly who are receiving both personal and practical help may be excluded from the public offer.

The Role of the Occupational Therapist

The occupational therapist (OT) as well as the other preventive home visitors are expected to be updated on social and health aspects in general and are able to assess, at a certain qualified level, the older person's general condition, housing conditions, finances, and social conditions. Thus, visitors should be acquainted with the availability of technical aids that can ease daily life, such as communication aids, assistance with home refurbishment (e.g., changed toilet and bathing arrangements or removal of doorsteps), personal and practical assistance, and personal financial assistance (Vass, et al., 2007a). Furthermore, the preventive staff must be well informed of the local authority's and voluntary associations' activity and visiting programs, have general knowledge on aging, and also be competent communicators.

Results

Clinical Application

Organization and Target Group

There is scarce evidence on how visitation programs are best organized and managed. Feasibility may be associated with local and national health and social care cultures. Considerable differences in structure make it difficult to know which part of the management process and medical assessment of most value. It is evident that the follow-up element is of crucial importance, but the optimal number of visits to offer per year is not known. It seems relevant to individualize the program according to the client's personality, and functional and social status, but after the age of 80 assessments once a year should catch the increasing rate of geriatric problems.

The Home Visit

Preventive home visits are an offer that the elderly may choose to accept or refuse. The person accepting the offer decides what he or she wants to divulge or discuss. However, the interview is supposed to focus on the client's general needs, and is always conducted on the client's premises (Vass et al., 2006).

Particular matters such as how the client copes with daily activities, social contacts, housing conditions, finances, physical performance, and general health are natural subjects for discussion. The interview gives the visitor a basis for providing information on and referrals to preventive and activating programs while also advising on the availability of social service, housing, or health services.

If such advice cannot immediately solve existing problems, the local authority is required to launch the necessary initiatives, such as providing technical aids that can ease the daily life; personal and practical help; or, contingent on the client's acceptance, medical assistance.

Education of Home Visitors

The educational program includes the following:

• Initial interdisciplinary introduction of what is accepted to be the best practice for all professionals involved in preventive home visits.

- Ongoing education of two key persons (e.g., occupational therapists, nurses, physiotherapists, and social workers) from each municipality, and followed up twice a year.
- Small group-based education of the local general practitioners.

The educational training focuses on relevant gerontologic and geriatric problems. It is based on updated preventive tasks for elderly people (Williams et al., 2002). The main content of the education for the key persons are as follows:

- To emphasize the importance of psychological, social, as well as health factors at the home visits. It is important to include the health dimension in the assessment during the visit, but no specific physical or mental examination is recommended.
- To focus on early signs of disability. Systematic and unexplained fatigue in daily activities (Avlund et al., 2007b) should be seen as an early trigger of functional decline. This measure is a strong predictor of later dependency on health and social services (Avlund et al., 2006). Two easily administered tests of functional ability are recommended (Avlund et al., 1996; Podsiadlo and Richardson, 1991).
- To support the client's resources and facilitate empowering strategies and social relations with respect to the individual's autonomy.
- To stress the importance of physical activity and stimulate the communities to facilitate participation in physical activities through convenient transportation and sports for elderly people.
- To focus on relevant geriatric problems, such as prevention of falls, mental problems, medication, incontinence, and nutrition.
- To inform the client about local services, such as gardening help, meals on wheels, and other social or health services if relevant.
- To encourage interdisciplinary follow-up in relation to the other social and health professionals at the local level, including the general practitioners.
- To inform about the relevance of practicing good communication techniques with the elderly relating to the personal contacts with the home visitors.

The main content of the general practitioners' education is recommended to do the following:

- Avoid ageism.
- Take any encounter initiated by the home visitors seriously.
- Use a short geriatric assessment strategy (Vass et al., 2005).

How the Intervention Eases Impairments, Activity Limitations, and Participation Restrictions

Results from a Danish effectiveness study have shown that the above-listed education points delayed functional decline in the elderly living in the intervention municipalities (Avlund et al., 2007c; Vass et al., 2005). The strongest effects were seen among the oldest and among the women, and even 1½ years after the end of the intervention (Avlund et al., 2007a). Eighty-year-old men and women who lived in the intervention municipalities were more likely to recover after early signs of activity limitations, measured as fatigue in daily activities (Avlund et al., 2007a; Vass et al., 2005). Varying patterns of change in activities were found after 4½ years, such as progressive, catastrophic, or reversible decline. The intervention had the largest effect on progressive activity limitation (Vass et al., 2007b). Furthermore, intervention was associated with change in physical activity among the inactive 80-year-old women. A larger proportion of these inactive women became more physically active during the intervention period, if they lived in an intervention municipality compared with living in a control municipality (Poulsen et al., 2007).

A qualitative study of the organization of the preventive home visits identified three distinct strategies for preventive home visitation programs. Municipalities' management styles could be categorized as framework management or management by rules. Smaller municipalities were associated with the framework management type. Management by rules municipalities had smaller population densities and their overall expenses for older people were higher. Framework management municipalities used more resources on preventive home visits, communicated better, experienced less staff turnover, and had higher social capital than management by rules municipalities (Vass et al., 2007c).

The cost-effectiveness of the educational intervention showed that intervention was cost-neutral, that is, that the intervention was associated with improved life expectancy for the same costs (Kronborg et al., 2006).

Evidence-Based Practice

During the last 20 years several randomized efficacy trials have shown that preventive home visits have beneficial effects on mortality, hospital admissions, and functional ability (Stuck et al., 2002).

Preconditions for effects are that the visit includes a multidimensional approach, that is, social, psychological, and health aspects and multidimensional interdisciplinary follow-up (Huss et al., 2008).

Discussion

The basis of the described results from the Danish effectiveness study on preventive home visits must be kept in mind. First, the Danish health care system fully finances hospitals, general practices, and community services through taxation. Second, the national in-home preventive assessment programs were usually conducted by skilled district nurses, occupational therapists, physiotherapists, and social workers who focused on establishing a trustful relationship, and who were encouraged to raise issues of everyday life relevance and to offer general health-promoting advice and guidance. If appropriate, health or social problems were identified so that practical or personal support could be established in the local setting. Follow-up visits were able to assess changes over time. Third, municipalities were motivated and had at least a fair possibility of promoting rehabilitation. They all agreed to uphold the legislation, and to join a scientific study, and they had the political support to act on clients' relevant needs, and to solve identified problems that turned up during the home visits.

The findings may have widespread application, because of the highly feasible nature of the intervention and the use of structured guidelines that paved the way for easy implementation in regional education.

The intervention effect was clearly stronger in the 80-year-old age group. The effects increased when home visitors, as well as general practitioners were presented with the assessment tools and instructed how to use and interpret them. This underlines the often claimed need for qualified interdisciplinary education, and is fully in agreement with recent research (Beswick et al., 2008; Huss et al., 2008) and with our intention of testing a simple tool for managing problems often occurring among older people.

It is important to be alert to clients' fatigue in daily activities because it triggers activity limitations in the individual assessment situation. It is also important to promote a common language for primary care professionals.

Education of the staff is a key factor in obtaining better practice settings. Targeting the nondisabled with preventive home visits that are followed-up in an integrated preventive primary care program may be an efficient way of organizing the prevention of functional decline in older people. Multifactorial and complex interventions can be tailored to meet individuals' needs and preferences, and might help the elderly live safely and independently (Beswick, 2008).

References

Avlund, K., Kreiner, S., and Schultz-Larsen, K. (1996). Functional ability scales for the elderly. A validation study. Eur J Public Health, 6, 35–42.

Avlund, K., Rantanen, T., and Schroll, M. (2006). Tiredness and subsequent disability in older adults. The role of walking limitations. J Gerontol A Biol Sci Med Sci, 61, 1201–1205.

Avlund, K., Rantanen, T., and Schroll, M. (2007a). Factors underlying tiredness in older adults. Aging Clin Exp Res, 19, 16–25.

Avlund, K., Vass, M., and Hendriksen, C. (2007b). Education of preventive home visitors. The effect on tiredness in daily activities. Eur J Ageing, 4, 125–131.

Avlund, K., Vass, M., Kvist, K., Hendriksen, C., and Keiding, N. (2007c). Educational intervention toward preventive home visitors reduced functional decline in community-living older women. J Clin Epidemiol, 60, 954–962.

Beswick, A.D., Rees, K., Dieppe, P., et al. (2008). Complex interventions to improve physical function and maintain independent living in elderly people: a systematic review and meta-analysis. Lancet, 371, 725–735

Danish Ministry of Social Affairs. (1995). Law 1117.

Gill, T.M. (2005). Education, prevention, and the translation of research into practice. J Am Geriatr Soc, 53, 724–726.

Huss, A., Stuck, A.E., Rubenstein, L.Z., Egger, M., and Clough-Gorr, K.M. (2008). Multidimensional preventive home visit programs for community-dwelling older adults: a systematic review and meta-analysis of randomized controlled trials. J Geront A Biol Sci Med Sci, 63, 298–307.

Kronborg, C., Vass, M., Lauridsen, J., and Avlund, K. (2006). Cost effectiveness of preventive home visits to the elderly. Economic evaluation alongside randomized controlled study. Eur J Health Econ, 7, 238–246.

Podsiadlo, D., and Richardson, S. (1991). The timed "Up and Go": A test of basic functional mobility for frail elderly persons. J Am Geriat Soc, 39, 142–148.

Poulsen, T., Elkjaer, E., Vass, M., Hendriksen, C., and Avlund, K. (2007). Promoting physical activity in older adults by education of home visitors. Eur J Ageing, 4, 114–124.

Stuck, A.E., Egger, M., Hammer, A., Minder, C.E., and Beck, J.C. (2002). Home visits to prevent nursing home admission and functional decline in elderly people. Systematic review and meta-regression analysis. JAMA, 287, 1022–1028.

Vass, M., Avlund, K., and Hendriksen, C. (2006). Older people and preventive home visits. AgeForum, 1–45. http://www.aeldreforum.dk.

Vass, M., Avlund, K., Hendriksen, C., Philipson, L., and Riis, P. (2007a). Preventive home visits to older people in Denmark: Why, how, by whom, and when? Z Gerontol Geriatr, 40(4), 209–216.

Vass, M., Avlund, K., Lauridsen, J., and Hendriksen, C. (2005). A feasible model for prevention of functional decline in older people. A municipality-randomised controlled trial. J Am Geriatr Soc, 53, 563–568.

Vass, M., Avlund, K., Paner, E.T., and Hendriksen, C. (2007b). Preventive home visits to older home-dwelling people and different functional decline patterns. Eur J Ageing, 4, 107–113.

Vass, M., Holmberg, R., Nielsen, H.F., Lauridsen, J., Avlund, K., and Hendriksen, C. (2007c). Preventive home visitation programmes for older people: The role of municipality organisation. Eur J Ageing, 4, 133–140.

Williams, I.E., Junius, U., Jones, D., et al. (2002). An evidence-based approach to assessing older people in primary care. The Royal College of General Practitioners, Occasional Paper 82. http://www.rcgp.org.uk/services__publications/history_heritage__archives/history__chronology/chronology/chronology_by_subject/publications.aspx.

Chapter 53
Issues Related to the Use of In-Vehicle Intelligent Transport Systems by Drivers with Functional Impairments

Marilyn Di Stefano and Wendy Macdonald

The parking aid helped Sam to position the vehicle appropriately in the parking space, despite his neck range of movement restrictions.

Abstract The use of in-vehicle intelligent transport systems (ITSs) by drivers undertaking driver evaluation and rehabilitation with occupational therapy driver assessors (OTDAs) is discussed. Key issues related to the use of ITSs by drivers with functional impairments are outlined, and general principles to guide practice in this field are proposed.

Keywords Driving • Driver evaluation and rehabilitation • Intelligent transport systems • ITSs

Background

Prior to any on-road assessment, occupational therapy driver assessors (OTDAs) undertake a range of clinical evaluations to understand clients' abilities and limitations relevant to driving. Such assessments establish that clients' sensorimotor and perceptual/cognitive abilities, along with their more general psychological characteristics, are adequate for driving. Also, the client must meet medical and licensing prerequisites as specified in applicable guidelines (e.g., American Medical Association and National Highway Traffic Safety Administration, 2003; Austroads, 2003; Canadian Medical Association, 2006). Then the OTDA usually conducts an in-car evaluation of driving performance.

In-car assessment is usually required because (1) there is typically a significant degree of variation in the performance abilities of clients within any particular medical diagnostic category, so that diagnosis alone cannot be relied upon in establishing exclusion criteria (for example, see Di Stefano and Macdonald, 2003a; Lovell and Russell, 2005); (2) the capacity of clinical assessments to predict on-road driving performance is not high (Bedard et al., 2008; Molnar et al., 2006); and (3) driving errors can have fatal consequences (Di Stefano and Macdonald, 2006a).

I. Söderback (ed.), *International Handbook of Occupational Therapy Interventions*,
DOI: 10.1007/978-0-387-75424-6_53, © Springer Science+Business Media, LLC 2010

An emerging issue for OTDAs is the possible use by their clients of in-vehicle intelligent transport systems (ITSs). Such systems may play a positive role by reducing the difficulty of the driver's task, but their impact is likely to be negative if they add to task complexity or distract attention from more important aspects of driving.

Definitions

In broad terms, ITSs include any computer-based system that permits advanced sensing, processing, communications, or control technologies to be applied to any system component related to the driver controlling a vehicle on a road within a road-traffic environment (Regan et al., 2001).

The ITSs of most immediate relevance to OTDAs are those that require some allocation of driver attention while driving. They may be either customized (applied postproduction) or available as standard vehicle devices supporting driver performance and offering safety benefits. Common examples include cruise control systems, navigation systems, parking assistance devices, alternative steering devices (such as joystick or multifunction steering wheel systems), and electronic secondary control systems for indicators, lights, horn, and environmental controls (Kalina and Green, 2006; Whelan et al., 2006).

Purpose

Consideration of the potential ways in which use of an ITS may impact upon the person–activity–environment fit will help occupational therapists (OTs) appreciate how such devices might aid or hinder the achievement of driving independence by a client.

The purpose of this chapter is to explore the issues that OTDAs need to consider when evaluating an individual client's use of an ITS and prescribing related interventions.

Method

Candidates for the Intervention

Any person of driving age with impairments or functional limitations who otherwise meets required medical standards and has the potential to be an independent driver may be considered for ITSs prescription. ITSs may eliminate, overcome, or compensate for the driver's restrictions. For example, they may reduce the effects of major motor-sensory or minor visual or cognitive impairments on performance in monitoring the traffic situation, or in maintaining good control of the vehicle. Drivers with amputations, reduced limb or spine function, or some mild cognitive limitations may be suitable candidates.

Frequency of Use

Although OTDAs commonly consider the application of vehicle modifications including ITSs during assessments (Wheatley and DiStefano, 2008), little is known about the nature or extent of the uptake of these technologies by people with disabilities. It is likely, however, that as ITSs become more popular and are increasingly included as standard features in domestic vehicles, their availability and use will increase in the future. Further, as greater numbers of people look upon driving as their main form of transportation and as the proportion of people who are older and have disabilities increase (OECD, 2001), the application of customized devices to support driving independence is likely to gain in popularity.

Settings

Consideration of ITS applications most commonly occurs during the initial phases of an occupational therapy assessment, when impairments and functional limitations are discussed and evaluated in relation to the client's driving needs and vehicle characteristics.

The Role of the Occupational Therapist

Occupational therapists play a major role in assisting individuals with performance limitations to achieve or resume independence in personal and community mobility. For some clients, this may include assistance to commence or resume driving a motor vehicle. Generalist OTs consider a broad range of mobility options and issues with their clients, while specialist OTDAs, who have particular expertise in driver evaluation and rehabilitation, consider in more detail the requirements of this very important instrumental activity of daily living (Stav, 2004).

Results

Clinical Application

An Assessment Framework: Human Information Processing

In evaluating the fit between a particular client and a specific ITS, it is useful to conceptualize the driving task as one of processing information. A simple model of the human as a processor of information is depicted in Fig. 53.1. This shows an

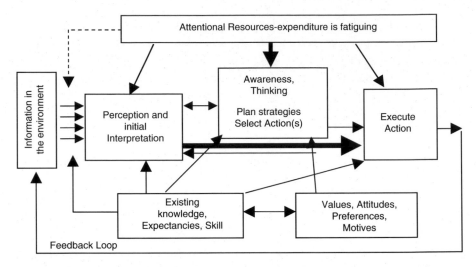

Fig. 53.1 A generic depiction of how people "process" information during activities such as driving. (From Macdonald, 2004, with permission.).

individual's sensory uptake and subsequent perception of information from the environment, leading to the execution of vehicle control actions, from which there is feedback that is then available for perception, and so on. It can be seen that between perception and action, there might be very little demand for expenditure of attentional resources (shown by the large arrow bypassing conscious awareness), or, if there is a need for conscious decision-making, a large amount of attention might be needed (Macdonald et al., 2006).

Such a model can help the OT to identify the critical aspects of a client's interactions with an ITS. Driver deficits affecting any stage of information perception, cognition, and subsequent response processes can affect the quality of driver interaction with the ITS, with consequent impacts on their driving performance. There are various possible means of addressing deficits in one or more aspects of a driver's information processing abilities, including driver remediation, training such as in compensatory strategies, customized (re)design of the ITS interface, or modifications to the task or environment such as by route planning to avoid complex intersections.

Assessment Issues: Evaluating Quality of the Fit Between Driver Abilities and the Demands of Interacting with an ITS

The OTDAs need to consider the client's preexisting driving experience and skills, their presenting limitations, and how effects of these limitations might be either ameliorated or exacerbated by use of an ITS (Di Stefano and Macdonald,

2006b). In addition, the client's access to vehicles and available funding for modifications needs to be considered in relation to their driving requirements and expectations (Di Stefano and Macdonald, 2003b). For example, consider the use of an advanced technology steering system by someone with reduced motor control. The client's successful performance will be dependent on the following:

- *Human factors*: whether or not the driver has adequate attentional resources to cope with the demands of the concurrent subtasks that comprise the overall driving task, including the demands of interacting with the ITS (Regan, 2004).
- *Interface design factors*: the fit between the driver's hand and the ITS control; the quality of feedback information from the device to the driver, whether proprioceptive, auditory, or visual, which determines whether degree of movement can be easily perceived with sufficient accuracy.
- *Task and environmental complexity:* affect the difficulty of various driving subtasks, such as steering an appropriate path, including avoidance of contact with other road users; maintaining an appropriate speed; obeying all road laws.

Table 53.1 depicts some common health/disability conditions, and their possible implications for ITS use. The examples given here illustrate that the process of matching driver needs and abilities to the characteristics of an ITS can be quite complex.

Evidence-Based Practice

Much of the recent research examining ITSs has drawn upon the theory and body of literature examining cognitive information processing. For example, there is now a considerable body of research evidence demonstrating the information processing demands and consequent road safety risks of using a mobile phone while driving (Patten et al., 2004; see McCartt et al., 2006 for a recent review).

There is also research demonstrating distraction effects, attentional resource demands, and more general impact upon driving behaviors of some in-vehicle communication and information devices (see Blanco et al., 2006, and Young et al., 2003, for a review). Some studies have considered these issues in relation to older drivers (Horberry et al., 2006; Strayer and Drews, 2004; Vrkljan and Miller, 2007).

However, there is still relatively little evidence specifically on the use of ITSs by drivers with various disabilities. Current publications in the disability literature referring to ITS use typically take the form of descriptive accounts, viewpoints, or reviews (Baldwin, 2002; Bouman and Pellerito, 2006; Landau, 2002; Murray-Leslie, 1997; Pellerito and Burt, 2006). There is a paucity of more targeted research examining ITS issues for drivers with particular types of impairment. In this context, OTDAs must keep up to date with new research developments, as well as being guided in their practice by applicable standards relating to ITSs (see Abram, 2004, for an outline of current international standards).

Table 53.1 Examples of common health/disability issues, related impairments, and their impact upon the use or need for intelligent transport systems (ITSs)

Health condition/disability	Example of long-term impairment	Possible functional impact of disability on driving	Potential difficulties/benefits of common ITSs
Spinal cord injury	Limited hand and upper limb function	May impact upon use of steering wheel	Difficulty using standard steering wheel, but potential to use alternative steering devices (e.g., hand controls, joy stick)
Dementia	Reduced/variable memory	May forget to apply seat belt, check to rear of vehicle when reversing	Seat-belt reminder and vehicle reversing systems may provide visual and auditory cues to support appropriate behaviors
Acquired brain injury	Reduced information processing, arousal and executive functions	Automatic vehicle systems that demand a significant level of driver attention may degrade other aspects of driving performance	Application and use of cruise/speed control and vehicle positioning systems need to be carefully evaluated
			Need to evaluate driver tendency to multitask (e.g., use mobile phone, in-vehicle entertainment), since this reduces the drivers capacity to attend to core components of the driving task
Arthritis	Joint stiffness in neck/upper spine	Difficulty with neck/trunk rotation required for checking external mirrors and performing head check	Parking aid and vehicle reversing systems used in conjunction with internal mirrors may compensate for physical restriction

Conclusion

Many technologies are being applied to the domestic motor vehicle. Those that interact directly with the driver may simplify the driving task, or, conversely, may make it more complex, particularly for drivers who may be accommodating new impairments, be unfamiliar with the specific interface requirements, or have limited experience with problem solving when such systems break down. Further, there may be a greater need for interdisciplinary collaboration around ITS prescription and training as greater choice and complexity complicates product specification.

As more vehicles equipped with ITSs become available, there will be an increasing need for both generalist and specialist driver assessor OTs to be cognizant of, and evaluate, the potential risks and benefits these technologies present for drivers with functional limitations. This chapter has discussed some of the key factors that need to be considered by OTs responsible for considering driving-related issues with their clients.

References

Abram, F. (2004). Safe driving. ISO Focus: The Magazine of the International Organization for Standardization, March, 7–10.

American Medical Association and National Highway Traffic Safety Administration. (2003). Physician's Guide to Assessing and Counseling Older Drivers. http://www.amassn.org/ama/pub/category/10791.html.

Austroads. (2003). Assessing Fitness to Drive: For Commercial and Private Vehicle Drivers: Medical Standards for Licensing and Clinical Management Guidelines, 3rd ed. Sydney: Austroads.

Baldwin, C. (2002). Designing in-vehicle technologies for older drivers: application of sensory-cognitive interaction theory. Theoret Issues Ergonom Sci, 3(4), 307–329.

Bedard, M., Weaver, B., Darzins, P., and Porter, M.M. (2008). Predicting driving performance in older adults: we are not there yet! Paper presented at the International Conference on Aging, Disability and Independence, St. Petersburg, FL.

Blanco, J., Biever, W.J., Gallagher, J.P., and Dingus, T.A. (2006). The impact of secondary task cognitive processing demand on driving performance. Accid Anal Prevent, 38(5), 895–906.

Bouman, J., and Pellerito, J. (2006). Preparing for the On-Road Evaluation. St. Louis, MO: Elsevier Mosby.

Canadian Medical Association. (2006). Determining Medical Fitness to Operate Motor Vehicles. http://www.cma.ca/multimedia/CMA/Content_Images/Inside_cma/WhatWePublish/Drivers_Guide/Contents_e.pdf.

Di Stefano, M., and Macdonald, W. (2003a). Assessment of older drivers: relationships among on-road errors, medical conditions and test outcome. J Saf Res, 34(5), 415–429.

Di Stefano, M., and Macdonald, W. (2003b). Intelligent transport systems and occupational therapy practice. Occup Ther Int, 10(1), 56–74.

Di Stefano, M., and Macdonald, W. (2006a). On-the-road evaluation of driving performance. In: Pellerito, J., ed. Driver Rehabilitation and Community Mobility: Principles and Practice (pp. 255–274). St. Louis, MO: Elsevier Health Sciences.

Di Stefano, M., and Macdonald, W. (2006b). In-vehicle intelligent transport systems. In: Pellerito, J., ed. Driver Rehabilitation and Community Mobility: Principles and Practice (pp. 373–390). St Louis, MO: Elsevier Health Sciences.

Horberry, T., Anderson, J., Regan, M.A., Triggs, T.J., and Brown, J. (2006). Driver distraction: The effects of concurrent in-vehicle tasks, road environment complexity and age on driving performance. *Accid Anal Prevent*, 38, 185–191.

Kalina, T.D., and Green, E.L. (2006). Developing a driver rehabilitation program. In: Pellerito, J., ed. Driver Rehabilitation and Community Mobility: Principles and Practice (pp. 521–537). St. Louis, MO: Elsevier Mosby.

Landau, K. (2002). Usability criteria for intelligent driver assistance systems. *Theoret Issues Ergonom Sci*, 3(4), 330–345.

Lovell, R., and Russell, K. (2005). Developing referral and reassessment criteria for drivers with dementia. *Aust Occup Ther J*, 52, 26–33.

Macdonald, W. (2004). Human error: causes and countermeasures. In: Proceedings of the Safety in Action Conference 2004. Victoria: Safety Institute of Australia, Victorian Division.

Macdonald, W., Pellerito, J., and Di Stefano, M. (2006). Introduction to driver rehabilitation and community mobility. In: Pellerito, J., ed. Driver Rehabilitation and Community Mobility: Principles and Practice (pp. 5–35). Philadelphia: Elsevier.

McCartt, A.T., Hellinga, L.A., and Bratiman, K.A. (2006). Cell phones and driving: review of research. *Traffic Injury Prevent*, 7, 89–106.

Molnar, F.J., Patel, A., Marshall, S., Man-Son-Hing, M., and Wilson, K.G. (2006). Clinical utility of office-based cognitive predictors of fitness to drive in persons with dementia: A systematic review. *J Am Geriatr Soc*, 54, 1809–1824.

Murray-Leslie, C. (1997). Driving Independently. In: Goodwill, C.J., Chamberlain, M.A., and Evans, C., eds. Rehabilitation of the Physically Disabled Adult, 2nd ed. (pp. 709–726). Cheltenham, UK: Stanley Thornes.

Organization for Economic Co-Operative Development. (2001). Aging and Transport: Mobility Needs and Transport Issues: OECD Report. Geneva, Switzerland: Organization for Economic Co-Operative Development.

Patten, C.J.D., Kircher, A., Ostlund, J., and Nilsson, L. (2004). Using mobile telephones: cognitive workload and attention resource allocation. *Accid Anal Prevent*, 36, 341–350.

Pellerito, J., and Burt, C.J. (2006). The Adapted Driving Decision Guide. St. Louis, MO: Elsevier Mosby.

Regan, M.A. (2004). A sign of the future II: human factors. In: Castro, C., and Horberry, T., eds. The Human Factors of Transport Signs (pp. 225–238). USA: CRC.

Regan, M.A., Oxley, J.A., Godley, S., and Tingvall, C. (2001). Intelligent Transport Systems: Safety and Human Factors Issues (Literature Review). Victoria, Australia: Royal Automobile Club of Victoria.

Stav, W.B. (2004). Driving Rehabilitation: A Guide for Assessment and Intervention. San Antonio: PsychCorp.

Strayer, D., and Drews, F. (2004). Profiles in driver distraction: effects of cell phone conversations on younger and older Drivers. *Hum Factors*, 46(4), 640–649.

Vrkljan, B.H., and Miller, P.J. (2007). Driving, navigation and vehicular technology: experiences of older drivers and their co-pilots. *Traffic Injury Prevent*, 8, 403–410.

Wheatley, C., and Di Stefano, M. (2008). Individualized assessment of driving fitness for older individuals with health, disability and age-related concerns. Traffic Inj Prev 9 (4), 320-327.

Whelan, M., Langford, J., Oxley, J., Koppel, S., and Charlton, J. (2006). The Elderly and Mobility: A Review of the Literature. http://www.monash.edu.au/muarc/reports/muarc255.html.

Young, K., Regan, M., and Hammer, M. (2003). Driver Distraction: A Review of the Literature. Melbourne: Monash University Accident Research Centre.

Chapter 54
Work-Related Health: Organizational Factors and Well-Being

Gudbjörg Linda Rafnsdottir and Thamar Melanie Heijstra

There is a connection between poor work organization and distress among employees.

Abstract Today a large proportion of the population in Western societies is in the labor market. As absenteeism due to illness has reached such a level that it is now perceived as an economic problem, it is of major importance to map out the causes of, prevent future absenteeism, and improve the health of employees. By discussing the job strain model and the effort-reward imbalance model, this chapter provides some insight into the connection between the work organization and the well-being of its employees. The importance of risk assessment is discussed, as it provides a method for staff members to become aware of the organizational factors that affect their well-being. If absenteeism due to illness among workers can be reduced, it will have positive effects for everyone involved, not only for workers and their organizations but for society as well.

Keywords Burnout • Organizational risk factors • Risk analysis • Well-being • Work-related stress

Background

This chapter discusses the connection between the work organization and the well-being of employees. Too high a work load and a lack of psychosocial well-being are two of the biggest health and safety challenges that we face in the Western labor market today.

Job stress affects the well-being of millions of people throughout the world, and absence from work due to sickness has been defined as an economic problem. The lack of well-being and the use of sick leave are partly related to the employees' work situation (Rafnsdottir et al., 2004; Siegrist and Marmot, 2004; Virtanen et al., 2005). Stress may also threaten workplace safety. The changing world of work is making increased demands on workers, through downsizing and outsourcing, increasing use of temporary contracts, increasing job insecurity, higher workload, more pressure, and poor work–life balance.

I. Söderback (ed.), *International Handbook of Occupational Therapy Interventions*,
DOI: 10.1007/978-0-387-75424-6_54, © Springer Science+Business Media, LLC 2010

A study on work organization and well-being in the field of geriatric care showed, for example, that mental exhaustion and finding work mentally difficult were associated with a number of factors that related to the organization of work, such as time pressure, bad communication with supervisors, and difficulty in harmonizing demands and expectations of patients, employees, and supervisors (Rafnsdottir et al., 2004).

The organization of work and the psychosocial work environment can even be risk factors for musculoskeletal disorders. Gunnarsdottir et al. (2003) showed that mental exhaustion and having been exposed to harassment, violence, or threats at work are workplace factors that are associated with discomfort in the neck and back of the head, shoulders, and lower back among women working in geriatric care. Dissatisfaction with supervisors, lack of information at work, failure to be consulted about intended changes, and lack of solidarity in the workplace also played an important role for one or more musculoskeletal symptoms.

Purpose

Taking the organization of work into account leads not only to healthier work forces but also to workplaces that are more productive and thus results in a better economy. Workplace illness leaves everybody involved disadvantaged. There is the human cost for workers and their families and the cost of reduced productivity for organizations. There are costs for governments as well, as illness and accidents place a burden on health care systems. Workplace health is therefore also a public health issue (European Network for Workplace Health Promotion [ENWHP], 2008; Siegrist and Marmot, 2004; Virtanen et al., 2005).

Method

Candidates for the Intervention

Different from many other risk factors, organizational and psychosocial factors are found in any sector and in any size of work organization. The focus on the organizational work environment has become stronger as the world of work is undergoing change, due to factors like globalization, increasing use of information technology, changes in employment practice, and the increasing importance of the service job sector in Western countries. This has led to new methods for analyzing organizational risk factors at work.

A frequently used method is risk *assessment*. It can be used to evaluate systematically the risks to workers' health and safety. If used correctly, it can enable employers and employees to identify and understand the action they need to take to eliminate or minimize the risks at the workplace. It looks at all aspects of the workplace and the work itself, considering what could cause harm, whether hazards, accident risks, longer term health risks, or illness can be eliminated, and, if not, what preventive or protective measures should be put in place [European Network for Workplace Health Promotion (ENWHP), 2008 a].

Epidemiology

According to the Health and Safety Laboratory (HSL) (2008), 2.3 million people in United Kingdom (UK) were suffering from an illness in 2001 and 2002, which they believed was caused or made worse by their current or past work. This prevalence estimate includes long-standing as well as new cases. Moreover, over half a million people in UK experience work-related stress and at a level that was making them ill. In addition, up to 5 million people in the UK feel, their work is very or extremely stressful, and in 2004 and 2005, 12.8 million working days were lost to stress, depression, or anxiety. Stress has also surpassed musculoskeletal disorders as the biggest contributor to absenteeism because of work-related stress illnesses. This can have major impact on other elements of business, such as productivity, organizational image, health and safety, and morale.

According to the European Agency for Safety and Health at Work (2008), stress was the second most reported work-related health problem in 2005 in Europe, affecting 22% of the workers.

A telephone survey among 1003 American employees showed that 54% of the participants had at least sometimes felt overworked in the past 3 months. About 90% agreed somewhat or strongly that they had been feeling time pressure relating to having to work faster or harder, and in order to be able to finish a job. Sixty percent of the participants often, or very often, had difficulties focusing on their work, experienced frequent work interruptions, and felt they had to handle too many tasks at the same time (Galinsky et al., 2001).

Where gender differences are concerned, women were found to feel more overworked than men did, and women were reported to have more jobs that are demanding. They were more frequently interrupted at work, and had to perform multiple tasks, without receiving appropriate time to do so. However, when men and women with these same complaints were compared to each other, the gender difference in feeling overworked disappeared (Galinsky et al., 2001).

In this study, the consequences of being overworked became clear as well. Not only are overworked employees likely to experience more work–family conflict, to neglect themselves, and to sleep less, but they are also significantly less likely to report their health as very good or excellent (Galinsky et al., 2001).

The Role of the Therapist

Traditional occupational health and safety methods are used by labor inspectorates and social insurance institutions to ensure that the laws of health and safety in the workplace and regulations are followed. Such inspections are important and have improved health in the workplace by reducing accidents and preventing occupational diseases and illnesses. However, in recent decades it has become clearer that sustainable health promotion and prevention calls for collaboration across different professions and policy fields, especially when working with organizational factors. Cooperating partners can be experts from public health sciences working in research institutions or academia, as well as experts representing the field of occupational health and safety, labor inspectorates, social insurance institutions, and consulting services (ENWHP, 2008b). The attempt to mainstream occupational health into the daily life of management is of importance, a part of the new Agency Strategy 2009–2013 and on the agenda of European Agency for Safety and Health at Work (2008).

Results

Clinical Application

Theories about the relationship between work conditions and the well-being of the employees are still under formulation. Research on the organizational work environment has increased, and the factors that should be taken into account in measuring organizational factors and psychosocial strain are discussed and debated (Cox et al., 2005).

When discussing organizational factors at work, two concepts come up repeatedly: stress and burnout.

Stress

The experience of stress arises from an imbalance between the perceived demands of the environment and the perceived resources available to the individual to cope with those demands. Some studies suggest that psychologically demanding jobs that allow employees little control over the work process even increase the risk of cardiovascular disease (Niedhammer et al., 1998).

Reducing work-related stress and psychosocial risks is not only a moral but also a legal imperative. There is a strong business case as well. In 2002, the annual economic cost of work-related stress in the European Union (EU-15) was estimated at 20 billion euros. The good news is that work-related stress can be dealt with in the same logical and systematic way as other health and safety issues (European Agency for Safety and Health at Work, 2008).

Burnout

Burnout is related to stress. Tracy (2000) points out that understanding burnout to be personal and private is problematic because burnout is largely an organizational issue caused by long hours, little down time, and continual peer, customer, and employer surveillance. Mental exhaustion is considered the most obvious manifestation of the burnout syndrome and the basic individual stress dimension of it (Schaufeli and Enzmann, 1998; Van Emmerik, 2002). Researchers have studied quantitative job demands, and the findings support the general notion that burnout is a response to overload and time pressure.

Coping with Stress and Burnout

Two models are presented here that have been developed to better understand the connection between the organizational factors at work and the well-being of the workers. These are the job strain model and the effort-reward imbalance model.

The Job Strain Model

The job strain model, also called the demand-control model, proposes that strain, such as distress or adverse health effects, occurs when an employee is exposed to a combination of high demands and low control. According to this model, high demand and little control give rise to dangerous levels of stress. Stress increases if the social situation is poor, that is, support from fellow workers and managers is lacking. A high level of demand by itself does not necessarily lead to stress if it is accompanied by sufficiently good control over the work situation. The *control* concept relates to autonomy, to what extent individual workers can structure and control how and when they should do their particular tasks; and to participation in planning and decision-making, that is, to what extent the workers are given opportunities to control or influence their job environment outcome. Control may act as a buffer for job demands, and improvement in control may improve the perceived quality of the work environment (Karasek and Theorell, 1990).

According to Levi (2000), it soon became evident that a third component was needed in the model, namely *social support*. Several different aspects of social support can be relevant, but it became clear that the addition of social support makes the demand-control perspective more useful in *job redesigning*.

The Effort-Reward Imbalance Model

The rewards we receive from work play a decisive role in our social status. Therefore, the relationships between the efforts invested in work and the rewards are central. High levels of effort combined with no, or random, gratification will adversely affect workers' health. Research has shown that workers who put forth a high amount of effort but receive low rewards and have low job security and low status, have a 2- to 4½-fold higher risk for coronary heart disease compared to workers who report a satisfactory effort-reward balance (Siegrist, 1996).

Risk Assessment

As mentioned before, many studies show a clear connection between work organization and well-being of the employees (Gunnarsdottir et al., 2003; Rafnsdottir and Gudmundsdottir, 2004; Siegrist and Marmot, 2004). Therefore, it is important to consider these organizational factors in management and when working with prevention and rehabilitation. Risk assessment, an examination of what, in the work environment, could cause harm to people, psychosocially or physically, is an example of a useful method for most organizations to create a good work environment, both physically and mentally.

Risk can be assessed in the workplace by a few steps. It is necessary to identify the hazards and decide who might be at risk and how. Then it is important to evaluate the risks and decide on precautions, recording the findings, and implementing them. Last but not least, it can be useful to review the assessment and update it if necessary (Frostberg et al., 2003).

In many organizations, the risks are well known and the necessary control measures are easy to apply. In other organizations, it is more complicated. People who run a small organization and are confident they understand what is involved can sometimes do the assessment themselves. However, employers in a larger organization often need to ask a health and safety adviser for help. In all cases, the staff or their representatives must be involved in the process (Health and Safety Executive [HSE], 2008).

Evidence-Based Practice

Management Standards

The management standards for stress (HSE, 2008) are an example of a method, *related to risk assessment,–* that makes it possible to identify the gap between preferable conditions at work and the current performance. These standards may help employers develop their own solutions to close this gap. The standards contain tools to analyze the workplace performance in six areas:

- Demands: workload, work patterns, and the work environment.
- Control: how much influence employees have in the way they do their work.
- Support: encouragement, sponsorship, and resources provided by the organization, line management, and colleagues.
- Relationship: promoting positive work to avoid conflict and dealing with unacceptable behavior.
- Role: whether people understand their role within the organization and whether the organization ensures that the person does not have conflicting roles.
- Change: How organizational change (large or small) is managed and communicated in the organization.

Together with any existing data, this information can be used in focus-group discussions with employees to determine what is happening locally and what should be done to close the gap.

When promoting workplace health, it can be useful to learn about the good practices in other companies or institutions and compare them to some of the good practices at the European Network Education and Training Occupational Safety and Health (ENETOSH) and on HSE (2008).

Discussion

The workplace and the work organization can affect the health and well-being of the employees in various ways, and workers and others have a legal right to be protected from harm or illness caused by failure in the work organization or the work environment. Therefore, all workplace health promotion is important, for the employees, the companies and the society. To increase well-being among employees, it is necessary to analyze the characteristics of the work and the conditions that are perceived as risks. Therefore, employers, managers, and occupational consultants must consider the organizational factors that affect the employees' well-being. These factors include time pressure, qualitative job demands, role conflict, lack of adequate information for completing tasks, lack of feedback, inequality, and lack of latitude for making work-related decisions. Absence of job resources such as social support from supervisors and coworkers is also of significance. As the labour market is widely gender segregated and women and men in many families have partly different roles in their homes, it is always of importance to consider gender when analyzing well-being at work.

References

Cox, T., Tisserand, M., and Taris, T. (2005). The conceptualization and measurement of burnout. Questions and directions. Work and Stress, 19(3), 187–191.

European Agency for Safety and Health at Work. (2008). Stress. http://osha.europa.eu/topics/stress.

European Network for Workplace Health Promotion. (ENWHP). (2008a). Work and health—an important but often neglected relationship in public health reporting. http://www.enwhp.org/index.php?id=509.

European Network for Workplace Health Promotion. (ENWHP). (2008b). Healthy workplaces—a top priority in Europe. http://www.enwhp.org/index.php?id=578.

European Network Education and Training on Occupational Safety and Health (ENETOSH). (2008). Network. http://www.enetosh.net/webcom/show_article.php/_c-29/i.html.

Frostberg, C., Bengtsson, B., Cardfelt, M., et al. (2003). Investigation and risk assessment in systematic work environment management—a guide. SOLNA Work Environment Authority publication services. The Swedish Work Environment Authority (Arbetsmiljöverket). http://www.av.se/dokument/nenglish/books/h375eng.pdf.

Health and Safety Executive. (2008). The management standards. http://www.hse.gov.uk/stress/standards/standards.htm.

Galinsky, E., Kim, S., and Bond, J. (2001). Feeling Overworked: When Work Becomes Too Much. New York: Families and Work Institute.

Gunnarsdottir, H.K., Rafnsdottir, G.L., Helgadottir, B., and Tomasson, K. (2003). Psychosocial risk factors for musculoskeletal disorders among personnel in geriatric care. Am J Ind Med, 44, 679–684.

Health and Safety Executive. (2008a). Risk management. http://www.hse.gov.uk/risk/index.htm.

Health and Safety Executive. (2008b). Work-related stress—good practice. http://www.hse.gov. uk/stress/experience.htm.

Health and Safety Laboratory. An agency of the Health and Safety Executive. (2008). Centre for Workplace Health. http://www.hsl.gov.uk/cwh/index.htm.

Karasek, R., and Theorell, T. (1990). Healthy Work: Stress Productivity and the Reconstruction of Working Life. New York: Basic Books.

Levi, L. (2000). Stressors at the workplace. Theoretical models. Occup Med, 15(1), 69–105.

Niedhammer, I., Goldberg, M., Leclerc, A., David, S., Bugel, I., and Landre, M.-F. (1998). Psychosocial work environment and cardiovascular risk factors in an occupational cohort in France. J Epidemiol Community Health, 52, 93–100.

Rafnsdottir, G.L., and Gudmundsdottir, M.L. (2004). New technology and its impact on well-being. Work, 22, 31–39.

Rafnsdottir, G.L., Gunnarsdottir, H.K., and Tomasson, K. (2004). Work organization, well-being and health in geriatric care. Work, 22, 49–55.

Schaufeli, W., and Enzmann, D. (1998). The Burnout Companion to Study and Practice. A Critical Analysis. London: Taylor & Francis.

Siegrist, J. (1996). Adverse health effect of high effort-low reward conditions. J Occup Health Psychol, 1, 27–37.

Siegrist, J., and Marmot, M. (2004). Health inequalities and the psychosocial environment—two scientific challenges. Soc Sci Med, 58, 1463–1473.

The Health and Safety Laboratory (HSL). (2008). http://www.hsl.gov.uk/about-us/index.htm.

Tracy, S. (2000). Becoming a character for commerce emotion. Manag Commun Q, 14, 90–128.

Van Emmerik, I. (2002). Gender differences in the effects of coping assistance on the reduction of burnout in academic staff. Work Stress, 13(3), 251–263.

Virtanen, M., Kivimaki, M., and Eloviainio, M. (2005). Local economy and sickness absence. Prospective cohort study. J Epidemiol Community Health, 59(11), 973–978.

Chapter 55
Functional Capacity Evaluation: An Integrated Approach to Assessing Work Activity Limitations

Libby Gibson

Being able to perform the physical demands of work entails more than being physically able to perform the tasks, and assessing this performance entails more than seeing what a client can do physically.

Abstract Occupational therapists (OTs) have an established role in assessing readiness for return to work. Functional capacity evaluation (FCE) is one method frequently used for this purpose. This chapter describes the new *Gibson approach to functional capacity evaluation (GAPP FCE)*. The assessment was developed by OTs. It provides an evidence-based and integrated framework for OTs to assess comprehensively the many aspects of performance of the physical demands of work. These aspects include key psychosocial variables known to influence physical performance and return to work. The *GAPP FCE* is described, including the eight-step process and a summary of evidence to date.

Keywords Disability evaluation • Employment • Vocational rehabilitation • Work capacity evaluation

Background

Traditionally occupational therapists (OTs) have had a professional role in the process of evaluation of workers' capacity for returning to work (Velozo, 1993). *Functional capacity evaluation* (FCE) is an *objective assessment* and one of the most common services provided by vocational and occupational rehabilitation professionals in this process (Deen et al., 2002; Jundt and King, 1999; Lysaght, 2004). This chapter describes the *GAPP FCE*.

The FCEs are widely used in workers compensation markets (1) to guide decisions about injured workers' capacity for returning to work, (2) in vocational rehabilitation to guide decisions about people with disabilities returning to new jobs, (3) in medicolegal settings for determinations of compensation, and (4) increasingly by employers

I. Söderback (ed.), *International Handbook of Occupational Therapy Interventions*,
DOI: 10.1007/978-0-387-75424-6_55, © Springer Science+Business Media, LLC 2010

preplacement or after job offers are made to match workers' abilities to job demands and identify reasonable job accommodations (Innes, 2006).

Definition

Functional capacity evaluation is a method used to assess the capacities of people with disabilities and occupational injuries to perform the physical demands (or activities) of a job or work in general (Gibson and Strong, 2003; Innes, 2006). FCE is an evaluation of an activity performance and activity limitation.

The GAPP FCE (Gibson et al., 2005) provides a method for detailed evaluation of difficulties an injured worker or client with a disability may have in performing a range of physical activities that may be required at work, such as sitting, standing, walking, reaching, lifting, and carrying.

Background

The GAPP FCE was developed because of recognized limitations of many existing assessment approaches, including (1) in general, a focus on biomechanical factors with limited attention to the psychosocial factors, despite evidence that these factors can affect physical performance and therefore need to be incorporated into to the assessments (Gibson et al., 2005); and (2) limited research into the reliability and validity of existing approaches, with many assessment instruments being used in the absence of such research (Innes and Straker, 1999a,b). Velozo (1993) called for research by OTs into "the relationship between components of functioning and occupational performance" (p. 206) among injured workers. The following recommendations to improve the work evaluations were stated:

(a) Improve measurement of constructs hypothesized to be relevant to work, (e.g., pain, personality, effort, physical and work capacity); (b) determine whether these constructs are actually related to work or return to work; and (c) develop new theoretical models and constructs related to work. (p. 207).

In response to these calls, the GAPP FCE research program was begun (Gibson et al., 2005).

Purpose

The aims of the GAPP FCE are to provide (1) an evidence-based and integrated framework for OTs administering the FCE; and (2) a method for the OTs to consider the various aspects that affect performance of the physical work demands included in the FCE, such as evaluation of biomechanical, physiologic, and psychosocial aspects of performance.

Method

Candidates for the Intervention

The GAPP FCE is primarily used with men and women of working age (ages 16 to 65) who have mild to moderate impairments of body function and structure and have the cognitive and psychological capacity to participate in the evaluation and cope with the other demands of the FCE, such as following instructions.

The FCE is most often undertaken when there is uncertainty about clients' capacity to perform the demands of their job or the demands of a new vocation if they need to work in a new area of employment. The FCE can help guide decisions about the readiness of the client for work, or the safety of return to work.

The GAPP FCE research has been primarily conducted with people living with chronic back pain. However, the clinical application of GAPP FCE would include (1) injured workers with musculoskeleletal disorders or disease of the musculoskeletal system and connective tissue (International Classification of Diseases [ICD-10] codes M00 to M99) (World Health Organization, 2007) such as upper extremity musculoskeletal disorders, and acute low back pain; and (2) workers with physical disabilities who are independently mobile and where their physical capacity to perform the physical demands of the work is not known and needs to be determined.

Epidemiology

According to a recent report by the Australian Safety and Compensation Council (2007), 17% of the working age population of Australia (one in six workers) have a disability, and the labor force participation rate is lower for people with disability compared to the rate of the general Australian population. Further, the majority of these people (72%) have physical restrictions, which is the most common reason for requiring an FCE.

Settings

The GAPP FCE is conducted with a range of equipment that assesses each of the items of the evaluation set up in an area dedicated to this purpose and large enough to allow adequate space to observe the use of all the items. This equipment includes a table and adjustable seating, a standing workstation, adjustable shelving with crate and weights, balance beam, and equipment for light assembly tasks. A flat, level area for assessing walking and a set of stairs should also be easily accessible nearby. Ancillary testing equipment is also needed including a stopwatch, heart rate monitor, blood pressure monitor, scales, tape measure, and calculator. The GAPP FCE recommends use of existing questionnaires and instruments to measure psychosocial variables, including the Spinal Function Sort (Matheson and Matheson, 1989).

The Role of the Occupational Therapist

The OT administers each item in the GAPP FCE, using the standard procedure and provided instructions, and observes and records how the client performs the physical activities included in the GAPP FCE, using the score sheets provided. Based on this performance, the OT makes recommendations about the client's capacity to perform work tasks. OTs use the framework provided by the GAPP FCE to guide their observations of the client's performance and decision-making about the client's physical capacity for return to work, including any major limiting factors and the barriers and facilitators for return to work. A key aspect of the GAPP FCE is its incorporation of evaluation of the worker's perceived capacities for return to work, found to be crucial for the outcome of returning to work (Schult et al., 2000).

Results

Clinical Application

The Content of GAPP FCE

There are 20 items in the GAPP FCE, each with a specific procedure to evaluate the following physical demands, based on the physical demands from the Dictionary of Occupational Titles (United States Department of Labor, 1991):

1. Sitting
2. Standing
3. Walking
4. Lifting waist to waist
5. Lifting floor to waist
6. Lifting above waist
7. Carrying bilateral
8. Carrying unilateral
9. Pushing and pulling
10. Climbing stairs
11. Balancing
12. Sustained semisquatting
13. Kneeling repetitively
14. Kneeling sustained
15. Crouching repetitively
16. Crouching sustained
17. Crawling
18. Reaching overhead
19. Handling
20. Fingering

Each of the 20 items does not need to be evaluated each time. The OT can decide which items need to be evaluated. When the client has a specific job to which he or she can return, the physical demands required on the job can be used to determine which items are evaluated. The GAPP FCE procedure recommends a set of core items to be evaluated with clients with back pain that have been trialed (Gibson et al., 2005).

The client also undertakes a number of steps before and after performance of the physical demands listed above. These steps are outlined below (see The Process of Performing GAPP FCE).

Purpose

The primary purpose of the GAPP FCE is to assist the improvement of injured workers' occupational performance for their worker role by determining their safe and accurate abilities to perform the physical demands of work activities using a comprehensive, reliable, and valid evaluation. The GAPP FCE may also assist in prevention of workplace injury if used for matching the client's capacities for the physical demands of a job after selection for a job.

Application

The GAPP FCE can be used in a number of ways and in a number of settings, as outlined above. Where the injured worker is being evaluated for a particular job, the GAPP FCE is best used in conjunction with a job analysis conducted through a worksite assessment so that the client can be evaluated in relation to the demands of the client's job. Where clients have no job to which they can return, or are looking at a new area of work because of their physical disability, the results of the GAPP FCE can assist the vocational counseling process of considering alternative occupations that match clients' physical functional capacities.

The Process of Performing GAPP FCE

The GAPP FCE provides standard instructions and score sheets to evaluate each of the 20 items in the GAPP FCE, and an accompanying user's manual that outlines each step of the GAPP FCE process.

The GAPP FCE process involves the following eight steps:

1. Preparation for the GAPP FCE
2. Collection of clients' background information
3. Physical screening
4. Evaluation of perceived functional capacity and other psychosocial variables
5. Physical demands performance testing
6. Post-FCE and follow-up measures
7. Scoring and rating
8. Using and reporting the results

Step 1: Preparation for the GAPP FCE

After the OT receives the referral for the FCE, the OT needs to establish that the client is medically stable and physically ready to participate in the GAPP FCE, which is done by obtaining medical clearance for the client to undertake the FCE. The GAPP FCE user's manual provides detailed guidelines to assist the OT suitably to (1) prepare the client for the FCE, (2) obtain informed consent from the client to undertake the FCE, and (3) establish medical readiness for the FCE.

Step 2: Collection of Background Information

The OT interviews the client about his or her injury or disability and its effects on returning to work and collects relevant demographic and other information, such as length of work disability and employment status and history.

Step 3: Physical Screening

The OT conducts further testing to confirm that the client is medically and physically suitable to undergo the FCE and obtains basic health information for baseline data, such as resting heart rate and blood pressure. This step is important to screen for any major precautions or contraindications for undertaking the FCE.

Step 4: Evaluation of Perceived Functional Capacity
and Other Psychosocial Variables

Before the OT observes clients' performance of the physical demands, the OT asks clients for their perception of their capacity, including their perceived capacity to perform the physical demands. This step includes administration of a battery of recommended questionnaires that measure a number of variables including pain intensity, location and description, perceived disability, fear of pain and or reinjury, and self-efficacy (Gibson et al., 2005). This process is valuable (1) to establish the client's perceived capacity prior to performance of the physical demands, (2) to establish a rapport with the client, and (3) to allay any fears that the client may have about the FCE.

Step 5: Physical Demands Performance Testing

This is the main step of the GAPP FCE process where the client performs the physical demands under the instruction and supervision of the administering OT. Each of the 20 items in the GAPP FCE has a specific procedure including guidelines for the therapist about the screening procedure for the item, the procedure to be used to evaluate the physical demand, and the required positioning of the client or equipment for evaluating that item. Each procedure also includes standard instructions that the OT uses with the client. The GAPP FCE user's manual provides instructions for measuring perceived capacity throughout the evaluation of the physical demands and provides recommendations for the sequence of testing of items. The OT uses the GAPP FCE score sheets, tailored specifically for each item, to record observations and client report during the performance of the physical demand and to determine when to end the task performance if indicated.

Step 6: Post–GAPP FCE and Follow-Up Measures

After evaluation of the last item in the GAPP FCE, the OT completes a range of measurements, such as the client's heart rate, blood pressure, and pain intensity and location to compare to values obtained before and during the FCE. The OT also provides the client with follow-up questionnaires to complete. This is done in the subsequent 2-day follow-up to measure the aftereffects, if any, of the FCE.

Step 7: Scoring and Rating the GAPP FCE

On completion of the administration of the GAPP FCE, the OT then rates each item of the GAPP FCE, and the final ratings and recommendations about return to work are provided in the score sheets.

Step 8: Using and Reporting the Results

In the final step of the GAPP FCE process, the OT interprets and reports the results in relation to the specific purpose of the FCE. The OT uses clinical reasoning skills to make recommendations about the clients' capacity to perform the physical demands of work, including the safety of such performance and any restrictions that may be required for short or long term.

The Results of the GAPP FCE Assessment

The GAPP FCE provides a framework for OTs to consider the interrelationships between the client's body functions and structures, performance of activities (physical demands), and participation in life roles, particularly work, and environmental, and client factors. The FCE is best used in conjunction with a job analysis (US Department of Labor, 1996) or a detailed job description, i.e., a criterion-referenced multidimensional work assessment (CMVA) (Söderback, et al., 2000).

The GAPP FCE (1) provides recommendations about performance of the activities or physical demands in the work context and work environment; and (b) contributes to the review of possible barriers and facilitators in the client's physical, social, and attitudinal environment for participation in the activities of work. This framework can help identify the major limiting factors affecting the client's performance of the physical demands of work and guide recommendations for how this performance can be improved to facilitate participation in the workforce.

Evidence-Based Practice

Development of the GAPP FCE has followed the standard test development and research processes under the guiding criteria of safety, reliability, validity, utility, and practicality/feasibility. The results of several studies give support for the approach in terms of its safety, feasibility, and utility, aspects of its content validity and item validity, and interrater reliability of OTs' recommendations for return to work based on performance in the GAPP FCE (Gibson and Strong, 2002, 2005; Gibson et al., 2005; Kersnovske et al., 2005). The GAPP FCE would benefit from undergoing larger-scale studies than those possible to date, including rare but much needed longitudinal predictive validity research (Innes, 2006).

Discussion

The FCE is a service commonly provided around the world by OTs. The GAPP FCE provides an approach to FCE that is strongly linked to both occupational performance models of practice and the International Classification of Functioning, Disability, and Health (ICF) model of functioning, disability, and health (Gibson and Strong, 2003). The GAPP FCE puts the emphasis on the observation and reasoning skills of the OT administering the evaluation, making it potentially amenable to tailoring to workplace-based evaluations and other emerging uses (Innes and Straker, 2002).

It provides a comprehensive and thorough evaluation process that can last for up to 3 hours.

The ongoing development of the GAPP FCE may provide an evidence-based approach to this growing area of occupational therapy practice.

References

Australian Safety and Compensation Council. (2007). Are People with Disability at Risk at Work? A Review of the Evidence. Commonwealth of Australia. Canberra: Australian Safety and Compensation Council.

Deen, M., Gibson, L., and Strong, J. (2002). A survey of occupational therapy in Australian work practice. Work, 19, 219–230.

Gibson, L., and Strong, J. (2002). Expert review of an approach to functional capacity evaluation. Work, 19, 231–242.

Gibson, L., and Strong, J. (2003). A conceptual framework of functional capacity evaluation for occupational therapy in work rehabilitation. Aust Occup Ther J, 50, 64–71.

Gibson, L., and Strong, J. (2005). Safety issues in functional capacity evaluation: findings from a trial of a new approach for evaluating clients with chronic back pain. J Occup Rehabil, 15, 237–251.

Gibson, L., Strong, J., and Wallace, A. (2005). Functional capacity evaluation as a performance measure: evidence for a new approach for clients with chronic back pain. Clin J Pain, 21, 207–215.

Innes, E. (2006). Reliability and validity of functional capacity evaluations: an update. Int J Disabil Manag Res, 1(1), 135–148.

Innes, E., and Straker, L. (1999a). Reliability of work-related assessments. Work, 13(2), 107–124.

Innes, E., and Straker, L. (1999b). Validity of work-related assessments. Work, 13(2), 125–152.

Innes, E., and Straker, L. (2002). Workplace assessments and functional capacity evaluations: current practices of therapists in Australia. Work, 18, 51–66.

Jundt, J., and King, P.M. (1999). Work rehabilitation programs: a 1997 survey. Work, 12, 139–144.

Kersnovske, S., Gibson, L., and Strong, J. (2005). Item validity of the physical demands from the Dictionary of Occupational Titles for functional capacity evaluation of clients with chronic back pain. Work, 24, 157–169.

Lysaght, R. (2004). Approaches to worker rehabilitation by occupational and physiotherapists in the United States: factors impacting practice. Work, 23, 139–146.

Matheson, L.N., and Matheson, M. (1989). Spinal Function Sort. Rancho Santa Margarita, CA: Performance Assessment and Capacity Testing.

Schult, M.-L., Söderback, I., and Jacobs, K. (2000). Multidimensional aspects of work capability. Work, 15(1), 41.

Söderback, I., Schult, M.L., and Jacobs, K. (2000). Work 15(1), 25–39.

United States Department of Labor. (1991). Dictionary of Occupational Titles, 4th ed. Washington, DC: U.S. Government Printing Office. U.S. Department of Labor (1991). The revised handbook for analyzing jobs. Washington, D.C.: Government Publishing Office.

Velozo, C.A. (1993). Work evaluations: critique of the state of the art of functional assessment of work. Am J Occup Ther, 47, 203–209.

World Health Organization. (2007). International Statistical Classification of Diseases and Related Health Problems Version for 2007. http://www.who.int/classifications/apps/icd/icd10online/.

Chapter 56
Prevention of Workers' Musculoskeletal Disorders: A Four-Stage Model

Navah Z. Ratzon and Tal Jarus

A four-stage prevention model for workers incorporating motor learning principles is aimed at enhancing safe work performance.

Abstract Prevention programs for musculoskeletal disorders are aimed at assisting workers in preventing musculoskeletal disorders, allowing restoration of function, and recovering the capacity to return to work. Over the past few decades, the number of work-related injuries has remained the same or even increased. Therefore, a four-stage prevention model incorporating principles of motor learning enables occupational therapists (OTs) to facilitate prevention programs for workers was suggested. The four-stage prevention model consists of on-site analysis and examination, basic intervention, progressive intervention, and follow-up.

Keywords Motor learning prevention programs • Musculoskeletal disorders (MSD) • Work-related musculoskeletal disorders (WRMSD) • Workplace

Background

Prevention programs concern primary and secondary prevention (Jones and Kumar, 2001; Linton and van Tulder, 2001). Primary prevention focuses on reducing the incidence of new episodes of injury. Secondary prevention programs are designed primarily to reduce disability or work absenteeism for people who already suffer from a disability (Carrivick et al., 2005; Frank et al., 1996a,b; Wessels et al., 2007).

Occupational therapists (OTs) offer services to workers in the workplace to prevent musculoskeletal disorders (primary prevention), to help the injured worker restore function, and to recover capacities needed to return to work (secondary prevention).

Prevention programs for work settings vary and often include education, exercise and flexibility training, fitness body mechanics, lifting ergonomics, and supervised practice sessions with individual feedback (Feuerstein et al., 2000; Linton and van Tulder, 2001).

Only a few prevention programs have produced a clear reduction in the incidence of musculoskeletal injuries when evaluated by rigorous scientific criteria (Frank et al., 1996a,b; Tveito et al., 2004). Moreover, despite prevention attempts, the overall trend for work-related injuries has been relatively stable over the past several decades (Occupational Health and Safety Agency for Healthcare in British Columbia [OHSAH], 2004; Ratzon et al., 1998, 2000; Silverstein et al., 2002). It is proposed that the four-stage prevention model combined with principles of motor learning may assist OTs in structuring prevention programs in order to facilitate workers' acquisition of correct movement patterns (Jarus and Ratzon, 2005).

Definitions

Motor learning refers to a set of internal processes associated with practice or experience, leading to relatively permanent changes in motor behavior (Magill, 2004; Schmidt and Lee, 2005; Schmidt and Wrisberg, 2000). The three main phases of *acquisition, retention, and transfer* can be demonstrated with ergonomic principles in the following example:

A worker learns to lift a box correctly (acquisition phase), then performs this task a week later (retention phase), and transfers this learning to correctly lift different items at the workplace (transfer phase) (Jarus and Ratzon, 2000; Magill, 2004; Schmidt and Lee, 2005).

Purpose

The purpose of the four-stage prevention model, based on motor learning and ergonomic principles, is to facilitate workers' acquisition of correct movement patterns, thus contributing to prevention of work injuries and work absenteeism.

Method

Candidates for the Intervention

The four-stage prevention model is designed for men and women of working age, both healthy workers (aimed for prevention of work injuries) and among those with a musculoskeletal disorder.

Epidemiology

Musculoskeletal disorders have far-reaching consequences for people in all occupational areas. These disorders are ranked as the leading cause of disability among the work force (Bernard and Fine, 1996; Centers for Disease Control and

Prevention, National Institute for Occupational Safety and Health [CDC NIOSH], n.d.; Luz and Green, 1992). Since it has been found that many musculoskeletal problems are connected, among other things, to risk factors related to a person's work environment and derived from biomechanical and psychosocial factors, the literature refers to them as WRMSDs (Skov et al., 1996; Trinkoff et al., 2002; Vroman and Macrea, 2001; Warren, 2001). In the United States, Canada, and Europe, the number of WRMSDs is estimated to be above 30% of the working population. These numbers vary for different occupations, depending on different risk factors in different jobs and workplaces. Yet it is agreed that data on exact percentages are not always available because there is a great deal of underreporting of these types of injuries, and therefore it does not represent the magnitude of the problem (Bernard, 1997; Canadian Centre for Occupational Health and Safety [CCOHS], 1997; Gauthy, 2005).

Settings

The four-stage prevention model is offered for implementation at the workplace, emphasizing the need to relate to the specific type of task and the specific structure of practice while referring to the characteristics of the worker.

The Role of the Occupational Therapist

Occupational therapists conduct the four-stage prevention model including the use of knowledge and skills aimed at analyzing the work task, evaluating the worker and the work environment, and planning and implementing the prevention program and the follow-up stage (see below).

The OT acts as a coordinator with the worker, the employer, and other coworkers. Observations, interviews, and evaluations are used as tools for conducting the model.

Results

Clinical Application

Based on motor learning principles (Jarus and Ratzon, 2000; Magill, 2004; Schmidt and Lee, 2005), a four-stage prevention model aims at enhancing sustainability of ergonomic intervention programs. The four stages are as follows:

- *Stage I* comprises an *on-site work task analysis* performed at the client's workplace as well as examination of the worker and the work environment. This stage is essential for building a proper prevention program matched to the worker, the tasks the worker performs, and the workstation (U.S. Department of Labor, 1991).
- *In stage II* the individual is *taught proper body mechanisms* to perform work in a safe manner based on an analysis of stage I. The prevention program at this stage is based on principles of motor learning to ensure that the worker will be able to retain and transfer the task to the work setting, and be guided by ergonomic principles used to prevent injuries and disabilities (this stage can be done individually or in a group).
- *Stage III* provides an opportunity for the worker to *apply skills learned* in stage II, and further upgrade such skills. Stage III is an ongoing individualized program designed to fit the specific worker at his or her specific workstation.
- In *stage IV,* the efficacy of the prevention program is evaluated in terms of the worker's retention and transfer performance. On-site work evaluation and long-term follow-ups are recommended for this stage.

An Example

The four-stage prevention model and the role the OT has for conducting the model is exemplified among nurses working in a general hospital:

- *Stage I.* Nurses who were invited to attend the prevention program were evaluated while performing their ordinary work tasks at their ward workstations. The OTs used assessment tools such as the Rapid Entire Body Assessment (REBA) to assess the level of the biomechanical workload during work (Hignett and McAtamney, 2000).
- *Stage II.* This stage takes place within the hospital ward. A nurse administers the assessments. The OTs role is to conduct the organization of the work environment, teach the nurses how to perform proper body postures during work that avoid rotational movements, and usage of aid accessories. Ergonomic solutions are recommended to be used during performance of the work tasks (Collins et al., 2004; Evanoff et al., 1999; Gatty et al., 2003; Owen et al., 2002). The nurses practiced motor learning principles, such as type of feedback or use of external focus of attention, is performed within the work environment, and OTs encourage the staff to increase work awareness through cooperation among themselves (Devereux et al., 1999).
- *Stage III.* During this progressive intervention phase, OTs teach the clients special techniques like segmental stabilizing exercises (SSEs) and a list of stress-releasing exercises to be performed after being in an uncomfortable position for a while (Gundewall et al., 1993; Skargren and Oberg, 1996). The exercises are taught according to motor learning principles that are suited to the individual complaints and the work situations in the specific ward.

- *Stage IV* is a follow up that contains long-term individual assessments. During this stage the OT has to check if the clients have or have not assimilated the prevention principles. If not, the OT has to step down to a lower stage and repeat the intervention approaches.

Evidence-Based Practice

Evidence suggests that outcomes of current work-related prevention programs do not demonstrate good retention, as indicated by longer follow-up studies, nor good transfer of training to the work site (Bohr, 2002; Jensen et al., 2006; Solberg, 2007). Most prevention programs are based on an *educational* model. The teaching stresses the distribution of printed guidance material or coaching (Lahad et al., 1994).

Some of the programs investigated the efficacy of *physical exercise* for prevention of musculoskeletal complaints (Delin et al., 1981; Skargren and Oberg, 1996).

However, few of the evaluation studies focus on the *interaction between workers and their work environment* while observing the person's performance within that work environment (Linton and Van Tulder, 2001).

Since there seems to be a scarcity of evidence on the efficacy of these comprehensive prevention programs, the four-stage prevention model suggests a prevention program that focuses on *occupational performance* and in addition to the above-mentioned program also consists of the on-site analysis and examination, the basic intervention, the progressive intervention, and the follow-up. The four-step prevention model is currently being implemented in several workplaces in Israel.

Discussion

An analysis of prevention programs for workers is presented using a four-stage prevention model that is based on motor learning principles. The authors proposed that the model has clinical relevance and applicability for actual clinical ergonomic settings. The program is suitable for people with symptoms of the motor functions as well as for those who do suffer from a musculoskeletal syndrome. In addition, the program allows a better participation at the workplace while taking into consideration not only medical or biologic dysfunction, but also the social aspects of work function and the context of work environment.

Conclusion

Analyzing both the characteristics of the task involved and the worker, and planning the structure intervention that apply practice based on motor learning principles, would be beneficial for improved long-term effects among workers. This certainly coincides with the broad perspective suggested in current OT models viewing the person, the environment, the occupation, and their effect on occupational performance (Christiansen et al., 2005).

It can be learned from this chapter that prevention programs could benefit from targeting the worker, the task, and the environment, while incorporating all four stages presented in the model. Further studies are warranted to establish evidence-based data for this model.

References

Bernard, B.P., ed. (1997). Musculoskeletal Disorders and Workplace Factors: A Critical Review of Epidemiologic Evidence for Work-Related Musculoskeletal Disorders of The Neck, Upper Extremity and Low Back. Washington, DC: National Institute for Occupational Health and Safety (NIOSH). http://www.cdc.gov/niosh/docs/97–141/.

Bernard, B.P., and Fine, L.J. (1996). Musculoskeletal disorders and workplace factors. A critical review of epidemiologic evidence for work related musculoskeletal disorders of the neck, UE and low back. U.S. Department of Health and Human Services. Orthop Clin North Am, 27, 679–709.

Bohr, P.C. (2002). Office ergonomics education: a comparison of traditional and participatory methods. Work, 19, 185–191.

Canadian Centre for Occupational Health and Safety (CCOHS). (1997). OSH Answers: Work-Related Musculoskeletal Disorders (WMSDs). http://www.ccohs.ca/oshanswers/diseases/rmirsi.html#1_3.

Carrivick, P.J., Lee, A.H., Yau, K.K., and Stevenson, M.R. (2005). Evaluating the effectiveness of a participatory ergonomics approach in reducing the risk and severity of injuries from manual handling. Ergonomics, 48, 907–914.

Centers for Disease Control and Prevention, National Institute for Occupational Safety and Health (CDC NIOSH). (n.d.). Ergonomics and Muscular Disorders. http://www.cdc.gov/niosh/topics/ergonomics/#nio.

Christiansen, C.H., Baum, C.M., and Bass-Haugen, J. (2005). Occupational Therapy: Performance, Participation, and Well-Being. Thorofare, NJ: Slack.

Collins, J.W., Wolf, L., Bell, J., and Evanoff, B. (2004). An evaluation of a "Best Practice" musculoskeletal injury prevention program in nursing homes. Injury Prevention, 10, 206–211.

Delin, D., Andersson, G., and Grimby, G. (1981). Effects of physical training and ergonomic councelling on the psychological perception of work and on the subjective assessment of low back insufficiency. Scand J Rehabil Med, 13, 1–9.

Devereux, J.J., Buckle, P.W., and Vlachonikolis, I.G. (1999). Interaction between physical and psychosocial work risk factors increase the risk of back disorders: an Epidemiological Study. Occup Environ Med, 56, 343–353.

Evanoff, B.A., Bohr, P.C., and Wolf, L.D. (1999). Effects of a participatory ergonomics team among hospital orderlies. Am J Ind Med, 35, 358–365.

Feuerstein, M., Marshall, L., Shaw, W.S., and Burrell, L.M. (2000). Multicomponent intervention for work related upper extremity disorders. J Occup Rehabil, 10, 71–83.

Frank, J.W., Brooker, A.S., DeMaio, S.E., et al. (1996a). Disability resulting from occupational low back pain. Part II: what do we know about secondary prevention? A review of the scientific evidence on prevention after disability begins. Spine, 21, 2918–2929.

Frank, J.W., Kerr, M.S., Brooker, A.S., et al. (1996b). Disability resulting from occupational low back pain. Part I: what do we know about primary prevention? A review of the scientific evidence on prevention before disability begins. Spine, 21, 2908–2917.

Gatty, C.M., Turner, M., Buitendrop, D.J., and Batman, H. (2003). The effectiveness of back pain and injury prevention programs in the workplace. Work, 20, 257–266.

Gauthy, R. (2005, June). Musculoskeletal disorders: where we are, and where we could be. Newsletter of the Health and Safety Department of the ETUI-REHS. http://hesa.etui-rehs.org/uk/newsletter/files/Newsletter-27-EN.

Gundewall, B., Liljeqvist, M., and Hansson, T. (1993). Primary prevention of back symptoms and absence from work: a prospective randomized study among hospital employees. Spine, 18, 587–594.

Hignett, S., and Mctamney, L. (2000). Rapid entire body assessment (REBA). Appl Ergonom, 31, 201–205.

Jarus, T., and Ratzon, N. Z. (2000). Can you imagine? The effect of mental practice on the acquisition and retention of a motor skill as a function of age. Occup Ther J Res, 20, 163–178.

Jarus, T., and Ratzon, N. Z. (2005). The implementation of motor learning principles in designing prevention programs at work. Work, 24, 171–182.

Jensen, L.D., Gonge, H., Jors, E., et al. (2006). Prevention of low back pain in female eldercare workers: randomized controlled work site trial. Spine, 31, 1761–1769.

Jones, T., and Kumar, S. (2001). Physical ergonomics in low-back pain prevention. J Occup Rehabil, 11, 309–319.

Lahad, A., Malter, A., Berg, A.O., and Dayo, R. (1994). The effectiveness of four interventions for the prevention of low back pain. JAMA, 272:1286–1291.

Linton, S.J., and van Tulder, M.W. (2001). Preventive interventions for back and neck pain problems: what is the evidence? Spine, 26, 778–787.

Luz, J., and Green, M.S. (1992). Sickness absence in 21 industrial plants in Israel (1986–87)—the Cordis Study. Isr J Med Sci, 28, 650–658.

Magill, R.A. (2004). Motor Learning: Concepts and applications. Dubuque, IA: W.C. Brown.

Occupational Health and Safety Agency for Healthcare in British Columbia (OHSAH). (2004). Trends in Workplace Injuries, Illnesses, and Policies in Healthcare Across Canada. http://www.ohsah.bc.ca/index.php?section_id = 441&section_copy_id = 400.

Owen, B.D., Keene, K., and Olson, S. (2002). An ergonomic approach to reducing back/shoulder stress in hospital nursing personnel: a five year follow up. Int J Nurs Stud, 39, 295–302.

Ratzon, N., Jarus, T., Baranes, G., Gilutz, Y., and Bar-Haim Erez, A. (1998). Reported level of pain of upper extremities related to multi-factorial workloads among office workers during and after work hours. Work, 11, 363–369

Ratzon, N.Z., Jarus, T., Mizlik, A., and Kanner, T. (2000). Musculoskeletal symptoms among dentists in relation to work posture. Work, 15, 153–158.

Schmidt, R.A. and Lee, T.D. (2005). Motor Control and Learning: A Behavioral Emphasis, 4th ed. Champaign, IL: Human Kinetics.

Schmidt, R.A., and Wrisberg, C.A. (2000). Motor Learning and Performance: A Problem-Based Learning Approach, 2nd ed. Champaign, IL: Human Kinetics.

Silverstein, B., Viikari-Juntura, E., and Kalat, J. (2002). Use of a prevention index to identify industries at high risk for work-related musculoskeletal disorders of the neck, back, and upper extremity in Washington state, 1990–1998. Am J Ind Med, 41, 149–169.

Skargren, E., and Oberg, B. (1996). Effects of an exercise program on musculoskeletal symptoms and physical capacity among nursing staff. Scand Med Sci Sport, 6, 122–130.

Skov, T., Borg, V., and Orhede, F. (1996). Psychosocial and physical risk factors for musculoskeletal disorders of the neck, shoulders, and lower back in salespeople. J Occup Environ Med, 53, 351–356.

Solberg, S.M. (2007). The LiftTrainer programme was not more effective than a video for reducing back injury in jobs with repetitive lifting. Evidence-Based Nurs, 10, 77.

Trinkoff, A.M., Lipscomb, J.A., Geiger-Brown, J., and Brady, B. (2002). Musculoskeletal problems of the neck, shoulder, and back and functional consequences in nurses. Am J Ind Med, 41, 170–178.

Tveito, T.H., Hysing, M., and Eriksen, H.R. (2004). Low back pain interventions at the workplace: a systematic literature review. Occup Med, 54, 3–13.

U.S. Department of Labor. (1991). The Revised Handbook for Analyzing Jobs. Indianapolis, IN: JIST Inc.

Vroman, K., and Macrea, N. (2001). Non-work factors associated with musculoskeletal upper extremity disorders in women: beyond the work environment. Work, 17, 3–9.

Warren, N. (2001). Work stress and musculoskeletal disorder etiology: the relative roles of psychosocial and physical risk factors. Work, 17, 221–234.

Wessels, T., Ewert, T., Limm, H., Rackwitz, B., and Stucki, G. (2007). Change factors explaining reductions of "interference" in a multidisciplinary and an exercise prevention program for low back pain. Clin J Pain, 23, 629–634.

Chapter 57
Motivational Interviewing: Enhancing Patient Motivation for Behavior Change

Robert J. Shannon

Despite our telling the client about the need to change his behavior, he just wouldn't do it.

Abstract The success of many therapies depends to a large degree on the extent to which patients engage with their treatment and adhere to the lifestyle changes that are recommended to them. However, this usually requires a high degree of effort and motivation on the part of the patient, and poor adherence is a common problem. A key task for occupational therapists (OTs), therefore, is enhancing motivation for behavior change. This is especially important given the increasing emphasis on helping patients to take more responsibility for their own care (Department of Health, 2004; Pill et al., 1998). Motivational interviewing has been shown to be an effective and efficient method for building motivation for behavior change in a number of problem areas (Hettema et al., 2005).

Keywords Behavior • Counseling • Motivation

Definition

Adherence: agreement between the patient's actual behavior and what was agreed to or prescribed.

Ambivalence: the experience of being of two minds about behavior change. It is a conflict between two courses of action, each of which has perceived costs and benefits. Unresolved ambivalence is a key barrier to sustained behavior change.

Change talk: patient's expressions of desire, ability, reasons, or need for change and commitment language (intentions, obligations, or agreements about change).

Motivation: incentives or driving forces that encourage behavior change.

Motivational interviewing (MI): a person-centered, counseling method designed to build motivation for behavior change by exploring and resolving ambivalence.

Resistance: arguments or disagreements about change; can be viewed as patients' attempts to have their ambivalence understood in the face of the therapist's

I. Söderback (ed.), *International Handbook of Occupational Therapy Interventions*,
DOI: 10.1007/978-0-387-75424-6_57, © Springer Science+Business Media, LLC 2010

arguments for change; can take a passive form, such as agreeing to change without an intention or commitment to do it.

Background

Traditional approaches to motivating patients to change behavior involve the provision of advice or education. When we see something that patients would benefit from, our "righting reflex" is to step in and "set things right" (Miller and Rollnick, 2002, p. 20). In an attempt to facilitate change, we often explain the benefits and importance of change, and the consequences of no change. The *righting reflex* reflects a genuine desire to help the patient. However, the problem is that many patients are of two minds (ambivalent) about change, and giving advice does little to resolve this. Indeed, giving advice to someone who is ambivalent can be detrimental to the change process. It is part of being human to want to be understood by others. So if patients are ambivalent about change and a therapist takes up the change side of patients' ambivalence, the natural response from them is to give voice to the other side of their ambivalence: "Yes, but I'm worried about ...." This is commonly labeled *resistance*, and is often interpreted as a sign of poor motivation, but in fact it simply represents patients' attempts to have their ambivalence understood. The more a therapist ignores aspects of the patient's ambivalence, or assumes greater importance or confidence for change than actually exists, the more the patient will resist (Rollnick et al., 1999). The problem with this is that our attitudes, beliefs, and intentions regarding behavior change are influenced by what we say (Bem, 1972). Therefore, if patients are counseled in a way that results in their defending their reasons not to change, they will become committed to that side of their ambivalence and talk themselves out of change.

A basic tenet of MI is that patients are more likely to be persuaded by their own arguments than by those of the therapist (Miller and Rollnick, 2002).

In health care settings, particularly when patients feel vulnerable, resistance is often displayed passively by apparently listening and agreeing to change, but without intention or commitment. This can also undermine change.

Motivational interviewing represents an alternative approach to advice giving. Rather than installing perceived deficits in knowledge, skills, or attitude, MI views patients as having an inherent motivation and capacity for change, which can be evoked (Miller and Rollnick, 2002). To resolve ambivalence (and thereby trigger change), the therapist provides a supportive, empathic atmosphere while selectively eliciting and strengthening the patient's own reasons for change (Miller, 2004). Once the patient is committed to change, a plan of action can be negotiated, itself increasing the likelihood of change.

Purpose

The goal of MI is to explore and resolve a patient's ambivalence about behavior change.

Method

Candidates for the Intervention

Motivational interviewing was originally developed for people with alcohol problems (Miller, 1983), but has since been used in a variety of different settings and with a broad range of behaviors. Examples of the different contexts in which MI has been studied and in which an occupational therapist (OT) may be involved include (1) alcohol abuse treatment, (2) asthma/chronic obstructive pulmonary disease, (3) brain injury rehabilitation, (4) cardiovascular health/hypertension, (5) chronic pain management, (6) diabetes risk reduction and treatment, (7) drug abuse treatment, (8) dual diagnosis (substance abuse and mental illness), (9) eating disorders and obesity, (10) emergency department/trauma/injury prevention, (11) employment readiness, (12) gambling treatment, (13) health promotion (e.g., physical activity), (14) HIV/AIDS risk reduction, (15) mental health treatment, and (16) tobacco use (Rollnick et al., 2008).

Settings

Motivational interviewing can be used as a motivational prelude to other active clinical interventions. For example, an OT offering a treatment program for patients with chronic pain based on principles of cognitive behavior therapy might use MI initially to build patients' motivation to make better use of the self-regulatory strategies that they will learn in the treatment program. There is good evidence that people who receive MI at the beginning of treatment are likely to stay in treatment longer, engage with the treatment to a greater degree, and experience better outcomes following the treatment than do people who receive the same intervention without the MI prelude (Hettema et al., 2005; Miller and Rollnick, 2002). One or two brief sessions of MI is often enough to provide the motivational catalyst to promote adherence to the treatment that follows.

Motivational interviewing has also been used as a stand-alone intervention, and most studies showing significant effects have generally involved relatively brief MI (one to four sessions). The mean dose of MI delivered in the Hettema et al. (2005) meta-analysis was about two sessions (mean 2.24 hours).

Another common application of MI is to *blend* it with other treatments, in other words to use MI *throughout* treatment. There is evidence that therapists' adherence to the collaborative, evocative, and autonomy-respecting spirit of MI is a strong predictor of behavior change beyond the technical components (Moyers et al., 2005). *Integrating* the spirit of MI with other interventions often improves outcome. To continue the pain management program example from above, a therapist delivering aspects of a cognitive behavioral therapy program in an MI style might ask for the patient's perspective on ways to problem solve rather than teach those things. The therapist might discuss the relevance of maladaptive cognitions but then carefully draw from patients their own perception of their thought patterns without labeling them as problematic or implying that the patient has to change; this is the MI style (Miller and Rollnick, 1991).

The Role of the Occupational Therapist

Developing Proficiency in Motivational Interviewing

In MI, the client and the OT bring different types of expertise to the consultation and work together to discuss the possibility of behavior change. The OT provides direction and support and elicits the client's thoughts about change. The therapist also provides information where necessary or when requested. However, the client is the active decision maker (Rollnick et al., 1999).

An important step in developing proficiency in MI involves suppressing the righting reflex (Miller and Moyers, 2007), that is, all temptation to tell clients that they must change should be avoided. This is the case if the client shows signs of resistance, but in reality the client will decide whether to change or not. The reason is that the signals that the client must change send a clear message of nonacceptance, which inhibits the change process. Like other psychological interventions and clinical procedures that OTs use, MI requires specific knowledge. It is a skilled counseling style that represents a fundamental departure from traditional approaches to encouraging behavior change. The most common form of training is a one-off workshop, but for most, this is insufficient in itself to promote clinically meaningful changes in MI proficiency. Additional coaching and feedback on practice is necessary (Miller and Mount, 2001; Miller and Moyers, 2007; Miller et al., 2004; Walters et al., 2005). A frequent occurrence, however, is that follow-up training is seldom well attended despite initial expressions of enthusiasm.

Results

Clinical Application

The Use of Motivational Interviewing

Motivational interviewing may be delivered in the following ways:

- Prior to another active intervention as a motivational prelude to improve engagement with the treatment
- In conjunction with another treatment
- As a stand-alone treatment

Miller (2004) has argued that because the outcomes of MI are generally realized after brief amounts of counseling, it may be appropriate to consider MI as a first intervention in stepped care. If behavior change does not occur after a reasonable amount of MI, a more intensive intervention can be used.

Motivational interviewing can also be used as a brief opportunistic intervention in circumstances where the patient has sought help or assistance for a problem but not specifically for help with behavior change (Rollnick et al., 1999). An example of this is talking about diet and exercise with patients who have diabetes and poor control of their blood sugar. The consultation provides a good opportunity to raise gently the subject of behavior change, even though it was not the patient's principal issue for discussing.

Motivational Interviewing: Theoretical Underpinning

Motivational interviewing was not founded on theory; rather, the original description was based on principles derived from its founder, William Miller's, intuitive practice (Miller, 1983). MI has been logically linked with a number of influential theories:

- It is grounded in Rogers's (1959) patient-centered counseling approach, which maintains that given the therapeutic conditions of empathy, acceptance, and support, people will draw on their own wisdom and desire to realize their potential, and as a consequence will change in ways that benefit their health and well-being.
- It is linked to Bem's (1972) self-perception theory, which holds that people's attitudes, thoughts, and beliefs are influenced by how they talk. In the context of discussions about behavior change, patients who spend most of the time engaged in change talk rather than defending their current behavior are most likely to talk themselves into change.
- Motivational interviewing was originally tied to Festinger's (1957) cognitive-dissonance theory, but Miller and Rollnick (2002) have since used the more general term *discrepancy* to describe mechanism by which motivation is developed. As clients talk loudly about their own reasons for change, a discrepancy develops in their mind between what they say they want and what they are currently doing. The bigger the discrepancy, the stronger the motivation is for behavior change.

Conducting Motivational Interviewing

The method of MI has been described in detail elsewhere (Miller and Rollnick, 2002; Rollnick et al., 2008). Therefore, a brief overview is presented here.

The Spirit

The essence of MI lies in its spirit. It is not a simple method to get patients to do things they do not want to do. Rather, it is a way of being with patients that draws on their motivations and values (Miller, 2004). While MI advocates specific skills and strategies, they need to be used in the context of a spirit that is collaborative, evocative, and respectful of the patient's autonomy (Miller and Rollnick, 2002).

The Key Guiding Principles

The key guiding principles of MI practice are to (1) resist the righting reflex; (2) understand and explore the patient's motivations; (3) listen with empathy; and (4) empower the patient, encouraging optimism and hope (Rollnick et al., 2008). The basic skills that are used to manifest the principles of MI are (1) asking open-ended questions, (2) affirming the patient, (3) expressing empathic reflective listening statements, and (4) providing summaries. These skills help create a nonjudgmental, supportive, empathic atmosphere, which frees patients to consider the possibility of change (Miller and Rollnick, 2002; Rogers, 1959. It draws on these skills to build motivation, strengthen, and commitment, and foster confidence for change by evoking and reinforcing the patient's own reasons for change (change talk) and responding to resistance (arguments against change) in a way that diffuses it.

The Change Talk

Change talk is a key-component in MI. It is elicited when OTs suppress their righting reflex. The correct way is (1) to ask questions that evoke the patient's own views about why change may be beneficial, (2) to ask what is wrong with the way things are, and (3) to ask how the patient might go about it in order to succeed. Examples of such questions are:

"In what ways would it be good for you to ____?" "What do you hope will be different? "How does [the behavior] fit into that?" "How might you go about it in order to succeed?"

Steve Rollnick's motivation and confidence rulers provide another way of evoking change talk (Rollnick et al., 2008, pp. 58–60). It begins with two open ended questions (here the example of regular exercise is used to illustrate):

On a scale from 0 to 10, how motivated are you right now to exercise on a regular basis, where 0 on the scale is not motivated at all and 10 is very motivated?

Then patients are asked how confident they are that they can make the change:

How confident are you that you could stick to a new level of exercise if you decided to do so, where 0 is not confident at all and 10 is very confident?

After getting scores for motivation and confidence, patients are asked to justify their scores: "Thinking about the motivation scale, why did you say X and not 0 (or a lower number)?" The responses will be change talk. This exercise can be repeated for the confidence scale.

Once change talk emerges, empathic reflective listening statements, which capture what was said, encourage further exploration. Asking for examples and elaboration ("In what ways?" "When was the last time?" "Can you give me an example?" What concerns you most about ____?") encourages patients to develop their arguments.

The resistance in a consultation may reflect that the therapist has misjudged some aspect of the patient's confidence or motivation for change and is a clear signal for a shift in communication. A simple reflective listening statement that acknowledges the patient's thoughts and feelings is often enough to diffuse the resistance.

For example, this dialogue might occur in a pain management context:

Patient: I tried that pacing thing in the last program I was in, but sometimes there are things that you have to do and it just goes out of the window.

> Therapist: You've got responsibilities and so far have not found a way to incorporate those into your pacing plan.

The following example uses a complex reflective listening statement to acknowledge what the patient has said but reframes it in a more positive way without undermining the patient's experience:

> Patient: I can't stand this. Just when things were going so well, I get this flare-up. You know, I was walking nearly a mile every day and I was able to bathe my son. And now I find it hard to move. It's like I'm back at the beginning. What's the point?

> Therapist: You've noticed by staying active, you've been able to do things that are important to you, but it's really hard to see the progress in light of this setback.

Other ways to respond to resistance involve different types of complex reflective listening statements and strategies such as *shifting focus and emphasizing personal control*. These are discussed in Miller and Rollnick (2002).

Motivational interviewing also draws on specific strategies for providing information and developing a plan of action.

Evidence-Based Practice

Recent meta-analyses of controlled trials of MI show that it is effective for enhancing *health behavior change in general* and for reducing drug and alcohol consumption in particular (Burke et al., 2003; Hettema et al., 2005). In the most recent meta-analysis of MI, the mean, short-term, between-group effect size was $d = 0.70$ decreasing to $d = 0.30$ at up to 1-year follow-up (Hettema et al., 2005). The change in effect size over time in the studies was generally because the control group got better or changed and started to catch up with the MI group, rather than the MI group relapsing. People also make better use of treatment after MI; when MI is used as a prelude to other proven interventions, attendance and engagement improve, as does long-term treatment outcome. A mean effect size of $d = 0.6$ (which persists over time) was observed across studies where MI is added to other active treatments. The Hettema meta-analysis was based on 72 clinical trials of MI. Now there are over 160 randomized trials of MI (Rollnick et al., 2008).

Motivational interviewing is considered an efficient method for effecting behavior change too. Most of the MI interventions in the Hettema meta-analysis were relatively brief, with the average dose of MI being about two sessions (mean = 2.24 hours). A large multicenter randomized controlled trial (Project MATCH Research Group, 1997) designed to assess how people respond to different treatment approaches for alcohol problems compared four sessions of an adaptation of MI (Motivational Enhancement Therapy, MET) with 12 sessions of 12-step facilitation or cognitive behavioral coping skills training. The outcomes for each of the three interventions were similar, but those randomized to receive MET reduced their drinking with less therapist contact time.

Discussion

The challenge of motivating patients to change behavior is a common one. Many of the patients with whom OTs work have conditions that can be improved, controlled, or managed through a change in behavior. While most, if not all, patients are motivated to achieve the outcome of behavior change, many are less motivated to engage in the behaviors necessary to achieve those benefits. In general, MI has been shown to be an effective and efficient method for achieving change in many of the health behaviors studied.

We are also beginning to understand the mechanisms involved in the effectiveness of MI. There is good evidence to support its relational component, specifically the use of patient-centered counseling skills and its spirit (Moyers et al., 2005). Process evaluation has also shown the importance of the selective eliciting and reinforcement of patient change talk as well as the importance of responding to resistance in a way that does not reinforce or prolong it. The level of resistance in a consultation is inversely related to behavior change (Miller et al., 1993), and change talk has been shown to be predictive of behavior change (Amrhein et al., 2003).

In its pure form, MI involves a number of sessions, often of long duration. Not all therapists have the luxury of such extended contact time, and for this reason adaptations of MI have been developed to manifest the spirit of MI but in a briefer format (Rollnick and Miller, 1995; Rollnick et al., 1992, 1999). A recent text (Rollnick et al., 2008) provides guidance on how MI might be blended into consultations when an OT has a number of tasks to undertake simultaneously.

References

Amrhein, P.C., Miller, W.R., Yahne, C.E., Palmer, M., and Fulcher, L. (2003). Client commitment language during motivational interviewing predicts drug use outcomes. J Consult Clin Psychol, 71(5), 862–878.

Bem, D.J. (1972). Self-perception theory. In: Berkowitz, L., ed. Advances in Experimental Social Psychology, Vol. 6 (pp. 1–62). New York: Academic Press.

Burke, B.L., Arkowitz, H., and Menchola, M. (2003). The efficacy of motivational interviewing: a meta-analysis of controlled clinical trials. J Consult Clin Psychol, 71, 843–861.

Department of Health [Richmond, England] (2004). Publications policy and guidance: choosing health: making healthy choices easier.
http://www.dh.gov.uk/en/Publicationsandstatistics/Publications/PublicationsPolicyAnd Guidance/DH_4094550. Retrieved 10/03/2009.

Festinger, L. (1957). A Theory of Cognitive Dissonance. Stanford, CA: Stanford University Press.

Hettema, J., Steele, J., and Miller, W.R. (2005). Motivational interviewing. Annu Rev Clin Psychol, 1(1), 91–111.

Miller, W.R. (1983). Motivational interviewing with problem drinkers. Behav Psychother, 11(2), 147–172.

Miller, W.R. (2004). Art of health promotion: motivational interviewing in service to health promotion. Am J Health Promot, 18(3), 1–10.

Miller, W.R., Benefield, R.G., and Tonigan, J.S. (1993). Enhancing motivation for change in problem drinking: a controlled comparison of two therapist styles. J Consult Clin Psychol, 61, 455–461.

Miller, W.R., and Mount, K.A. (2001). A small study of training in motivational interviewing: Does one workshop change clinician and client behavior? Behav Cogn Psychother, 29(4), 457–471.

Miller, W.R., and Moyers, T.B. (2007). Eight stages in learning motivational interviewing. J Teaching Addict, 5, 3–17.

Miller, W.R., and Rollnick, S. (1991). Motivational Interviewing: Preparing People to Change Addictive Behavior. New York: Guilford Press.

Miller, W.R., and Rollnick, S., eds. (2002). Motivational Interviewing: Preparing People for Change, 2nd ed. New York: Guilford Press.

Miller, W.R., Yahne, C.E., Moyers, T.B., Martinez, J., and Pirritano, M. (2004). A randomized trial of methods to help clinicians learn motivational interviewing. J Consult Clin Psychol, 72(6), 1050–1062.

Moyers, T.B., Miller, W.R., and Hendrickson, S.M. (2005). How does motivational interviewing work? Therapist interpersonal skill predicts client involvement within motivational interviewing sessions. J Consult Clin Psychol, 73(4), 590–598.

Pill, R., Rees, M.E., and Rollnick, S. (1998). Can nurses learn to let go? Issues arising from an intervention designed to improve patients' involvement in their own care. J Adv Nurs, 29, 1492–1499.

Project MATCH Research Group. (1997). Project MATCH secondary a priori hypotheses. Addiction, 92, 1671–1698.

Rogers, C.R. (1959). A theory of therapy, personality, and interpersonal relationships as developed in the client-centered framework. In: Koch, S., ed. Psychology: The Study of a Science: Vol. 3. Formulations of the Person and the Social Contexts (pp. 184–256). New York: McGraw-Hill.

Rollnick, S., Heather, N., and Bell, A. (1992). Negotiating behaviour change in medical settings: the development of brief motivational interviewing. J Mental Health (UK), 1(1), 25–37.

Rollnick, S., Mason, P., and Butler, C. (1999). Health Behaviour Change: A Guide for Practitioners. London: Churchill Livingstone.

Rollnick, S., and Miller, W.R. (1995). What is motivational interviewing? Behav Cogn Psychother, 23, 325–334.

Rollnick, S., Miller, W.R., and Butler, C.C. (2008). Motivational Interviewing in Health Care: Helping Patients Change Behavior. New York: Guilford Press.

Walters, S.T., Matson, S.A., Baer, J.S., and Ziedonis, D.M. (2005). Effectiveness of workshop training for psychosocial addiction treatments: a systematic review. J Substance Abuse Treat, 29(4), 283–293.

Part VI
Evaluation of Occupational Therapy Interventions

Chapter 58
Basic Elements for Conducting Evidence-Based Occupational Therapy

Ingrid Söderback

Abstract This chapter reports on methodology for evaluating the effectiveness of the interventions discussed in this handbook. The content and the four steps that compose evidence-based interventions are described as well as the various methods for conducting quality assurance. Assessment instruments represent the prerequisites for conducting evaluations of intervention effectiveness. Therefore, their possible aims, psychometric functions, and the process of collecting data and interpreting the results are reported in broad terms. An overview of the various available methods, such as the Goal Attainment Scale for evaluating a single client's progress when participating in therapeutic sessions, is presented. The terminology of outcome statements is discussed. Finally, recommendations for future advances in occupational therapy are suggested.

Keywords Assessment instruments • Effectiveness • Evaluation • Evidence-based interventions • Goal Attainment Scale • Outcome statements • Psychometric theory • Quality assurance • Single Case Research Design

Introduction

The interventions discussed in this handbook were presented based on the role of the occupational therapist (OT) in *managing, teaching, enabling, and promoting the clients' potential to be occupied with wanted and meaningful occupations, activities, and tasks.* The expectation of the clients, the profession, and society (Soderback, 1995) is that this *main goal* of occupational therapy—to be occupied—should be attained through the *occupational therapy interventions. The four main subgoals of these interventions are adaptation*, that is, the clients' internal, temporal, and environmental adaptations are improved; *teaching*, that is, the clients *learn* or *relearn* to perform daily activities; *recovery, that is,* the clients experience themselves as being occupied through participation in meaningful activities and tasks that influence their physiological and psychological healing; and *health and wellness*, that is, accidents in traffic, home, and work are prevented so as to promote clients' health.

The interventions discussed in this handbook are commonly used worldwide in clinical practice and have scientific evidence of their *effectiveness*. However, there

I. Söderback (ed.), *International Handbook of Occupational Therapy Interventions*,
DOI: 10.1007/978-0-387-75424-6_58, © Springer Science+Business Media, LLC 2010

are great variations of the extent of the interventions being evidence based, as was discussed in each intervention under the heading Evidence-Based Practice, which provides a foundation for clinical decisions and practical use.

This chapter discusses the following components: (1) *assessments,* (2) *research design,* and *(3) outcomes* of occupational therapy interventions. These components are necessary if the knowledge base of evidence-based interventions should increase in the future, to increase and ensure the *quality* of occupational therapy. The concepts of evidence-based interventions and quality assurance of occupational therapy should be investigated in parallel in clinical practice.

Evidence-Based Interventions

The term *evidence-based medicine* originated at McMaster Medical School in Canada in the 1980s to label this clinical learning strategy. The term was introduced to the database Medline in 1997, and was first identified in connection with occupational therapy through Ottenbacher's and Maas's (1999) post hoc power statistical analysis of 30 research interventions, demonstrating that the occupational therapy interventions "produced a potentially useful treatment effect, but the effect was not detected as significant."

Evidence-based medicine means that interventions include "the process of systematically finding, appraising, and using contemporaneous *research findings* as the basis for clinical decisions. Evidence-based medicine asks questions, finds and appraises the relevant data, and harnesses that information for everyday clinical practice". Evidence-based medicine follows four steps: "(1) formulate a clear clinical question from a patient's problem; (2) search the literature for relevant clinical articles; (3) evaluate (critically appraise) the evidence for its validity and usefulness; (4) implement useful findings in clinical practice" (Rosenberg and Donald, 1995). Applied to occupational therapy, these four steps are exemplified below.

Clear Formulated Clinical Questions

A study aimed at providing evidence of an intervention should include clear formulated clinical questions based on the clients' occupational problem. These questions originate from the clients', the professional, and the stakeholders perspectives.

It might be preferable to conduct these studies from the *clients' viewpoint.* For example, Hale and Cowls (2005) (see chapter 24) evaluated: Which are the eight clients' opinions about participating in psychoeducational groups? Their views were that voluntary attendance and the supportive milieu of the groups were the most appreciated.

Evaluation of the quality of the hospital discharge process, as outlined in a system-oriented approach, investigated: Which is frail elderly's perception of their satisfaction with and trust in the quality of care after discharge from the hospital to home, (Söderback, 2008). However, there are relatively few studies with this client-originated viewpoint.

It is much more common that research questions are originated from the occupational therapy *professional perspective* as treatment outcome studies, implying evaluation assessments of the results or the consequences of conducting a specific intervention. The results are expected to show efficacy of interventions, safety of interventions, program evaluations, or efficacy assessments. For example, a common research question is: "Is the new routine for the use of this specific intervention more effective than the routine ordinarily used?"

Studies originated from the *stakeholder perspective*, include cost-benefit analysis. These studies are conducted with the research question: "Is the cost of an intervention program defensible compared to its expected benefits or cost-effectiveness. In other words, alternative ways to achieve effectively results are investigated. For example, occupational therapy interventions conducted in ten sessions were more cost-effective for patients with dementia and their caregivers, compared to those who did not participate in occupational therapy (Graff et al., 2008) (see chapter 19).

Search Literature for Relevant Clinical Articles

Occupational therapists working as clinicians may find information about evidence-based occupational therapy interventions through the following specific databases:

- *OT seeker* (McKenna et al., 2008) is a valuable discipline-specific, online database and an excellent way of making research accessible for OTs' decision-making. The OT seeker is proved to be of clinical value, as demonstrated in a study in which 62% of OTs (n = 309), who used the source during a 30-day period had improved their ability to locate evidence-based interventions (Bennett et al., 2007).
- *The database Cochrane reviews* (Collaboration Cochrane Library, 2008) provides practitioners with up-to-date information as a base for relevant evidence in their field of interest. For example, the Cochrane Library was used to identify the strategies for dealing with clinical heterogeneity of interventions of occupational and physiotherapy. The results showed limitations in the number and type of outcome measures and the lack of quantitative data synthesis (van den Ende et al., 2006).
- *Entrez-PubMed* is the general database for medicine with representation of most of the profession-specific occupational therapy journals presented in the English language (National Library of Medicine, 2008a).

Evaluating the Evidence for Validity and Usefulness of Occupational Therapy Interventions

The scientific methods used for studies expected to prove or reject the evidence of the effectiveness of occupational therapy interventions include the following:

- Results of well-reported randomized controlled trials (RCTs).[1] The quality of these studies may be analyzed according to the Nelson-Moberg Expanded Consort assessment instrument. However, the primary psychometric data that results from this instrument showed that there is a need for greater sophistication if it is to be a valid tool for evaluation of RCTs (Moberg Mogren and Nelson, 2006).
- Systematic reviews performed according to the Cochrane Review Guidelines or the best evidence synthesis review (van der Velde et al., 2007).
- Other ways for determining the evidence of the effectiveness of interventions include, for example, qualitative case methodology, results from consensus conferences, focus groups, the Delphi method, reports from peer review groups, and a best evidence synthesis review.[2] Using one of these methods should result in a guideline for determining the evidence of the effectiveness of an occupational therapy intervention.

Implement Useful Findings in Clinical Practice

If research is to be optimally used to provide clinicians with evidence for the interventions applied, the following recommendations should be observed: (1) contextualize the research and clinical practice by outlining the research results that it is easy to access and understand; (2) establish a researcher–stakeholder partnership; (3) provide professional–peer support (Koch et al., 2006); and (4) provide clinicians with knowledge through targeted workshops, and provide follow-up support aimed at implementing new routines of evidence-based practice (McCluskey and Lovarini, 2005).

Quality Assurance in Occupational Therapy

In health care, quality assurance is a continuing process using measures aimed at improving the quality of the occupational therapy interventions that the clients are offered. These measures assess quality and effectiveness, and identify the shortcomings, which should result in recommendations for improvement and follow-up monitoring (National Library of Medicine, 2008b). The quality of occupational therapy interventions is expected to be acceptable, accessible, accredited, comprehensive, cost-effective, equitable, effective, efficient, relevant, and reliable (Wright and Whittington, 1992).

Several methods are available for ensuring the quality of occupational therapy interventions: (1) The *Donabedian method* (1980/1982) is aimed at identifying the quality and problems in health care through investigation of structure (resources and administration), process (culture and professional cooperation), and outcome (competence development and goal achievement) (Kunkel et al., 2007). This method is sparsely used in occupational therapy. (2) "A chart-stimulated recall (CSR)

---

[1] For information on research design see, Stein and Cutler, 2000.

[2] For an explanation of these methods, see a textbook containing scientific methodology (Polit and Hungler, 1999).

peer-review process and the interview tool were revised, implemented, and evaluated...
to assess the clinical competence of occupational therapy staff" (Salvatori et al., 2008),
and the same method was used to outline clinical guidelines for occupational therapy
interventions in patients with burn injuries (Simons et al., 2003). (3) *Evaluation of
intervention programs* is a commonly used approach in studies evaluating effectiveness. For example, Goodman et al. (2005) (see chapter 6) demonstrated that 74%
of all ergonomic recommendations regarding improvement of computer stations had
been implemented by an engineer company. (4) The *DySSy-model* (Kitson, 1989)
uses an eight-step process for ongoing assessments; for example, an evaluation of
occupational therapy case-record documentation showed that only 21 of 100 of the
records were complete (Backman et al., 2008).

Assessment Instruments

All health services in Sweden are expected to be based on scientific evidence, meaning that *effectiveness* (that is if the intended goals are reached) and *efficiency* (that is
the amount of resources required to reach the goal) (Söderback, 1995) of an occupational therapy intervention are demonstrated. In other words, the intervention should
be effective for improving the clients' functioning (World Health Organization, 2007,
p. 11). Therefore, assessment instruments with guaranteed reliability and validity
constitute an absolute prerequisite for (1) making well-founded evidence-based clinical decisions, (2) evaluating, planning, goal setting in occupational therapy interventions, (3) conducting RCT scientific studies, and (4) investigating the effectiveness,
efficiency, and cost-benefit analysis of clinical interventions' outcomes.

   Assessment is a process of collecting objective and relevant data. These data are
measured, scored, and interpreted according to standardized criteria, which includes
psychometric reliability and validity and an adequate performance procedure (Stein
and Cutler, 1998). The assessment process requires analysis of the critical factors of
the client's continuum of functioning and impairment, related to the significance and
meaning of task performance, the tools used, and the environment where the task or
occupation will occur. An assessment instrument provides quantity measures expressed
in scores, frequencies, time, percent, or physical measures such as length or temperature.
Assessments are used with emphasis on different functional dimensions depending on
the client's disease and disability. For example, the assessment for clients with chronic
fatigue syndrome emphasizes the amount of energy needed to perform the actual tasks
related to the functional capacity of the client (Barrows, 1995).

Selection of an Instrument for Assessment

The rationale for selecting an adequate assessment instrument for a client and situation, as well as the procedure for gathering data, is based on a problem-solving
process that is both continuous and dynamic. The following sections discuss the

OTs' decision-making in selecting appropriate assessment instruments through a systematic review of their psychometric properties, feasibility, and viability. This review may be useful in determining the appropriateness of assessment instruments for a client's unique situation. For this purpose, the appendix provides a blank form for evaluation of assessment instruments.

Available Types of Assessment Instruments

The OT should make a choice of which type of assessment instrument would be appropriate for use in relation to the individual client's status, diagnosis and functioning, expected occupational therapy goal, and present environment. The choice might be between:

Global assessment instruments are used to compare the client's results with those of a normative group.

Diagnosis-specific instruments are used for clients who suffer from the same medical diagnosis or disabilities.

Domain-specific instruments are used for assessing impairments, activity limitations (e.g., related to work capacity), or age or participation restrictions. The results of this assessment determine the characteristic patterns of clients' who belong to a specific domain.

The Aims of Assessment Instruments

There are assessment instruments aimed at (1) *describing,* (2) *predicting,* or (3) *evaluating outcome* (Law and Letts, 1989). A *descriptive* assessment instrument is used to establish clients' occupational characteristics, symptoms, or patterns of occupational performances aimed at determining the choice of occupational therapy interventions. A *predictive* assessment instrument is used to determine the future need for support for performing activities of daily living (ADL) and generalization effects (see Chapter 22). The *evaluating* outcome assessment instruments are used in RCT studies and to determine clients' goal attainment and other expected results after that clients have participated in an intervention.

Content of the Assessment Manual

Every assessment instrument should include a manual for conducting the assessment, a computer program for interpreting the results, and a form for recording the results. The required contents of a manual are (1) administration instructions; (2) the assessment instrument's aim (describe, predict, evaluate) and focus; (3) the theoretical base of the assessment; and (4) the psychometric functions (see below). The administration instructions are the guiding principles for conducting the specific assessment. The focus may be intended for a diagnosis, or a domain, or related to age, or combinations of these. The psychometric functions are data regarding the validity, that is, that the measure determines what it really is intended to measure, and the reliability, that is, how exact the measure is.

Psychometric Functions: Types of Measurement Scales

The items represent measures that are constructed with scales of *nominal* (*category*), *ordinal, interval,* or *quota.* The sensitivity of an assessment instrument is determined by the types of the assessment scale, that is, for which clinical situations the assessment instrument is appropriate, such as to describe function, predict future functioning, or evaluate outcome.

Nominal and ordinal measurement scales are used to differentiate between categories. Assessment instruments constructed with nominal scales are appropriate to use for *describing clients' occupational characteristics* and give an indication the range of the disability and occupational dysfunction, but are not useful for evaluation of effectiveness.

Measurements based on an *ordinal measurement scale* (e.g., the Likert scale, Guttman cumulative scale, and Goal Attainment Scale [GAS][3]) define the order of ranks that make comparisons between people with the same prerequisites and over time. The results give a summarized assessment of the client's present status and predict the outcome of participation in an intervention (how *effective* the intervention will be for this client).

Assessments based on an *interval measurement scale* show a continuum, such as a range of motion, size difference in centimeters or minutes, and include the exact distance between the measurement points, but without an absolute zero point. The standardized scale type, based on the interval scale, shows the client's divergence from the mean value, and is used for measuring intelligence, for example.

A *quote measurement scale* has the same prerequisites as an interval scale measurement, but includes an absolute zero point. The interval and the quote measurement scales are preferable when determine intervention *effectiveness*.

Psychometric Functions: The Items

The *items* are composed the questions or observations of a performance of a specific task or parts of it. Several items constitute *variables*, also called factors, and these in turn constitute categories.

The items that constitute variables have their relative positioning order on a measurement scale. This order is determined by statistical methods, such as Chronbach's coefficient alpha (α). Such coefficients determine how exact the measure of an assessment instrument is; that is, it represents the *reliability*. The reliability statistics are used to understand for which clinical situations the assessment instrument is appropriate. The *internal consistency* of an assessment instrument is expected to be between $\alpha = 0.71$ and $\alpha = 0.80$ in order to have acceptable measurement properties useful for receiving *descriptive* information. The alpha (α) coefficient should be higher than 0.81 for measurement properties necessary for the *evaluation* of intervention effectiveness. However, assessment instruments to be used with a *predicative* aim should have an internal consistency of more than $\alpha = 0.95$ (Law and Letts, 1989).

---

[3]For complete information about these scale types, see Polit and Hungler, 1999.

Psychometric Functions: Validity of an Assessment Instrument

Logical reasoning and the construction of an assessment instrument are a matter of vital importance for its validity.

The *content validity,* representative validity, or face validity concerns the degree to which items represent the subject of measure, for example, that measures of daily activities really are the client's daily activities.

The *construct validity,* theory validity, or internal validity corresponds to the theoretical origin of the assessment instrument (convergent validity), or is distinct from it (divergent validity).

The *criterion validity* or empirical validity concerns the degree to which an assessment measures concurrent changes between two group members or predicts the client's changes over time among members of a group of clients.

Collecting Data Using an Assessment Instrument

The variations in collecting data are shown in Fig. 58.1.

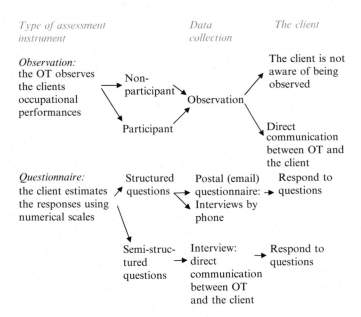

Fig. 58.1 Different ways of colleting data using assessment instruments.

Reporting Results of Assessments

Results of an assessment are determined in terms of the following:

- *Raw scores,* which seldom give useful information for goal setting or evaluation. Normally, raw scores should at least be converted to percentage.

- *Response patterns* or behavior outcome, which is used to compare and describe differences in function among people belonging to similar groups (e.g., clients with the same diagnoses, impairments, activity limitations, participation restrictions, or socioeconomic circumstances).
- *Derived scores* (e.g., standard scores, measures of central tendency, standard deviations or percentiles), which give OTs the opportunity to compare clients' function over time and between groups; that is, evaluation of intervention effectiveness is possible.
- *Index,* which is a ratio that compares two related measures. For example, the body mass index describes the relationship between a client's height and weight.
- *The degree of difficulty* in performing a task, which can be analyzed by using a Rasch analysis (Fisher, 1993; Kirkley and Fisher, 1999; Linacre and Wright, 1991–1996). This statistical measure indicates the client's estimated ability to perform tasks in relation to the degree of difficulty in performing the tasks. Thus, scoring occurs in two ways: (1) the difficulty level of the tasks, and (2) the way in which the results of a client are comparable to others having a similar disability. Use of the Rasch analysis enables the OT to plan interventions. For example, the *Evaluation of Daily Activity Questionnaire* (EDAQ) (Nordenskiöld et al., 1996) was used to describe how well women with rheumatoid arthritis ($n = 47$) could perform activities of daily living. Among 102 activities, the women indicated that grocery shopping was the hardest task to perform and walking indoors was the easiest task to perform. The Rasch analysis is used with the *Assessment of Motor Process Skills* (AMPS) (Fisher, 1993).
- *Method-time measurement* (MTM) scores (Farrell, 1993), which are criterion-referenced procedures that measure the time it takes for a client to complete a predetermined number of basic movements within a predetermined time standard (Jacobs, 1991). These results are used in determining job readiness by comparing the worker's performance to established job standards.
- *Modular Arrangement of Predetermined Time Standards* (Farrell and Muik, 1993), which is a version of MTM where the standard length of time is related to the area of work in which the specific movement is performed.

Outcome Assessments Aimed at Evaluating a Single Client's Participation in an Intervention

Evaluation of *one* client's participation in an occupational therapy intervention is not enough to determine evidence for the effectiveness of the intervention. However, evaluation of a client's development during a series of occupational therapy sessions should be a natural part of the intervention, because it (1) gives the OT valuable information about the necessity of changes in the intervention, (2) might be a motivation factor for the client, and (3) could be a useful base for conducting studies that might contribute to a decision based on evidence effectiveness.

The clinical evaluation of the client's progress is related to (1) the projected goals of the intervention, (2) the direction of the impairment or disability (improvement, maintenance, or deterioration) (Söderback, 1995), and (3) the focus of the evaluation (e.g., self-care, physical improvement).

Quantitative[4] evaluations are most often based on assessment instruments of the client's participation in an intervention. These evaluations are conducted as (1) *a summative assessment* including a testing before and after the intervention, or (2) *a formative assessment* or a series of assessments during the time an intervention is carried out. Pretesting identifies the client's need for occupational therapy intervention, while posttesting gives information about the client's change(s). The results of these summative or formative assessments are possible to determine by using the *reliability change index* (RCI) (Guidetti and Söderback, 2001; Ottenbacher et al., 1988).

Even if less represented in the literature, GAS (Chang and Hasselkus, 1998; Kiresuck et al., 1994) is a valuable method for determining a client's change during participation in interventions. For example, in a vocational training program, the results showed that three out of four patients had attained their predetermined goals ($T = >50$) (Gruwsved et al., 1996).

Finally, *Single Case Research Experimental Design* (Kazdin, 1982, or comparable textbook; see http://www.amazon.com/) is a scientific alternative for the OT to receive information about the effectiveness of an intervention that is newly applied to or modified for a small group of clients. See, for example, Campbell et al.'s (2007) multiple-baseline study that investigated the effectiveness of errorless learning applied to a client with severe traumatic brain injury. The results showed significance ($p < .001$) of memory lapses during a 3-month follow-up.

Outcomes

Outcomes are efforts aimed at "assessing the quality and effectiveness of health care as measured by the attainment of a specified end result or outcome," but the efficacy, safety, and practicability may also be investigated due to treatment evaluations (National Library of Medicine, 2008b). Outcome is an important dimension of health attribute of interventions, including ability to function, health perceptions, and satisfaction with care (American Occupational Therapy Association, 2002).

Reporting Outcome Evaluation of Interventions

The changes, or outcomes, that occur after a client has finished participation in an intervention is suggested to be evaluated using statements that concern the level of (1) the ability to perform occupations, (2) satisfaction with occupational perform-

---

[4]*Qualitative* methods for evaluating the effectiveness of occupational therapy interventions are greatly advocated but for the present without this frame of effectiveness evaluation.

ances, (3) independence in self-care activities, (4) quality of life, (5) well-being, (6) satisfaction with current health status, (7) internal adaptation to impairment or disability, (8) compliance with interventions, and (9) satisfaction with appropriateness, usefulness, and cost-effectiveness (Stein et al., 2006).

Such statements, used for evidence of the interventions' effectiveness, are of great importance for the credibility of outcome and for defining the profession. It might be suggested that the more the profession uses joint statements about outcome, the better respected will be the intervention. Of course, the opposite is also true: disparate statements of outcome will cause less evidence for its effectiveness. Therefore, the question is: *What are the most appropriate statements to be used to determine occupational therapy interventions?* In other words, *What outcome terms should be recommended for use?* The answers to these questions are beyond the scope of this handbook. However, a nonsystematic overview (Table 58.1) is presented, aimed at showing the current status of the intervention outcome statements presented in this handbook. Most of the examples used originated with the authors of this handbook. The content reflects a wide range between interventions in which no evaluation of outcomes were performed and other interventions conducted with RCT studies. A very wide range of outcome statements exists. Some of them seem to have less connection to the core content of occupational therapy. Other outcome statements concern occupations, such as the number of occupational performances errors, activities of daily living, or sustaining work performance. Many outcome statements originated from the International Classification of Functioning, Disability, and Health (ICF) terminology, for example, measures of impairments such as balance and anxiety.

The conclusion of this incomplete survey of outcome statements is that the occupational therapy profession would be more respected if these statements were congruently used by OTs.

Recommendations for the Future

This handbook is based on an extensive literature review and the expert knowledge the authors possess. The content gave me valuable information about the present state of the art of occupational therapy and is pros and corns. For the future, I would recommend:

- Further development and documentation of interventions.
- Teamwork for conducting more extensive RCT studies, which will result in greater numbers of clinical decisions being based on evidence.
- Continuously assessed quality assurance as a nature part of the clinical work.
- Arrangement of consensus conferences aimed at discussing outcome statements that are congruent. Such statements would facilitate communication among OTs worldwide, as they are working to meet their clients' occupational needs.

Table 58.1 Statements used for defining outcomes of occupational therapy interventions

Occupational therapy intervention	Medical diagnoses/impairments	Outcome statement	Reference
Environmental adaptations	General adaptations	Older adults and their families	Survival time	Gitlin et al. (2006)
	Housing adaptations	General	Accessibility; number of physical environmental barriers; usability	Fänge and Iwarsson (2005)
Accessibility	Ergonomic workplace interventions for computer users with cumulative trauma disorders	General	Number of resolved physical problems at the workplace	Goodman et al. (2005)
Accommodation	Wheelchair seating: pressure mapping	General	Not evaluated	
	Wheelchair prescription	General	Accident rate; extent of pressure sores; number and extent of repairs; reconditioning, adjustments; user satisfaction	Hansen et al. (2004)[a]
Electric prostheses: orthotics and splinting	Neuro-prosthesis	Quadriplegia	Measures of: independence; hand function	Popovic et al. (2006)
	Splinting:	Traumatic hand injury	Not evaluated	
	Splinting:	Burn injury	Not evaluated	
Prescription of assistive devices:		Children with disabilities	Not evaluated	
		Low-vision	Facilitating a supporting network; supports barrier-free low vision acquisition	Copolillo and Teitelman (2005)
Universal design	Universal design		Not evaluated	
	The design of hand tools:		Not evaluated	

Temporal adaptation	Temporal adaptation	Mental illness	Imbalance in temporal occupation: passive leisure activities; abnormally long sleep	Krupa et al. (2003)
Cognitive teaching approaches and the behavioral teaching approach	Problem solving:	Families caring for persons with dementia	Clients improved skills; less need for assistance; fewer negative behavioral occurrences	Gitlin et al. (2005)
	Teaching and supporting in daily functioning	Dementia	Daily functioning; reduced burden on the caregiver	Graff et al. (2006)
Cognitive teaching approaches the dialogue technique approach	Meta-cognitive occupation-based training	Traumatic brain injury	Facilitating participants' self-awareness; increased anxiety	Fleming et al. (2006)
	Meta-cognitive Mental Imagery Strategies The self-regulation	Brain damage	Better relearning of trained and untrained tasks	Liu et al. (2004)
	Strategies to compensate to apraxia	Stroke clients	Motor functioning ADL; generalization	Geusgens et al. (2006)
Energy conservation	Energy conservation education	Multiple sclerosis	Participants' valued participation in the therapeutic cooking group as effectively: functional activities; socialization	Hill et al. (2007)
			Number of new energy conservation strategies	Ip et al. (2006)
			Oxygen consumption: for shopping, for hanging laundry	Matuska et al. (2007)

(continued)

Table 58.1 (continued)

Occupational therapy intervention		Medical diagnoses/impairments	Outcome statement	Reference
Psychoeducation	Psychoeducational groups		Participants valued: voluntary attendance; supportive milieu	Cowls and Hale (2005)
	Illness management training	Acute psychiatric ward	Improving illness insight; lower re-admission rate	Chan et al. (2007)
	Psychosocial intervention	Schizophrenia	Combination of OT and clozapine more effective than the use of clozapine alone; occupational therapy represents an additional therapeutic option	Buchain et al. (2003)
	Treating alteration of lifestyle	Anxiety and panic disorder	Anxiety decrease	Lambert et al. (2007)
	Behavioral approach; 12-step program	Clients with substance use	Number of clients with no substance use	Chapter 28
Neuromusculoskeletal and movement-related learning	Trunk restraint function	Upper limb motor impairment	Decreased trunk movement; elbow extension	Michaelsen et al. (2006)
	Constraint-induced movement therapy (CIT)	Stroke	Motor function	Bowman et al. (2006)
	Strategies for cuing with self speech	Stroke	Motor performance of reaching velocity	Maitra et al. (2006)
	Joint protection	Rheumatoid arthritis	Joint protection adherence; early morning stiffness; activities of daily living; fewer hand deformities	Hammond and Freeman (2004)

Sensory functional training	Sensory integration	Children with Down syndrome	Balance	Uyanik et al. (2003)
	Constraint-induced movement therapy with botulinum toxin-A injection	Children with cerebral paresis upper-limb	Treatment effect	Hoare et al. (2007)
	Pain management: back schools		Level of disability; health-related quality of life	Vollenbroek-Hutten et al. (2004)
	Pain management		Not evaluated	
Learning approaches for participation in working life	Practice of work and ergonomics		Not evaluated	
	Reintegration to work	Depression	Reduction in time of work-loss; reduction of work stress	Schene et al. (2007)
	Supported employment	Severe mental illness	Sustain at work	Twamley et al. (2003)
	Individual placement and support (IPS)	Severe mental illness	Return to work	Burns et al. (2008)
	Conducting transitional strategies	Children with special needs	Not evaluated	
Engagement in occupations	Creating opportunities for participation in mental health day health services		Structured days; support networks; feelings: alienated; decisions of life influence	Bryant et al. (2004)
	Recreational activities	Clients with Alzheimer's disease	Behavioral symptoms; caregiver reaction to behavioral disturbances	Farina et al. (2006)
	Horticultural therapy	Elderly people	Impact of separation on couples	Martin et al. (2008)[a]
	Medical music therapy	Dementia	Mood state; heart rate	Wichrowski et al. (2005)[a]
			Mental representations of movement are influenced by the current state of nociceptive feedback	Schwoebel et al. (2002)
	Music as a resource for health and well-being	Cancer care	Not evaluated	

(continued)

Table 58.1 (continued)

Occupational therapy intervention	Medical diagnoses/impairments	Outcome statement	Reference
Preventing accidents in the home	Preventing falls	Older people	The effect education for primary care professionals is sustained in women – not in men	Avlund et al. (2007)
	Preventive home visits to people	Older people	Functional ability	
Preventing traffic accidents	Use of in-vehicle intelligent transport system		Driving errors made during license review tests	Di Stefano and Macdonald (2003)
Preventing work-related injuries	Work-related health. Organizational factors	Workers	Correlative studies	–
	Functional capacity evaluation	Back pain clients	Clinical feasibility; recommendations for return to work; performance of the physical demands of work	Gibson et al. (2005)
	A four stages intervention model	Workers with musculoskeletal disorders	Not evaluated	
	Motivational interviewing		Not evaluation	

Note: This table is a nonsystematic overview of the interventions that is presented in this handbook by the chapter authors. Not evaluated means that no evaluation study was found in the PubMed Database http://www.nslij-genetics.org/search_pubmed.html.) [a]The author has not contributed to this handbook.

Appendix   A Checklist aimed for the Choice of an Appropriate Assessment Instrument

1	The assessment instrument entitled: Version?
2	The source of the assessment instrument: Author(s)? Reference(s)?
3	References with: (a) clinical applications? (b) evidence of the psychometric functions of the assessment instrument?
4	Theory or model that constitutes the base of the assessment instrument?
5	Is a manual, a computer program, recording forms, and other equipment for administration of the assessment instrument available?
6	How is the assessment instrument administered? How are the data collected? How are results given to the client?
7	What is the focus of the assessment instrument? (global, diagnosis-specific, etc.)
8	For what is the assessment instrument intended? (diseases, diagnoses, disability, impairment, age, language)
9	What is the aim of the assessment instrument? (describe, predict, evaluate)
10	Describe the construction of the assessment instrument (e.g., number and titles of items and factors).
11	What measurement scale is used? (nominal, ordinal, interval, quote)
12	What type of scale is used for the assessment?
13	What is known about the reliability of the assessment instrument? (internal consistency, observer-/test-retest reliability)
14	How sensitive is the assessment instrument (suitable for application to describe, evaluate, predict)?
15	How appropriate (sensitive) is the assessment instrument for performing repeated measures?
16	What reliability coefficients are known that correspond to a group of people with the same prerequisites as the client who would take the assessment?
17	What standard deviation is known according to the group of people with the same prerequisites as the client who would take the assessment?
18	What is known about the validity of the assessment instrument? (content, concurrent, criterion)
19	With what method are the results calculated?
20	Is there enough psychometric information for calculating the results and is the specific formula for calculating the results stated?
21	Are guidelines for interpretation of the clients' performance available?
22	Are cut-off scores, criteria, or other limits for the clients' performance stated that make the result interpretable for making clinical decisions or evaluating intervention results?
23	What is known about the cost-benefit of the assessment instrument?
24	Does the administrator (therapist) need specific knowledge?
25	What are the positive and negative experiences of using the assessment instrument (preferably based on scientific publications) for similar situations as for the actual client?

References

American Occupational Therapy Association. (2002). Occupational therapy practice framework: domain and process. Am J Occup Ther, 56, 609–634.

Avlund, K., Vass, M., Kvist, K., Hendriksen, C., and Keiding, N. (2007). Educational intervention toward preventive home visitors reduced functional decline in community-living older women. J Clin Epidemiol, 60(9), 954–962.

Backman, A., Kåwe, K., and Bjorklund, A. (2008). Relevance and focal view point in occupational therapists' documentation in patient case records. Scand J Occup Ther, 15(4):212–220.

Barrows, D.M. (1995). Functional capacity evaluations of persons with chronic fatigue immune dysfunction syndrome. Am J Occup Ther, 49(4), 327–337.

Bennett, S., McKenna, K., Hoffmann, T., Tooth, L., McCluskey, A., and Strong, J. (2007). The value of an evidence database for occupational therapists: an international online survey. Int J Med Inform, 76(7), 507–513.

Bowman, M.H., Taub, E., Uswatte, G., et al. (2006). A treatment for a chronic stroke patient with a plegic hand combining CI therapy with conventional rehabilitation procedures: case report. NeuroRehabilitation, 2(21), 167–176.

Bryant, W., Craik, C., and McKay, E.A. (2004). Living in a glasshouse: exploring occupational alienation. Can J Occup Ther, 7(15), 282–289.

Buchain, P.C., Vizzotto, A.D., Henna, N.J., and Elkis, H. (2003). Randomized controlled trial of occupational therapy in patients with treatment-resistant schizophrenia. Rev Bras Psiquiatr, 25(1), 26–30.

Burns, T., Catty, J., White, S., Becker, T., Koletsi, M., Fioritti, A., Rössler, W., Tomoy, T., van Busschbach, J., Wiersma, D., and Lauber, C; For the EQOLISE group (2008). The impact of supported employment and working on clinical and social functioning: results of an international study of individual placement and support. Schizophr Bull Apr 21 [Epub ahead of print] PMID: 18403375 [PubMed - as supplied by publisher].

Campbell, L., Wilson, F.C., McCann, J., Kernahan, G., and Rogers, R.G. (2007). Single case experimental design study of Carer facilitated Errorless Learning in a patient with severe memory impairment following TBI. NeuroRehabilitation, 22(4), 325–333.

Chan, S.H., Lee, S.W., and Chan, I.W. (2007). TRIP: a psycho-educational programme in Hong Kong for people with schizophrenia. Occup Ther Int, 14(2), 86–98.

Chang, L.H., and Hasselkus, B.R. (1998). Occupational therapists' expectations in rehabilitation following stroke: sources of satisfaction and dissatisfaction. Am J Occup Ther, 52(8), 629–637.

Collaboration Cochrane Library (2008). The Cochrane Library. The reliable source of evidence in health care. http://www.cochrane.org/reviews/clibintro.htm.

Copolillo, A., and Teitelman, J.L. (2005). Acquisition and integration of low vision assistive devices: understanding the decision-making process of older adults with low vision. Am J Occup Ther, 59(3), 305–313.

Cowls, J., and Hale, S. (2005). It's the activity that counts what clients value in psycho-educational groups. Can J Occup Ther, 72(3), 176–182.

Di Stefano, M., and Macdonald, W. (2003). Assessment of older drivers: relationships among on-road errors, medical conditions and test outcome. J Safety Res, 34(4), 415–429.

Donabedian, A. (1980/1982). Explorations in Quality Assurance and Monitoring. Michigan: Health Administration Press.

Fänge, A., and Iwarsson, S. (2005). Changes in ADL dependence and aspects of usability following housing adaptation—a longitudinal perspective. Am J Occup Ther, 59, 296–304.

Farina, E., Mantovani, F., Fioravanti, R., et al. (2006). Efficacy of recreational and occupational activities associated to psychologic support in mild to moderate Alzheimer disease: a multi-center controlled study. Alzheimer Dis Assoc Disord, 20(4), 275–282.

Farrell, J.M. (1993). Predetermined motion-time standards in rehabilitation. A review. Work, 3(2), 56–72.

Farrell, W.J., and Muik, E.A. (1993). Computer applications that streamline test scoring and other procedures in occupational therapy. Am J Occup Ther, 47(5), 462–465.

Fisher, W.P. Jr. (1993). Measurement-related problems in functional assessment. Am J Occup Ther, 47(4), 331–338.

Fleming, J.M., Lucas, S.E., and Lightbody, S. (2006). Using occupation to facilitate self-awareness in people who have acquired brain injury: a pilot study. Can J Occup Ther, 73(1), 44–55.

Geusgens, C., van Heugten, C., Donkervoort, M., van den Ende E., Jolles, J., and van den Heuvel, W. (2006). Transfer of training effects in stroke patients with apraxia: an exploratory study. Neuropsychol Rehabil, 16(2), 213–229.

Gibson, L., Strong, J., and Wallace, A. (2005). Functional capacity evaluation as a performance measure: evidence for a new approach for clients with chronic back pain. Clin J Pain, 21(3), 207–215.

Gitlin, L.N., Hauck, W.W., Dennis, M.P., and Winter, L. (2005). Maintenance of effects of the home environmental skill-building program for family caregivers and individuals with Alzheimer's disease and related disorders. J Gerontol A Biol Sci Med Sci, 60(3), 368–374.

Gitlin, L.N., Winter, L., Dennis, M.P., Corcoran, M., Schinfeld, S., and Hauck, W.W. (2006). A randomized trial of a multicomponent home intervention to reduce functional difficulties in older adults. J Am Geriatr Soc, 54(5), 809–816.

Goodman, G., Landis, J., George, C., et al. (2005). Effectiveness of computer ergonomics interventions for an engineering company: a program evaluation. Work, 24(1), 53–62.

Graff, M.J., Adang, E.M., Vernooij-Dassen, M.J., et al. (2008). Community occupational therapy for older patients with dementia and their caregivers: cost effectiveness study. BMJ, 336(7936), 134–138.

Graff, M.J., Vernooij-Dassen, M.J., Thijssen, M., Dekker, J., Hoefnagels, W.H., and Rikkert, M.G. (2006). Community based occupational therapy for patients with dementia and their caregivers: randomised controlled trial. BMJ, 333(7580), 1196.

Gruwsved, Å., Fernholm, C., and Söderback, I. (1996). Evaluation of a vocational training programme in primary health care rehabilitation: a case study. Work, 7, 47–61.

Guidetti, S., and Söderback, I. (2001). Description of self-care training in occupational therapy: case studies of five Kenyan children with cerebral palsy. Occup Ther Int, 8(1), 34–48.

Hammond, A., and Freeman, K. (2004). The long-term outcomes from a randomized controlled trial of an educational-behavioural joint protection programme for people with rheumatoid arthritis. Clin Rehabil, 18(5), 520–528.

Hansen, R., Tresse, S., and Gunnarsson, R.K. (2004). Fewer accidents and better maintenance with active wheelchair check-ups: a randomized controlled clinical trial. Clin Rehabil, 18(6), 631–639.

Hill, K.H., O'Brien, K.A., and Yurt, R.W. (2007). Teaching energy conservation. Therapeutic efficacy of a therapeutic cooking group from the patients' perspective. J Burn Care Res, 28(2), 324–327.

Hoare, B.J., Wasiak, J., Imms, C., and Carey, L. (2007). Constraint-induced movement therapy in the treatment of the upper limb in children with hemiplegic cerebral palsy. Cochrane Database Syst Rev, 18(2), CD004149.

Ip, W.M., Woo, J., Yue, S.Y., et al. (2006). Evaluation of the effect of energy conservation techniques in the performance of activity of daily living tasks. Clin Rehabil, 20(3), 254–261.

Jacobs, K. (1991). Occupational Therapy. Work-Related Programs and Assessments. Boston: Little, Brown.

Kazdin, A.E. (1982). Single-Case Research Designs. Methods for Clinical and Applied Settings. New York: Oxford University Press.

Kiresuck, T., Smith, A., and Cardillo, J.E. (1994). Goal Attainment Scaling Applications, Theory, and Measurement. London: Lawrence Erlbaum Associates.

Kirkley, K.N., and Fisher, A.G. (1999). Alternate forms reliability of the assessment of motor and process skills. J Outcome Meas, 3(1), 53–70.

Kitson, A. (1989). A Framework for Quality. A Patient-Centred Approach to Quality Assurance in Health Care. Harrow, England: Royal College of Nursing.

Koch, L.C., Cook, B.G., Tankersley, M., and Rumrill, P. (2006). Utilizing research in professional practice. Work, 26(3), 327–331.

Krupa, T., McLean, H., Eastabrook, S., Bonham, A., and Baksh, L. (2003). Daily time use as a measure of community adjustment for persons served by assertive community treatment teams. Am J Occup Ther, 57(5), 558–565.

Kunkel, S., Rosenqvist, U., and Westerling, R. (2007). The structure of quality systems is important to the process and outcome, an empirical study of 386 hospital departments in Sweden. BMC Health Serv Res, 9(7), 104.

Lambert, R.A., Harvey, I., and Poland, F. (2007). A pragmatic, unblinded randomised controlled trial comparing an occupational therapy-led lifestyle approach and routine GP care for panic disorder treatment in primary care. J Affect Disord, 99(1–3), 63–71.

Law, M., and Letts, L. (1989). A critical review of scales of activities of daily living [see comments]. Am J Occup Ther, 43(8), 522–528.

Linacre, J.M., and Wright, B.D. (1991–1996). A User's Guide to Bigsteps (Manual). Chicago: MESA Press.

Liu, K.P., Chan, C.C., Lee, T.M., and Hui-Chan, C.W. (2004). Mental imagery for promoting relearning for people after stroke: a randomized controlled trial. Arch Phys Med Rehabil, 85(9), 1403–1408.

Maitra, K.K., Telage, K.M., and Rice, M.S. (2006). Self-speech-induced facilitation of simple reaching movements in persons with stroke. Am J Occup Ther, 60(2), 146–154.

Martin, L., Miranda, B., and Bean, M. (2008). An exploration of spousal separation and adaptation to long-term disability: six elderly couples engaged in a horticultural programme. Occup Ther Int, 15(1), 45–55.

Matuska, K., Mathiowetz, V., and Finlayson, M. (2007). Use and perceived effectiveness of energy conservation strategies for managing multiple sclerosis fatigue. Am J Occup Ther, 61(1), 62–69.

McCluskey, A., and Lovarini, M. (2005). Providing education on evidence-based practice improved knowledge but did not change behaviour: a before and after study. BMC Med Educ, 19(5), 40.

McKenna, K., Bennett, S., Strong, J., Tooth, L., and Hoffmann, T. (2008). OT-seeker.

Michaelsen, S.M., Dannenbaum, R., and Levin, M. (2006). Task-specific training with trunk restraint on arm recovery in stroke: randomized control trial. Stroke, 37(1), 186–192.

Moberg Mogren, E., and Nelson, D.L. (2006). Evaluating the quality of reporting occupational therapy randomized controlled trail by expanding the CONSORT criteria. Am J Occup Ther, 62(2), 226–235.

National Library of Medicine. (2008a). PubMed. http://www.ncbi.nlm.nih.gov/pubmed/ Retrieved 10/3/2009.

National Library of Medicine. (2008b). PubMed: MeSH is NLM's controlled vocabulary used for indexing articles in PubMed. http://www.ncbi.nlm.nih.gov/entrez/query.fcgi?db=PubMed Retrieved 10/3/2009.

Nordenskiöld, U., Grimby, G., Hedberg, M., Wright, B., and Linacre, J.M. (1996). The structure of an instrument for assessing the effects of assistive devices and altered working methods in women with rheumatoid arthritis. Arthritis Care Res, 9(5), 358–367.

Ottenbacher, K.J., Johnson, M.B., and Hojem, M. (1988). The significance of clinical change and clinical change of significance: issues and methods. Am J Occup Ther, 42(3), 156–163.

Ottenbacher, K.J., and Maas, F. (1999). How to detect effects: statistical power and evidence-based practice in occupational therapy research. Am J Occup Ther, 53(18), 181–188.

Polit, D.F., and Hungler, B.P. (1999). Nursing Research. Principles and Methods. Philadelphia: Lippincott.

Popovic, M.R., Thrasher, T.A., Adams, M.E., Takes, V., Zivanovic, V., and Tonack, M.I. (2006). Functional electrical therapy: retraining grasping in spinal cord injury. Spinal Cord, 44(3), 143–151.

Rosenberg, W., and Donald, A. (1995). Evidence based medicine: an approach to clinical problem solving. BMJ, 310(6987), 1122–1126.

Salvatori, P., Simonavicius, N., Moore, J., Rimmer, G., and Patterson, M. (2008). Meeting the challenge of assessing clinical competence of occupational therapists within a program management environment. Can J Occup Ther, 75(1), 51–60.

Schene, A.H., Koeter, M.W., Kikkert, M.J., Swinkels, J.A., and McCrone, P. (2007). Adjuvant occupational therapy for work-related major depression works: randomized trial including economic evaluation. Psychol Med, 37(3), 351–362.

Schwoebel, J., Coslett, H.B., Bradt, J., Friedman, R., and Dileo, C. (2002). Pain and the body schema: effects of pain severity on mental representations of movement. Neurology, 59(5), 775–777.

Simons, M., King, S., and Edgar, D. (2003). Occupational therapy and physiotherapy for the patient with burns: principles and management guidelines. J Burn Care Rehabil, 24(5), 323–335.

Soderback, I. (2008). Hospital discharge among frail elderly people: a pilot study in Sweden. Occup Ther Int, 15(1), 18–31.

Stein, F., and Cutler, S.K. (1998). Psychosocial Occupational Therapy: A Holistic Approach. San Diego: Singular Publishing Group.

Stein, F., and Cutler, S.K. (2000). Clinical Research in Occupational Therapy, 4th ed. San Diego: Singular Publishing Group/Thomson Learning.

Stein, F., Söderback, I., Cutler, S.K., and Larson, B. (2006). Occupational Therapy and Ergonomics. Applying Ergonomic Principles to Everyday Occupation in the Home and at the Work, 1st ed. London/Philadelphia: Whurr Publisher/Wiley.

Söderback, I. (1995). Effectiveness in rehabilitation. Crit Rev Rehab Med, 7(4), 275–286.

Twamley, E.W., Jeste, D.V., and Lehman, A.F. (2003). Vocational rehabilitation in schizophrenia and other psychotic disorders: a literature review and meta-analysis of randomized controlled trials. J Nerv Ment Dis, 19(8), 515–523.

Uyanik, M., Bumin, G., and Kayihan, H. (2003). Comparison of different therapy approaches in children with Down syndrome. Pediatr Int, 45(1), 68–73.

van den Ende, C.H., Steultjens, E.M., Bouter, L.M., and Dekker, J. (2006). Clinical heterogeneity was a common problem in Cochrane review of physiotherapy and occupational therapy. J Clin Epidemiol, 59(9), 914–919.

van der Velde, G., van Tulder, M., Côté, P., Hogg-Johnson, S., Aker, P., and Cassidy, J.D. (2007). The sensitivity of review results to methods used to appraise and incorporate trial quality into data synthesis. Spine, 32(7), 796–806.

Vollenbroek-Hutten, M.M., Hermens, H.J., Wever, D., Gorter, M., Rinket, J., and Ijzerman, M.J. (2004). Differences in outcome of a multidisciplinary treatment between subgroups of chronic low back pain patients defined using two multiaxial assessment instruments: the multidimensional pain inventory and lumbar dynamometry. Clin Rehabil, 18(5), 566–579.

Wichrowski, M., Whiteson, J., Haas, F., Mola, A., and Rey, M.J. (2005). Effects of horticultural therapy on mood and heart rate in patients participating in an inpatient cardiopulmonary rehabilitation program. J Cardiopulm Rehabil, 25(5), 270–274.

World Health Organization. (2007). ICF Introduction. http://www.who.int/classifications/icf/site/index.cfm (homepage) Retrieved 10/03/2009.

Wright, C.C., and Whittington, D. (1992). Quality Assurance. An Introduction for Health Care Professionals. New York: Churchill Livingstone.

Index